Contents

Exercises, Cases, Figures, Tables, Boxes, and Appendixes Used in This Publication

Exercises

Cases

Figures

Tables

Box

Appendixes

Acknowledgments

For all of their joint and individual efforts in the preparation of this book, we sincerely thank the faculty and staff of the Department of Occupational Therapy, Steinhardt School of Culture, Education, and Human Development, at New York University. Special thanks are extended to the authors and contributors to this work. Among those who contributed mightily to the book but whose names do not appear elsewhere is Alison Shona Fanous, who helped us edit and prepare the final manuscripts. We are in her debt. We also thank Christina A. Davis who, as director of AOTA Press, encouraged and supported all of our efforts.

Marie-Louise Blount profoundly appreciates the love and support of Elena and Wesley Blount and family members Barry Levinson, Meyer Levinson-Blount, and Ari Levinson-Blount, who have made all of her endeavors worthwhile. Jim Hinojosa thanks both of his parents, who instilled in him a love for engagement in purposeful, meaningful activity. He sincerely thanks Steven A. Smith for all his support. Additionally, he thanks Anne C. Mosey, who provided the insight that refined his thinking about activity and occupational therapy.

We are indebted to our clients because they reaffirm our beliefs about the value of active engagement and the meaningfulness of occupational therapy. Finally, we are indebted to our students, current and former, who provided the reason for writing this book. From them, we continually learn the value of what we do.

Contributors

Fran Babiss, PhD, OTR/L
Coordinator of Evidence-Based Practice
South Oaks Partial Hospital
Amityville, NY

Paulette Bell, MA, OTR
Occupational Therapist
DeKalb Medical Center
Decatur, GA

Marie-Louise Blount, AM, OT, FAOTA
Adjunct Clinical Professor
Department of Occupational Therapy
Steinhardt School of Culture, Education, and Human Development
New York University
New York, NY

Wesley Blount
Editor
New York, NY

Karen A. Buckley, MA, OT/L
Clinical Assistant Professor
Department of Occupational Therapy
Steinhardt School of Culture, Education, and Human Development
New York University
New York, NY

Lisa E. Cyzner, PhD, OTR
Private Pediatric Practitioner
Cyzner Institute
Charlotte, NC

Nancy Robert Dooley, PhD, OTR/L
Associate Professor and Occupational Therapy Program Director
New England Institute of Technology
Warwick, RI

Rita P. Fleming-Castaldy, PhD, OT/L, FAOTA
Assistant Professor
University of Scranton
Scranton, PA

Kristine Haertl, PhD, OTR/L
Associate Professor
Department of Occupational Science and Occupational Therapy
St. Catherine University
St. Paul, MN

Jim Hinojosa, PhD, OT, FAOTA
Professor
Department of Occupational Therapy
Steinhardt School of Culture, Education, and Human Development
New York University
New York, NY

Margaret Kaplan, PhD, OTR/L
Associate Professor
Occupational Therapy Program
State University of New York Downstate Medical Center
Brooklyn, NY

Lisette Kautzmann, EdD, OT, FAOTA
Professor Emerita
Department of Occupational Therapy
Eastern Kentucky University
Richmond, KY

Paula Kramer, PhD, OTR, FAOTA
Professor and Chair
Department of Occupational Therapy
College of Health Sciences
University of the Sciences in Philadelphia
Philadelphia, PA

Jane Miller, MA, OT
Occupational Therapist
Doctoral Candidate
Department of Occupational Therapy
Steinhardt School of Culture, Education, and Human Development
New York University
New York, NY

Deborah Moore, MA, OTR/L
Occupational Therapist
Visiting Nurse Service of New York
New York, NY
and
Adjunct Instructor
Department of Occupational Therapy
Steinhardt School of Culture, Education, and Human Development
New York University
New York, NY

Laurette Olson, PhD, OTR
Associate Professor
Graduate Program in Occupational Therapy
Mercy College
Dobbs Ferry, NY

Anita Perr, MA, OT, ATP, FAOTA
Clinical Assistant Professor
Department of Occupational Therapy
Steinhardt School of Culture, Education, and Human Development
New York University
New York, NY

Sally E. Poole, MA, OT, CHT
Clinical Assistant Professor
Department of Occupational Therapy
Steinhardt School of Culture, Education, and Human Development
New York University
New York, NY
and
Co-owner
Hands-On Rehab
Valhalla, NY

Ruth Segal, PhD, OTR
Professor and Chair
Department of Occupational Therapy
School of Health and Medical Sciences
Seton Hall University
South Orange, NJ

Jeff Tomlinson, MSW, OTR, FAOTA
Washington Heights Community Service
New York, NY
and
Adjunct Instructor
Department of Occupational Therapy
Steinhardt School of Culture, Education, and Human Development
New York University
New York, NY

Judy Urban Wilson, MA, OTR
Assistant Director
Department of Occupational Therapy
Bellevue Hospital Center
New York, NY

Foreword

Activity has been a part of the construct of occupational therapy since the profession's inception. Reflecting the views of the Arts and Crafts Movement, most activities consisted primarily of arts and crafts and resulted in objects made by hand. On the basis of observations, personal experience, testimonials, and anecdotal reports, the founders and early practitioners of occupational therapy developed a deep and abiding belief in the curative power of participation in activities.

The commitment to activity as a core component of occupational therapy's domain remained unchallenged until the late 1940s. Therapists at this time, particularly those working in physical rehabilitation, became enamored of the scientific, biomechanical approach practiced by other physical medicine professionals. To them, occupational therapy's use of arts and crafts seemed unscientific and naïve. A new dialogue grew within the profession as questions regarding which activities were therapeutic and what should be considered when prescribing activities for people were debated. The discussion was wide ranging, from those practitioners favoring a biomechanical approach to purists who believed that arts and crafts were the only authentic tools of the profession. Previously established beliefs about the profession's domain of practice were questioned, and the commitment to activities upheld by the profession's founders no longer seemed relevant. From the perspective of the literature, it looked as though the profession was coming apart at the seams.

Fortunately, several talented theorists emerged to help the profession reconstitute itself. Early writings by Gail Fidler and Anne Mosey were among the first modern attempts to define the profession and identify its legitimate tools. Focusing on purposeful activity, David Nelson and his colleagues reestablished its value. They reclaimed the role of activities through of several studies demonstrating that in improving performance, purposeful activities were superior to nonpurposeful activities and rote exercise. Additional studies by other authors led to the current understanding of activity, purposeful activity, and occupation. These understandings were formally articulated in the first and second editions of the *Occupational Therapy Practice Framework: Domain and Process* (American Occupational Therapy Association [AOTA], 2002, 2008).

It is exciting to see that there is enough new information to warrant a third edition of *The Texture of Life: Purposeful Activities in the Context of Occupation*. The editors and authors are to be commended for their splendid presentation of a variety of interesting chapters, covering a wide range of topics related to how occupational therapists think about purposeful activities and occupations and how they use them in practice. As in the previous editions, careful attention has been given to documentation of source material, and an extensive list of references is included. Most important, the text has been revised to include the new definitions and concepts presented in the second edition of the *Framework* (AOTA, 2008). The authors' commitment to systematic inclusion of this language is a generous gift to the profession. The definitions, examples, and case scenarios provide significant support for understanding and embracing the new language.

The importance of furthering the dissemination of a common language that can be articulated by students, practitioners, and faculty cannot be underestimated. In the AOTA (2007) *Centennial Vision,* one of the six barriers to moving forward as a profession was termed *unclear professional language and terminology* (p. 614). In concert with overcoming this barrier, one of the four strategic directions identified in the *Centennial Vision* moves us toward "people understanding who we are and what we do" (p. 614). If ever there was a time for members of the profession to speak in one voice, this is it. *The Texture of Life* gives the members of the profession the tools needed to achieve this goal.

—Lisette Kautzmann, EdD, OT, FAOTA
Professor Emerita
Department of Occupational Therapy
Eastern Kentucky University
Richmond, KY

References

American Occupational Therapy Association. (2002). Occupational therapy practice framework: Domain and process. *American Journal of Occupational Therapy, 56,* 609–639.

American Occupational Therapy Association. (2007). *Centennial Vision* and executive summary. *American Journal of Occupational Therapy, 61,* 613–614.

American Occupational Therapy Association. (2008). Occupational therapy practice framework: Domain and process (2nd ed.). *American Journal of Occupational Therapy, 62,* 625–683.

Preface

Rapid changes in the profession of occupational therapy required the writing of a third edition of *The Texture of Life: Purposeful Activities in the Context of Occupation*. The contributors to this edition have written chapters that address the changes in the profession and its priorities and present current and up-to-date information. They have struggled with ideas that are foundational to the profession's core and have written chapters that support clinical practice. A new CD-ROM contains exercises and other forms to enhance the text's educational and clinical use.

A major change in our profession is that occupational therapists and occupational therapy assistants have endorsed the use of the term *occupation*. As a result, the terms *activities* and *purposeful activities* are used less frequently. The expanded use of the term *occupation* has multiple implications for the profession. Do others understand the term *occupation*? Do the practitioners who use it understand occupation? Does the use of the term influence the profession's practices or not? How does it influence consumers' and society's acceptance of the profession? Finally, how has the endorsement of exclusive use of the term *occupation* influenced the profession's philosophical and theoretical development? In this text, the authors have addressed some of these issues. We hope that others will question these ideas and expand on them.

For this edition, we asked the authors to use the *Occupational Therapy Practice Framework: Domain and Process* (2nd ed.; American Occupational Therapy Association, 2008) and the *International Classification of Functioning, Disability and Health* (World Health Organization, 2001) as basic references. In addition, we asked them to address occupation as it is being used and developed within the profession. We also emphasize that the purpose of this text is to discuss the scope and depth of our profession with a focus on activities. For us, an important aspect of the profession is the value and meaning activities have in our lives.

We believe that our contributors have responded to our challenges. We hope that this text provides clarity with respect to the current language that we are using, and we hope that it provides a clear understanding of important concepts fundamental to occupational therapy. Finally, we hope it will serve as the foundation for continuing dialogue. We hope that others who agree and disagree will continue to help us refine our most fundamental ideas.

—Jim Hinojosa, PhD, OT, FAOTA
Marie-Louise Blount, AM, OT, FAOTA

References

American Occupational Therapy Association. (2008). Occupational therapy practice framework: Domain and process (2nd ed.). *American Journal of Occupational Therapy, 62,* 625–683.

World Health Organization. (2001). *International classification of functioning, disability and health.* Geneva, Switzerland: Author.

1

Occupation, Purposeful Activities, and Occupational Therapy

Jim Hinojosa, PhD, OT, FAOTA
Marie-Louise Blount, AM, OT, FAOTA

ctivities—what we do, the foundation of much of our routine, enterprise, and art—have a unique place in the context of occupational therapy. In fact, mapping the import of activities in occupational therapy shows a varied landscape, one with multiple meanings. Activities are foundational to human occupation. Occupations are specific to the people who are engaged in and experiencing them within their sociocultural context; they are grounded in place, social group, and cultural meaning (Pierce, 2001).

In this chapter, we focus on purposeful activities as they relate to the practice of occupational therapy today. We define and outline the relationships among the major constructs of the profession: *occupation, activity, purposeful activity,* and *occupational performance.* Moreover, we provide the framework for the rest of the book.

This chapter addresses some of the more fundamental of the meanings attributed to activities and establishes that occupational therapy's application of these meanings is the core of the profession and an integral part of practice. We discuss how occupational therapists and occupational therapy assistants apply these varying meanings in describing their reasoning and creating their practice. The labels used are not always the same, and the ideas behind them are not necessarily uniform. Our position is that these varying labels for and ideas regarding activities represent important vigor in the profession's thinking and the richness of the methods used. Occupational therapists and occupational therapy assistants should, therefore, take stock of these ideas and develop an understanding of their potential for practice.

In occupational therapy, the term *purposeful activity* is used rather than *activity* to highlight the fact that occupational therapists and occupational therapy assistants use activities that have a function and are therapeutically goal directed. In this text, we support the position that practitioners use

1

the term *occupation* to capture the scope of a fundamental construct of occupational therapy. Included in a person's occupations are the purposeful activities that he or she engages in as part of living. Some practitioners choose to use only the concept of occupation (American Occupational Therapy Association [AOTA], 2008; Nelson, 1997; Nelson & Jepson-Thomas, 2003). In fact, in the 2008 revision of the *Occupational Therapy Practice Framework: Domain and Process* (2nd ed., or *Framework–II*; AOTA, 2008), the authors concluded that although scholars in the field acknowledge differences between the terms *activity* and *occupation*, they have decided to use only *occupation*. In their definition, *occupation* includes activities.

Many practitioners strive for unambiguous personal definitions of *occupation, activity,* and *purposeful activity.* Although the distinctions among the three terms and their specific uses may be clear to many, to others the terms describe similar phenomena: the person's participation in daily life pursuits (AOTA, 2002). In this chapter, we propose distinct definitions that capture the essential characteristics distinguishing each definition. *Activities* encompass a wide range of actions that a person takes to accomplish or perform something. In occupational therapy, when a person participates in an action to realize a goal and this activity is personally important, the person is engaged in a *purposeful activity.* *Occupations* are purposeful activities that are personally meaningful to the person, who engages in them out of personal choice or sociocultural necessity. In other words, when a person engages in purposeful activities out of personal choice and values those activities, these clusters of purposeful activities form occupations (Hinojosa, Kramer, Royeen, & Luebben, 2003). Thus, occupations are unique to each individual, providing personal satisfaction and fulfillment as a result of engaging in them (AOTA, 2002; Pierce, 2001).

If *purposeful activity* refers to portions of occupations and encompasses a variety of behaviors and performances (AOTA, 1993), the need still exists to discuss, delimit, and understand the behaviors and tasks that are part of the activity and at the same time appreciate the occupations under which the activity is subsumed. In other words, having a definition for a phenomenon does not necessarily simplify one's understanding of it or of the issues it raises.

We suggest, therefore, an approach to these questions recommended by Mosey (1985), that is, a pluralistic approach. Henderson et al. (1991)

EXERCISE 1.1: REFLECTION ON DAILY LIFE ACTIVITIES

Reflect and list the actions in which you have engaged today. Classify them into activities, purposeful activities, and occupations. Identify those that were difficult to categorize. Why were they difficult to categorize? What criteria did you finally decide to use to categorize the unclear activities?

Sᴍᴀʟʟ Cᴀᴘꜱ EXERCISE 1.2: RANGE OF ACTIVITIES

Consider other aspects of activities that range from simple to complex, identifying not only the polar ends of a given continuum but also the various stages of complexity that exist along the continuum.

---

have also suggested that practitioners embrace a multidimensional view of purposeful activity as both an entity and a therapeutic modality. We support Mosey's (1985) and Henderson et al.'s (1991) acknowledgment that occupational therapy services can and do include approaches and methods other than purposeful activity. Because purposeful activity is fundamental to occupational therapy practice, practitioners need to understand the many modes in which the term is used.

In occupational therapy, some approaches use the term *purposeful activities,* and other approaches use substitute terms. However, all approaches include the belief that occupational therapists and occupational therapy assistants use activities in a specific manner. Henderson et al. (1991) also noted that practitioners use a wide range of types and levels of activity in practice. Activities may range from low level (e.g., reaching for an object) to high level (e.g., a simulated work activity). They may also range from simple to complex, for example, on a continuum from gross (e.g., an assembly toy in which a smaller plastic ring is placed on top of a larger plastic ring) to fine (e.g., attaching a small nut to a bolt and screwing it in place) or from very brief (performing a very time-limited activity once) to more lengthy (a demanding work or leisure activity carried out in a concentrated fashion for an hour or more).

As Henderson et al. (1991) pointed out, both purposefulness and the varied meanings invested in the term *purposeful activities* are "attributes of persons and not of activities" (p. 370). Henderson et al. were rightly concerned that occupational therapists and occupational therapy assistants realize that the meaning (purposefulness) of an activity is invested in it by the person performing the activity or, sometimes, by the practitioner, often with the client's collaboration. They identified the fact that in acute care settings and in any situation in which remediation of disability is the goal of intervention, activities or segments of activities may be a means of attaining that purpose or goal. Their view, which we share, is that all activities have the potential to be meaningful and purposeful. Many variables—such as the person performing the activity, the context in which it is used, and when in the course of a program or series of activities it is introduced—affect the activity's meaningfulness and purposefulness. Occupational therapists and occupational therapy assistants often use other techniques or tools, with or without activities, as part of their interventions. Often, these techniques or tools are not meaningful to the client. Nevertheless, the practitioner's concern and goal is to provide an intervention that will facilitate a person's ability to engage in meaningful daily life activities or occupations.

Henderson et al. (1991) identified the relevance to occupational therapy of the profession's historical and traditional applications of activity and its more contemporary expressions of choices or applications of activity. They were concerned not only with the ways in which occupational therapists and occupational therapy assistants view and use activities but also with the ways in which they investigate activity's therapeutic aspects.

We believe that activities represent the core and the texture of people's daily lives. Occupation, activity, and purposeful activities have additional manifestations for occupational therapists and occupational therapy assistants, giving rise to the multiple and varied meanings attributed to the concepts. We propose that no single definition is correct or absolute. In fact, we believe that discussion of the meanings of the terms adds to an understanding and appreciation of the concepts behind them. Ultimately, practitioners' increased understanding of these concepts improves their use of them within the context of therapeutic intervention.

Occupational Therapy: The Profession's Mandate

Before examining the tools that a profession uses, it is important to consider the profession's purpose and focus. Professions exist to apply knowledge for the benefit of the members of society (Kielhofner, 1992; Luebben, Hinojosa, & Kramer, 2010; Mosey, 1981, 1996). Although each profession has a unique purpose, professions often overlap in the services they provide and the tools they use as part of their interventions to benefit members of a society (Kramer, Luebben, & Hinojosa, 2010). Each profession's practice is grounded in the society in which it exists and therefore may vary depending on the region of the country, the city, or the culture in which it is practiced. These differences in a profession's practices sometimes create tension for those members of the profession who would like to believe that all members of the profession practice in the same manner with the same goals (Strauss, 2001).

Members of a distinct profession share a specialized training and a unique expertise. They also share a common philosophy and a code of ethics. Occupational therapists' and occupational therapy assistants' philosophical beliefs outline how they view the person, society, and people in the context of their environment. The tools practitioners use to intervene with clients are heavily influenced by occupational therapy's philosophical orientation.

In 1979, the AOTA Representative Assembly approved an association policy related to the philosophical base of occupational therapy (AOTA, 1979). In this statement, AOTA articulated the profession's basic beliefs about human nature and adaptation. Moreover, it stated that practitioners believe in the importance of purposeful activity to facilitate the adaptive process. Adoption of this statement highlights the importance of purposeful activity, which was then considered to be synonymous with *occupation*. The relationship between purposeful activities and occupation has been the focus of major philosophical discussion within the profession. The following definitions delineate the terms as they are used in this book.

ACTIVITY

Activities are the actions that people take to accomplish a physical or mental task. "Activities are a class of human actions that are goal directed" (AOTA, 2008, p. 669). "Activity is the execution of a task or action by an individual" (World Health Organization [WHO], 2001, p. 10). Activities suggest an active process and may involve engagement with others, although some are performed alone. Some activities involve specific objects and space.

People engage in activities because they are expected to do them, because they want to do them, or because they need to do them. Most of the activities that people engage in as a part of daily life are ordinary and mundane; as noted by Cynkin and Robinson (1990), there is nothing dramatic or glamorous about making a bed, fixing a faucet, taking a shower, or washing clothes. For the most part, people are unaware of the many activities they perform as part of their daily routines; most are performed automatically (Cynkin & Robinson, 1990). People do not even think about the importance of these daily activities until they can no longer perform them.

PURPOSEFUL ACTIVITY

People engage in purposeful activities as part of their daily routines. "Purposeful activity refers to goal-directed behaviors or tasks . . . that the individual considers meaningful" (AOTA, 1993, p. 1081). *Purposeful activities* are tasks or experiences in which the person actively participates. Although engaged in a purposeful activity, the person directs his or her attention to the task (AOTA, 1993).

Purposeful activities are one of the foundational elements of an occupation. Unique combinations of purposeful activities link together with the person's personal meanings to form his or her occupations.

Purposeful activities are goal directed in that they involve active participation and require coordination among a person's physical, emotional, and cognitive systems. *Goal directed* means that the person actively engages in actions to meet a personal purpose or need; it does not mean that the end product must be a physical outcome. In occupational therapy, purposeful activities are an important therapeutic tool. They are used alone to address a specific need, or they are used in patterns or groups to help a person develop meaningful occupations (AOTA, 1997).

Occupation

"Occupations are the ordinary and familiar things that people do every day" (AOTA, 1995, p. 1015). The meaningful groupings of activities that people engage in as part of their daily lives are *occupations*. These occupations give life meaning and have been broadly categorized by practitioners as work, self-care, and play or leisure. The range of activities included in any one occupation is defined by the person who is engaging in the activity and the circumstances around which the activity is performed. For example, eating can be pleasure at a state fair, work at a business lunch, or self-care at home.

The many important dimensions of an occupation make it a unique classification for occupational therapists and occupational therapy assistants. First and foremost, occupations have personal, specific meaning to the person. This personal meaning is variable and determined by contextual, temporal, psychological, social, symbolic, cultural, ethnic, and spiritual dimensions. Second, occupations involve mental abilities and skills, and they may or may not have an observable physical dimension. Third, the occupations in which a person engages define him or her. Fourth, as the person interacts with his or her environment, matures, or responds to life conditions, his or her preferred occupations are likely to change (AOTA, 1997).

The principal concern of occupational therapy is to maintain, restore, or facilitate a person's ability to function within his or her daily occupations. We have broadly defined *daily occupations* to include active participation in self-maintenance, work, leisure, and play activities.

Occupational Performance

"Occupational performance is the doing, the action, the active behavior, or the active responses exhibited within the context of an occupational form" (Nelson, 1988, p. 634). *Occupational form* refers to the context of action contributing to the meaning and purpose that the occupation brings to the person (Nelson, 1988). The occupational form includes the occupation's essential elements, such as its organizational structures, that influence the person's performance of the occupation. The occupational form has both objective and subjective dimensions. Aspects of the objective dimension may be the physical stimuli involved, the objects and their characteristics, the human context, and the temporal context. The subjective or perceived dimension is derived from the sociocultural reality that is independent of the specific person (Nelson, 1988).

Thus, *occupational performance* is a person's action in response to the occupation as the person perceives it. Occupational therapists and occupational therapy assistants are concerned with occupational performance; in other words, they focus on facilitating a client's ability to participate in occupations, taking into consideration the client's perception of the occupations.

Tools of the Profession

Occupational therapists and occupational therapy assistants use a wide variety of strategies and tools in their practice. These therapeutic tools are selected to be consistent with well-defined theoretical bases or rationales. We should note that occupational therapists and occupational therapy assistants do not conceptualize practice in one universally accepted way. Some view practice as based on a model, others suggest paradigms, and others use frames of reference. In this book, we do not address the issue of how practice is conceptualized. We accept the view that scholars use different organizational structures and view practice differently. What is important is that each of the models, paradigms, or frames of reference provides guidelines for the selection and use of therapeutic tools. Each practitioner selects from a wide assortment of tools with which he or she is both knowledgeable and competent and can use in practice. Specialization of practice has resulted in variations in the tools practitioners use. However, whatever tools they choose to use, they all share a common goal: the person's being able to engage in daily living, work, play, or leisure activities.

The practices and concerns of a profession change over time with the advancement of knowledge and technology. Thus, a profession changes its priorities and practices in response to changes in society. This continuous change ensures that the profession remains viable and is responsive to the needs of the society that it serves. Occupational therapy's evolution in response to changes in society, knowledge, and technology has indeed made it a viable, dynamic profession that continues to meet its mandate from society. Yet change has been difficult for some practitioners. For example, the extensive early use of crafts has been replaced with new modalities such as manual manipulation, computer adaptation, or physical activity. Changes in the importance and use of a modality are sometimes seen as not consistent with the profession's philosophical base. Using the previous example, some practitioners continue to believe that "true" occupational therapy must involve active engagement in an activity.

Occupational therapy's mandate has always been to enable people to engage and participate in their own daily life activities. Occupational therapy, as a health care profession, has been influenced by the trends and concerns of medicine (Baum & Christiansen, 1997). Although medicine continues to affect the profession's evolution, other, more recent changes in society seem to be having a greater influence. In response to societal change, occupational therapy has moved into education and community-based service delivery models. This change in society's priorities has led to an increase in the number of practitioners working in education-based practices and a change in the site of practice to schools and community settings (Kramer & Hinojosa, 1999). This shift in the site of practice and service delivery models is also evident in other areas of practice. The 1990s saw a shift from clinic settings to more integrated community, classroom, and home settings. These

---

EXERCISE 1.3: PERSONAL HIERARCHY OF NEEDS

An important concern of educators is what motivates people and how this interrelates with the development of human potential. Abraham Maslow (1970, 1971), the founder of humanistic psychology, proposed that a person's gratification of needs is the most important single principle underlying development. He proposed seven hierarchical levels of needs: physiological, safety, love and belongingness, esteem, self-actualization, knowing and understanding, and aesthetics. People fill these needs by engaging in meaningful activities. Reflect on the past 2 days and how you satisfied your personal needs in the categories identified in Maslow's hierarchy:

- Physiological needs (food, drink, sleep, survival)
- Safety (avoidance of danger and anxiety, desire for security)
- Love and belongingness (affection, feeling wanted, roots in a family or peer group)
- Esteem (self-respect, feelings of adequacy, competence, mastery)
- Self-actualization (striving for or using talents, capacities, potentialities)
- Knowing and understanding (curiosity, learning about the world)
- Aesthetics (experience and understand beauty for its own sake).

After completing the list, consider

- What needs were being met or not met?
- What activities contributed to the satisfaction of your needs?
- What does the list suggest about your health status?

Note. From *Educational Psychology: Principles and Applications* (p. 253) by Glover, J. A., Bruning, R. H., & Filbeck, R. W., 1983. Boston: Little, Brown. Copyright © 1993, by Little, Brown. Adapted with permission.

---

changes have been in response to numerous internal influences (e.g., growth in knowledge, advances in technology) and external influences (e.g., social and government policy, payment practices).

OCCUPATIONAL THERAPY'S INTERVENTION TOOLS

The application of any frame of reference (model, practice guidelines, paradigm) involves the use of a variety of intervention strategies and tools. *Tools* are those items, actions, means, modalities, methods, or instruments that are used in practice in a theoretically prescribed manner to bring about change. These tools become legitimate in a profession when the profession's members have expertise in their use (Mosey, 1996). Occupational therapists and occupational therapy assistants use a variety of tools, depending on their particular frame of reference (Mosey, 1986). Beyond purposeful activities, other legitimate tools discussed in the literature are the nonhuman environment, the conscious use of self, activity analysis and adaptation, activity groups, teaching–learning processes, stimulus–response interactions, atmospheric elements, physical agent modalities, and technology (Kramer et al., 2010; Mosey, 1986, 1996). In addition to these tools, the profession has others that are very specialized and often specific to one frame of reference (Kramer et al., 2010). A profession's tools change with evolving knowledge, technological advances, and clients' changing needs.

One of the major issues related to tools is that many practitioners consider the tools of the profession to be exceptionally significant. Some may even consider the tools to be symbolic of the profession as a whole (Kramer et al., 2010). This significance may be the result of the tangible aspects of legitimate tools and because practitioners use them daily as they interact with clients (Mosey, 1986). In addition, many practitioners view the tools of their profession as unique. In reality, however, the legitimate tools are not unique and are shared by many professions. What is unique is the way in which a specific profession applies them. In occupational therapy, this singularity lies in how the tools are used together in the application of the specific frame of reference or guideline for intervention.

ACTIVITIES AS A THERAPEUTIC MODALITY

Each day, people engage in numerous activities. They perform some activities to meet their self-care needs, some because they enjoy them, and others in response to others' expectations or to circumstances that require action. Thus, activities are the things that people do, and they are also the building blocks that people use to construct their lives. Occupational therapy evolved from this context—from the realized importance of how people occupy their time as human beings—and thus the concern with occupations is central to occupational therapists' beliefs. Activities are purposeful when they are goal directed and meaningful to the person who is completing the task or action. When practitioners view a pattern of daily activities together that have personal meaning to a client, they categorize them as *occupations*. Thus, *occupations* are fundamentally based on activities (Hinojosa et al., 2003; Kramer & Hinojosa, 1995).

From this perspective, both activities and the resulting occupations are a fundamental and essential aspect of life. People's daily activities and occupations define who and what they are; engagement in purposeful activities gives their lives meaning. Occupational therapists and occupational therapy assistants, in defining their domain of concern, typically view activities as part of occupations (e.g., they divide activities into activities of daily living [ADLs], work or productive activities, or play or leisure activities). By viewing activities in this manner, practitioners think about how they relate to the outcome for the person who engages in them. Thus, the same activities may fit into several occupations depending on the goal of the activity, the person's developmental status, and the specific circumstances and context in which the person performs the activity.

The following example illustrates this point: For a school-age child at camp, writing a letter to his or her parents may be work. For a young person, writing a letter to a girlfriend may be a leisure activity. For an adult, writing a shopping list may be an ADL. The occupations for which writing is a component activity thus include work, leisure, and ADLs. For the professional author, writing is an occupation in both the employment and the occupational therapy senses. In this scenario, the professional author engages in several writing activities that together are viewed as an occupation.

In the following discussion, we outline the unique view of purposeful activities and occupations that occupational therapists share.

ACTIVITIES OF DAILY LIVING

Each day, all people engage in a variety of *ADLs*. These occupations are composed of self-care activities, which are the means by which people interact with and respond to their personal demands and needs. Not all self-care activities are interesting or enjoyable; in fact, many basic self-care activities are boring, routine, and unexciting. These ordinary daily self-care activities, however, are basic to people's survival as social human beings and crucially important to their self-esteem and self-worth. The ability to feed oneself, dress oneself, or take care of one's own toileting needs provides valued independence. In sum, people's ability to take care of themselves and meet their daily needs is vital to their existence. The multitude of purposeful activities categorized as self-care are determined by a wide range of factors, including individual attributes and abilities, culture, context, developmental status, and socioeconomic status.

WORK OR PRODUCTIVE OCCUPATIONS

The occupations of *work or productive occupations* are composed of the numerous activities that people engage in to support themselves and their families, to fill time in a socially acceptable fashion, to give expression to their interests, to apply their education and training, to maintain important social status, to alleviate stress, to mitigate loneliness, or to avoid doubts about life's purposes, to name just a few possibilities. Work is an obligation for many people, but in our society it is not usually a requirement for children, some students, some people with disabilities, and many retirees.

Much of people's time is devoted to work and productive activities. In addition to time spent working, people often devote time to preparing for work and traveling to and from work. Many people have more than one job, and the activities involved in work are extremely varied. Many U.S. workers must adjust to the demands of large, formal organizations and complex technology. Also, and sometimes problematically, often because of the amount of time spent at work, work becomes for many a center of social life. Close friendships, groups with shared interests, loving relationships, and marriages often arise in work settings, leading the workplace to be a locale of many satisfactions and stresses. Work activities are central to the lives of most adult men and women and become a key focus of what makes many people's lives meaningful.

PLAY OR LEISURE OCCUPATIONS

Play or leisure occupations include a wide range of activities that one engages in for their intrinsic pleasure and enjoyment. They can range from solitary and sedentary activities, such as reading a book, to group activities such as sports. An important characteristic of play or leisure activities is that people engage in them because they want to. As with self-care activities, a wide range of factors—including individual attributes and abilities, culture, context, developmental status, and socioeconomic status—determines a person's play and leisure purposeful activities. Leisure occupations may call for little or a great deal of equipment, perhaps ranging from a pair of dice to complex fishing gear. Specific environments and sometimes large amounts of space can be involved in the pursuit of leisure. For certain leisure participants, fishing in a nearby lake might meet the same ends as playing golf on a vast golf course.

Occupational therapists and occupational therapy assistants are concerned with the wide range of activities in which people engage. Activities are fundamental and normal for all humans. Purposeful activities and their associated occupations define what and who people are, allow people to express feelings, and have personal and social meaning to people. People learn from engaging in purposeful activities and get satisfaction from them. Through purposeful activity, a person can explore interests, satisfy needs, determine and assess capacity and limitations, meet personal and interpersonal needs, and cope with life. Most important, from participating in purposeful activities, a person develops and acquires his or her own occupations.

Purposeful Activities as a Tool of Intervention

Occupational therapists and occupational therapy assistants use purposeful activities as tools of intervention. Therefore, it is crucial that they have more than just an appreciation of them. Not only must practitioners have in-depth knowledge of purposeful activities as the foundation of occupation, but they must also understand the value and benefit of purposeful activities as therapeutic media. Using purposeful activities as therapeutic tools requires an understanding of the component elements of purposeful activities. In addition, because of the larger goal of purposeful activities, occupational therapists must view them within the context of a person's life, abilities, and life circumstances. When using purposeful activities, in other words, one must always keep in mind the person's broader occupations.

Occupational therapists and occupational therapy assistants have always used activities as part of their interventions with clients, but why do they use purposeful activities? Although specific activities have changed and will continue to change, the six basic reasons for choosing to use purposeful activities are relatively constant:

1. Purposeful activity builds on a person's abilities and leads to the achievement of personal and functional goals. For an activity to be purposeful, it must have four qualities: First, the activity must be directed toward a goal that the participant considers important. Second, the participant must be actively engaged in it because he or she wants to be. Third, the activity must have personal meaning to the participant (Evans, 1987; Gilfoyle, 1984; Mosey, 1986; Nelson, 1988; Nelson & Jepson-Thomas, 2003). An activity's purposefulness is always grounded in the person who is doing the activity and the situational context in which it is done (Henderson et al., 1991). Fourth, the participant must be capable and have the knowledge, skills, and abilities to engage in the activity. Therefore, practitioners select purposeful activities because they are meaningful to the person and build on his or her capacities to bring about change. The person's ability to complete purposeful activities provides the foundation for his or her occupations. As described earlier, when a person engages in purposeful activities out of personal choice because they are meaningful and significant, these purposeful activities form occupations.

2. Purposeful activity offers the person opportunities for effective action and to achieve a goal. Therefore, the person must be an active participant. The completion of the activity has a result: a physical outcome such as finishing a chore or an intellectual achievement such as acquiring information from reading a book. An important factor is that the person is fully involved in the activity. Practitioners believe that successful accomplishment will lead to the person's development of abilities and skills and that with these improved skills and abilities, the person will then begin or continue to engage in occupations.

3. Purposeful activities provide opportunities for the person to achieve mastery of the environment and to perform something successfully, thus promoting feelings of personal competence. By skillfully selecting an appropriate activity, practitioners can match the person's capabilities, potential, and desires with particular tasks. Thus, an appropriate purposeful activity provides an opportunity for a person to master skills, accomplish something, and build self-confidence. Accomplishment of various tasks

leads to a successful experience and ultimately to the accomplishment of purposeful activities. These accomplishments, when grouped together, develop into successful achievement of occupations. For example, a person who can master washing his or her face (purposeful activity) and then bathing (purposeful activity) may gradually become capable of independently completing his or her own self-care (occupation). From the individual's perspective, the feeling of mastery of the environment is realized as he or she engages in purposeful activities (washing and bathing) as part of the intervention plan.

4. When engaged in a purposeful activity, the person directs his or her attention to the accomplishment of the activity's end goal. One major value of this engagement in a purposeful activity is that the person's attention is not on the specific tasks and actions required. For example, a child who is playing with a doll is less likely to attend to the increased upper-extremity range of motion, cognitive challenges, or psychosocial interaction sought by the practitioner; instead, the child's goal is to have fun while engaging in an imaginary activity. When an adult makes a sandwich, he or she may not focus on the pain or limited range of motion associated with arthritis, concentrating instead on the edible product.

5. Engagement in purposeful activity within the context of interpersonal, cultural, physical, and other environmental conditions requires and elicits coordination among the person's sensory, perceptual, motor, and cognitive systems and his or her emotions. The nature of being involved in an activity (which has a goal and an anticipated outcome and involves several tasks) leads to engagement in a purposeful activity and occurs in complex interactions between the person and his or her environment. Although a practitioner can control the degree of each factor to some extent, the nature of selecting an activity that is meaningful requires multiple levels of processing. The therapeutic value of purposeful activities is enhanced by the complex interaction of factors that stem from involvement in a specific purposeful activity.

6. Engagement in purposeful activity provides direct and objective feedback about performance to both the practitioner and the client. Feedback is gathered during the performance of the activity and from the result of the actions. Because the purposeful activities are part of real-life occupations, they provide additional insight into the person's potential to engage in occupations successfully. Feedback from real-life meaningful activities provides valuable information that cannot be obtained from simulated or fabricated tasks.

These six reasons provide the rationale that occupational therapists have always used to justify their use of purposeful activities. Although the types of activities have continually changed, occupational therapists and occupational therapy assistants are committed to using meaningful, real-life purposeful activities as the best tool for evaluation and intervention.

OCCUPATIONAL THERAPISTS' EXAMINATION AND USE OF PURPOSEFUL ACTIVITIES

To use purposeful activities as part of an intervention, occupational therapists examine their use from many perspectives. In the following sections, we outline some of the general characteristics of purposeful activities that occupational therapists and occupational therapy assistants consider as they use them as evaluation and therapeutic tools.

GOAL OF THE ACTIVITY FOR THE PERSON

Each person has goals that drive his or her engagement in an activity. These goals may be immediate or long term. The nature of the goals also varies depending on the person's reason for doing the activity and the time he or she has to complete it. For the occupational therapist or occupational therapy assistant, the person's goal for engaging in the activity is an important factor to consider when judging performance. Practitioners often assume that when the goal for engaging in the activity comes from the person, the person has greater investment in the activity and places more value on it. Likewise, practitioners often assume that if the person is completing the activity for someone else, he or she may not put forth the same effort or have the same investment in the activity. These assumptions, however, may not be true. When analyzing performance of a task or completion of an activity, one factor that a practitioner must consider carefully is the person's motivation to perform. The practitioner must consider what he or she knows about the person's occupations and, with the person, select purposeful activities that will support these occupations.

MEANING AND VALUE OF THE ACTIVITY TO THE PERSON

Occupational therapists and occupational therapy assistants use activities in evaluation and intervention that have personal value and meaning for the person. When practitioners select activities to use with a person, they choose those that are important to that person, based on factors such as his or her personal attributes, culture, lifestyle, and life situation. For example, when working with children, practitioners frequently choose play activities that are meaningful and appropriate to the child. For example, if the child has a physical limitation, comes from a Hispanic background, and lives in a large metropolitan area, practitioners carefully consider each of these factors when selecting a specific activity.

KNOWLEDGE, ABILITIES, AND SKILLS REQUIRED TO ENGAGE IN THE ACTIVITY

Every purposeful activity requires knowledge, abilities, and skills to produce an effective outcome. Occupational therapists and occupational therapy assistants use task analysis and their understanding of the activity to determine what is required to engage in it. On the basis of this analysis, they then select activities that match the person's capacities.

REQUIRED OBJECTS, ARTICLES, AND PARAPHERNALIA

Most purposeful activities involve the use of objects, articles, or paraphernalia to accomplish the various component tasks. A key point of an activity analysis is to determine what materials are actually required and to what extent. Practitioners examine the materials that are essential to the task, and at times they modify, adapt, or change the materials required. They try, however, to maintain the integrity of the purposeful activity.

ACTIONS REQUIRED TO ENGAGE IN THE ACTIVITY

Although many activities are carried out in specific ways, they can often be modified, adapted, or changed if needed. The actions of an activity include the structure, rules, organizational features, and timing that each task in the activity requires. Additionally, actions may have to be carried out in a specific way, in a specific order, or in a set amount of time. Occupational therapists and occupational therapy assistants examine activities in relation to the actions required to engage in and complete them. Such examination requires adept activity analysis skills. People often obtain satisfaction not just from the activity itself but also from the routine and the objects usually used in the performance.

REQUIRED LEVEL OF ENGAGEMENT WITH THE HUMAN ENVIRONMENT

Whereas all purposeful activities require that the person who is engaged in the activity participate, many necessitate others' participation. Depending on the activity, this other can be a specific person (e.g., mother, spouse, family member, friend), an acquaintance (e.g., peers, colleagues, health care providers), or a stranger. Sometimes the activity demands that the people involved have particular knowledge or skills. The specific activity and the context in which it is done may also influence each person's degree of participation. Practitioners carefully examine the degree and quality of participation required for the whole activity and its component tasks.

REQUIRED LEVEL OF ENGAGEMENT WITH THE NONHUMAN ENVIRONMENT

As discussed previously, most purposeful activities involve the use of objects, articles, or paraphernalia. Beyond these, the nonhuman environment may include pets and other animals that may be crucial to the activity. Purposeful activities that involve interaction between the nonhuman elements of the environment and the people included in the activity also vary in terms of degree of involvement. Again, as with the human environment, practitioners carefully examine the degree and quality of participation required for the whole activity and for its component tasks.

CONTEXT IN WHICH THE ACTIVITY IS PERFORMED

Performance of a task or an activity can be context dependent. The context within which an activity is done includes physical, social, cultural, and temporal factors. *Context* is, in some definitions, another word for *environment*. It can also be used to describe verbal situations or meanings. Both senses of this term are important to occupational therapists. *Context* may refer to the intervention setting itself as well as the environment in which the occupation may eventually be performed. It is a complex and multifaceted idea and, as such, calls for careful consideration by the practitioner.

PURPOSEFUL ACTIVITIES IN EVALUATION AND INTERVENTION

The person's actual performance in purposeful activities provides insight into his or her ability to engage in occupations and function in the real world. This information, along with other assessment data, is used to develop a comprehensive intervention plan. By definition, prescription of purposeful activity is client specific. Thus, activities are selected on the basis of the person's needs, the person's abilities and disabilities, and the activity's inherent characteristics. Once the activity has been selected, the practitioner grades or adapts the chosen activity to promote successful performance or elicit a particular response.

EXERCISE 1.4: DUNTON'S NINE CARDINAL PRINCIPLES FOR OCCUPATIONAL WORK

Following are Dunton's nine cardinal principles to guide the emerging practice of occupational therapy (Peloquin, 1991). Please read them and discuss how they relate to the previous discussion of the use of purposeful activities in occupational therapy. How appropriate are they today?

1. The work should be carried on with cure as the main object.
2. The work must be interesting.
3. The patient should be carefully studied.
4. One form of occupation should not be carried to the point of fatigue.
5. It should have some useful end.
6. It preferably should lead to an increase in the patient's knowledge.
7. It should be carried on with others.
8. All possible encouragement should be given the worker.
9. Work resulting in a poor or useless product is better than idleness. (pp. 733–734)

Purposeful activities have the potential to facilitate a client's mastery of a new skill, to restore a deficient ability, to provide a means for compensating for a functional disability, to maintain health, and to prevent dysfunction. During intervention, practitioners select activities or modify them in response to the crucial changes in the person to provide opportunities for gradual development of skills and other related therapeutic benefits. Aspects of the purposeful activity manipulated as part of the intervention include sequence; duration; task procedures; the person's position; the position of the tools and materials; the size, shape, weight, or texture of materials; the nature and degree of interpersonal contact; the extent of physical handling by the practitioner during the performance; and the environment in which the activity is attempted. All of these are discussed in detail in later chapters.

Summary

Occupational therapists and occupational therapy practitioners use purposeful activities to restore function and to compensate for functional deficits (AOTA, 1993). Before using a purposeful activity as part of an intervention plan, practitioners complete an analysis of the activity based on both the client and the context. This process is called *activity analysis,* which includes identifying the essential information, abilities, skills, and proficiencies necessary to complete each task. They also consider the person's age, occupational roles, cultural background, gender, interests, and preferences. Scrutinizing the context and circumstances surrounding the performance of the activity, practitioners skillfully select purposeful activities within the conditions of the frame of reference that has been selected to guide the intervention. Using activity synthesis, occupational therapists implement purposeful activities that are appropriate.

References

American Occupational Therapy Association. (1979). Philosophical base of occupational therapy, Resolution 531-79. *American Journal of Occupational Therapy, 33,* 785.

American Occupational Therapy Association. (1993). Position Paper—Purposeful activity. *American Journal of Occupational Therapy, 47,* 1081–1082.

American Occupational Therapy Association. (1995). Position Paper—Occupation. *American Journal of Occupational Therapy, 49,* 1015–1018.

American Occupational Therapy Association. (1997). Statement—Fundamental concepts of occupational therapy: Occupation, purposeful activity, and function. *American Journal of Occupational Therapy, 51,* 864–866.

American Occupational Therapy Association. (2002). Occupational therapy practice framework: Domain and process. *American Journal of Occupational Therapy, 56,* 609–639.

American Occupational Therapy Association. (2008). Occupational therapy practice framework: Domain and process (2nd ed.). *American Journal of Occupational Therapy, 62,* 625–683.

Baum, C., & Christiansen, C. (1997). The occupational therapy context: Philosophy–principles–practice. In C. Christiansen & C. Baum (Eds.), *Occupational therapy: Enabling function and well-being* (2nd ed., pp. 26–45). Thorofare, NJ: Slack.

Cynkin, S., & Robinson, A. M. (1990). *Occupational therapy and activities health: Toward health through activities.* Boston: Little, Brown.

Evans, K. A. (1987). Definition of occupation as the core concept of occupational therapy. *American Journal of Occupational Therapy, 41,* 627–628.

Gilfoyle, E. M. (1984). Transformation of a profession [Eleanor Clarke Slagle Lecture]. *American Journal of Occupational Therapy, 38,* 575–584.

Glover, J. A., Bruning, R. H., & Filbeck, R. W. (1983). *Educational psychology: Principles and applications.* Boston: Little, Brown.

Henderson, A., Cermak, S., Coster, W., Murray, E., Trombly, C., & Tickle-Degnen, L. (1991). The Issue Is—Occupational science is multidimensional. *American Journal of Occupational Therapy, 45,* 370–372.

Hinojosa, J., Kramer, P., Royeen, C. B., & Luebben, A. (2003). The core concept of occupation. In P. Kramer, J. Hinojosa, & C. B. Royeen (Eds.), *Perspectives in human occupation: Participation in life* (pp. 1–17). Philadelphia: Lippincott Williams & Wilkins.

Kielhofner, G. (1992). *Conceptual foundations of occupational therapy.* Philadelphia: F. A. Davis.

Kramer, P., & Hinojosa, J. (1995). Epiphany of human occupation. In C. B. Royeen (Ed.), *Human occupation* (AOTA Self-Study Series, Lesson 8). Bethesda, MD: American Occupational Therapy Association.

Kramer, P., & Hinojosa, J. (1999). Domain of concern of occupational therapy: Relevance to pediatric practice. In P. Kramer & J. Hinojosa (Eds.), *Frames of reference for pediatric occupational therapy* (2nd ed., pp. 9–26). Baltimore: Lippincott Williams & Wilkins.

Kramer, P., Luebben, A. J., & Hinojosa, J. (2010). Contemporary legitimate tools of pediatric occupational therapy. In P. Kramer & J. Hinojosa (Eds.), *Frames of reference for pediatric occupational therapy* (3rd ed., pp. 50–66). Baltimore: Lippincott Williams & Wilkins.

Luebben, A. J., Hinojosa, J., & Kramer, P. (2010). Domain of concern of occupational therapy: Relevance to pediatric practice. In P. Kramer & J. Hinojosa (Eds.), *Frames of reference for pediatric occupational therapy* (3rd ed., pp. 31–49). Baltimore: Lippincott Williams & Wilkins.

Maslow, A. H. (1970). *Motivation and personality* (2nd ed.) New York: Harper & Row.

Maslow, A. H. (1971). *The further reaches of human nature.* New York: Viking.

Mosey, A. C. (1981). *Occupational therapy: Configuration of a profession.* New York: Raven.

Mosey, A. C. (1985). A monistic or a pluralistic approach to professional identity? [Eleanor Clarke Slagle Lecture]. *American Journal of Occupational Therapy, 39,* 504–509.

Mosey, A. C. (1986). *Psychosocial components of occupational therapy.* New York: Raven.

Mosey, A. C. (1996). *Applied scientific inquiry in the health professions: An epistemological orientation* (2nd ed.). Bethesda, MD: American Occupational Therapy Association.

Nelson, D. L. (1988). Occupation: Form and performance. *American Journal of Occupational Therapy, 42,* 633–641.

Nelson, D. L. (1997). Why the profession of occupational therapy will flourish in the 21st century [Eleanor Clarke Slagle Lecture]. *American Journal of Occupational Therapy, 51,* 11–34.

Nelson, D. L., & Jepson-Thomas, J. (2003). Occupational form, occupational performance, and a conceptual framework for therapeutic occupation. In P. Kramer, J. Hinojosa, & C.

B. Royeen (Eds.), *Perspectives in human occupation: Participation in life* (pp. 87–155). Philadelphia: Lippincott Williams & Wilkins.

Peloquin, S. M. (1991). Occupational therapy service: Individual and collective understandings of the founders, Part 2. *American Journal of Occupational Therapy, 45,* 733–744.

Pierce, D. (2001). Untangling occupation and activity. *American Journal of Occupational Therapy, 55,* 138–146.

Strauss, A. L. (2001). *Professions, work, and careers.* New Brunswick, NJ: Transaction.

World Health Organization. (2001). *International classification of functioning, disability and health.* Geneva: Author.

2

⬧

Perspectives

Marie-Louise Blount, AM, OT, FAOTA
Wesley Blount
Jim Hinojosa, PhD, OT, FAOTA

As much as occupational therapy has always been defined by the use of purposeful activity and occupation, very little has been done to pull together the concepts of *purposeful activities* and *occupation* that theorists use to define the profession. Needless to say, many differing theoretical approaches have grown and transformed as the profession has grown and changed over the years. As theorists have added to the body of knowledge from different perspectives, these differing approaches have led to multiple realities regarding the ways in which occupational therapy is seen, with each relevant term taking on a different meaning with each new theorist. At the same time, to carve out unique vantage points, theorists will frequently ignore others' definitions or subtly redefine the scope of another's work.

The broadening range of occupational therapy's areas of practice has necessitated a continual need to expand the definitions that make up the very notion of the profession. What began as a limited range of arts and crafts activities has grown to include the rehabilitation of soldiers; pediatric therapy and the role of play; examination of self-care; and, recently, spirituality and nonactive occupations of different kinds. Each expansion has brought with it a reexamination of the very notion of what constitutes purposeful activities and occupation, and delicate nuances have separated terms that often seem similar, such as *occupation* and *purposeful activities*.

It would be difficult under any circumstances to present an overview of the development of theoretical terms in occupational therapy, which may explain why there have been few attempts to bring together the various contributions of the professions' important theorists and examine them one after another. Since the publication of this book's first edition, however, several books and articles have laid out similar historically based approaches to developing theories or practice models. Several new theorists have entered the fray with new conceptual approaches to the profession, definitions, and theoretical approaches underpinning the therapeutic models. Some of the theorists we originally discussed have refined their approaches, and occupational science has grown in ways that may often be beyond the scope of occupational therapy. What has become clearer in the years since the first edition is that theory in occupational therapy has become a synthesis of ideas relating to activity and performance.

No single correct answer to the question of "which theory?" exists, and that is why we still believe that nothing can substitute for reading the works of each of these distinguished contributors in their original form. Each theorist has, in some way, attempted to draw respectfully on earlier work to ground his or her approach; each definition of *activity* is, in some way, a refinement of past work. What we present here is an overview of the major theorists with summaries of their important contributions to the concepts of purposeful activities and occupation. We believe that with understanding of these differing approaches comes perspective and awareness of the important work already done in laying a theoretical basis for the profession.

We believe in developing a taxonomy that will afford consistency in referencing and add to the body of knowledge regarding occupational therapy. The profession is a dynamic entity, growing and changing even as we gather these ideas together. Any attempt at defining terms must reflect this continual dynamic change and the constant synthesis that persists in developing theoretical approaches. Some of the theoretical approaches we discuss are included primarily for their historical importance to the field rather than for their current applications; however, taken together these theories show the progression of thinking about occupational therapy practice.

Activities and Lifestyle Performance: Gail Fidler

As an occupational therapist, association leader, educator, and scholar, Gail Fidler had a powerful influence on the profession's knowledge and understanding of purposeful activities. Fidler's views and opinions about purposeful activities came from her conviction that doing activities is vitally important and therefore meaningful to people. For occupational therapy, activities have powerful therapeutic merit. From Fidler's (1996) perspective, *purposeful activities* and *occupation* are synonymous terms for the same construct.

Fidler recognized that if society is to value occupational therapy and the use of activities as authentic therapeutic modalities, occupational therapists need a conceptual rationale for using activities. In 1948, observing that the occupational therapy literature discussed only the appeal, interest factors, and popularity of activities, Fidler argued that occupational therapists needed a scientific method of empirically examining activities and analyzing their value. She proposed an activity analysis as one approach, giving therapists a means to examine activities by dividing them into component parts.

Understanding an activity's component parts provides the information that a therapist needs to match a specific activity to a client's need and treatment objectives (Fidler, 1948). This original activity analysis is the foundation for many activity analyses used today. Subsequently, Fidler (1969) turned her attention to the therapeutic value of active involvement in doing activities in task groups.

In 1954, with her husband Jay, Fidler published a book titled *Introduction to Psychiatric Occupational Therapy*. This text included extensive discussion of the use of activities in psychiatric settings and provided a conceptual rationale for using purposeful activities for all occupational therapists. Analyzing the component parts of an activity provides the information that therapists require to correlate the client's needs, interests, and abilities. Moreover, occupational therapy impels the person to develop skills through an action-oriented learning experience (Fidler & Fidler, 1954). Fidler and Fidler introduced occupational therapists to the psychodynamic properties of activities. Some aspects of the activity to be examined were related to then-contemporary psychodynamic beliefs, including motion, procedures, materials, creativity, symbols, hostile and aggressive components, control, predictability, narcissism, sexual identification, dependence, reality testing, and group relatedness. Fidler and Fidler also stressed the importance of human and nonhuman environments in understanding and performing activities.

In a 1978 article titled "Doing and Becoming: Purposeful Action and Self-Actualization," Fidler and Fidler provided a theoretical rationale for purposeful activities. They selected the word *doing*, saying that "doing is viewed as enabling the development and integration of the sensory, motor, cognitive, and psychological systems; serving as a socializing agent; and verifying one's efficacy as a competent, contributing member of one's society" (p. 305). Knowledge about activities allows an occupational therapist to select a particular activity that matches the client's therapeutic needs, learning readiness, intact functions, and values. The practitioner then plans and implements an action-learning experience to allow the client to develop skills (Fidler & Fidler, 1978). Purposeful activities provide opportunities and means for a person to achieve mastery and competence because all activities have social relevance; each person has individual activity interests, which have personal meaning and a place in the social construct, and these activities can remediate dysfunction and have therapeutic value (Fidler, 1981).

In the introduction to *Activities: Reality and Symbol*, Fidler and Beth Velde (1999) summarized the elements that define activity; in 2002, Velde and Fidler put forward the Life Style Performance Model to provide a comprehensive picture of a person's activities, abilities, needs, interests, capacities, and self-expectation of his or her human and nonhuman world. This model highlights the interrelatedness of person, environment, activity profile, and quality of life. The model describes four activity domains: (1) activities concerned with self-care and self-maintenance, (2) personally referenced pleasure and intrinsic gratification, (3) societal contribution, and (4) interpersonal engagement. The role of a practitioner in this model is to work with a client toward a healthy activity pattern. Quality of life is considered to be extremely important, and the practitioner needs to have a holistic view of practice—that is, getting direction from the client.

In this respect, Velde and Fidler's (2002) model closely resembles the work of Mary Law (1998) and the Person–Environment–Occupation Model developed out of the client-centered approach as presented in the first edition of *Occupational Therapy: Overcoming Human Performance Deficits* (Christiansen & Baum, 1991). As with Law (see the "Person–Environment–Occupation Model: Mary Law" section), the client interview is paramount, the client's needs are foremost, and the measures for successful intervention are on the personal rather than the scientific level.

Thus, the role of purposeful activity is, in many ways, individual and personalized. Focusing on the benefits of therapeutic intervention for the person is obviously an important part of practice; however, one also needs to recognize the difficulty of objective study of the roles and effectiveness of different activities within these client-centered performance models. Fidler's synthesis of the ideas she developed with her collaborators shows both how theoretical thinking evolves over time and that inclusive theories adapt well and new concepts arise.

Occupational Behavior: Mary Reilly

A seminal and critical writer and thinker in occupational therapy is Mary Reilly. Although she has not devoted all of her attention to issues of activity and occupation, her ideas, eventually subsumed under the title *occupational behavior* (Reilly, 1966), gave attention to these issues of activity and occupation, making concerns about these issues an underlying theme.

Among Reilly's concerns was the impetus to study and investigate the profession to establish its contributions to science clearly. Reilly (1960) therefore suggested that a major area for occupational therapy research should be the nature and meaning of activity. The presumption that people require activity to attain and maintain health is fundamental to the profession's beliefs, in Reilly's (1960) opinion: "We are becoming more aware of the fact that the interests of man emerge in the gratification of his senses" (p. 208). Indeed, she stressed that investigation of the need to engage in activity should move beyond traditional occupational therapy reliance on arts and crafts and into analysis of such activities as the appropriate level for the investigation (Reilly, 1960). She emphasized the physical, sensory, and psychic rewards inherent in activity and spoke against the idea that various approaches to the use of activity (e.g., separating dance from recreation from crafts) serve as the best approach to the application of therapeutic activity.

In her Eleanor Clarke Slagle Lecture, Reilly (1962) further affirmed the centrality of work to human existence. Her thesis in this presentation was that human productivity provides the most life satisfaction and that occupational therapy applies this principle to the maintenance and restoration of health. Occupational therapy intervention (*treatment,* in her words) requires that the therapist investigate and address problems people have in coping with "play, work, and school" (p. 7). She also expressed in this presentation her rejection of the word *activity* to describe how occupational therapists engage patients because she had become wary of the increasing use of terms such as *activity therapy* in treatment settings that moved occupational therapy away from seeking to enhance individual human productivity.

As Reilly's approach to the study of occupational therapy came to be called *occupational behavior* (Reilly, 1966), she referred back to the core ideas of early occupational therapy thinkers: that a satisfying life required a balanced approach to work, rest, and play. Occupational therapy, appropriately applied, would establish a setting in which all of these aspects of life could be addressed. In describing a model program that did address all of these, Reilly included exercise programs, required work activities, and learning recreational skills and included some group activities and social skills.

Reilly's interest in occupation and related activities later developed into a special concentration on the occupation of play as it applied to both children and adults (Reilly, 1974). She investigated, along with her students, the development of occupational behaviors during play and play's relationship to people's exploration of their environments, their development of competence, and their fulfillment of the drive to achieve.

Reilly's striving to understand the nature and functions of human occupation and to apply this knowledge to occupational therapy intervention led to the development of the Model of Human Occupation and eventually to the school of thought called *occupational science.*

Model of Human Occupation: Gary Kielhofner

As students of Reilly, Gary Kielhofner and Janice Burke have taken a theory of occupational behavior and expanded both its external framework and its organizing principles. Kielhofner (Figure 2.1) continued to refine this theoretical approach as a Model of Human Occupation (MOHO; Forsyth & Kielhofner, 2003; Kielhofner, 1995, 2008, 2009; Kielhofner & Burke, 1980), and he used the model to observe and explain most aspects of theory related to occupational therapy. Indeed, one of the central tenets of the model is that human occupation can be used for therapeutic benefit, which also advocates a balanced lifestyle that includes both work and leisure (thus expanding on Reilly's [1974] notion of play).

In Kielhofner's (1985) view, "Occupation is a multifaceted phenomenon that involves the simultaneous operation of biological, psychological, social, and ecological factors" (p. xvii). Like most of Kielhofner's definitions, his notion of *occupation* relies on multiple levels of explanation to allow for as

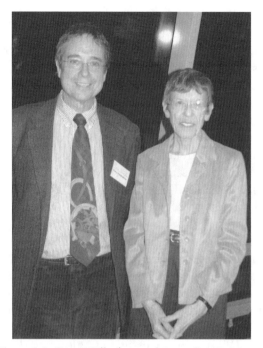

Figure 2.1. Gary Kielhofner and Anne Cronin Mosey.

many aspects within a framework as are needed to explain the multitude of possibilities inherent in human behavior.

Kielhofner (1995) began his model by developing historical perspectives on human behavior within the context of systems theory. From this, he posited that human beings are an example of an open system, that is, that human activity involves taking in information (or input), synthesizing the information, and then creating output. The important quality of an open system, he argued, is the opportunity for feedback, responses to the output that allow the person to make changes and, with the same input, create a different output.

Within the person, Kielhofner and Burke (1980) saw several components and determinants that affect human behavior. These include *volition*, *habituation*, and *performance*. *Volition* refers to the impulses that cause the person to value certain types of occupation, including *personal causation* (the knowledge of self), *values* (images of what is good, right, or important), and *interests* (the disposition to find particular occupations pleasurable). *Habituation*, in turn, refers to the normative definitions the person places on occupation, encompassing *roles* (publicly recognized positions or society's input) and *habits* (the private regulation of behavior). *Performance* deals with the person's skills in performing occupations, containing communication, process, and perceptual–motor skills (Kielhofner, 1995).

After laying down the internal structures that make up individual behavior, Kielhofner (1985) then dealt with the external aspects of human occupation, including determining whether the person is functional or dysfunctional and thus in need of therapeutic intervention. Just as function in his view has three levels—exploration, competence, and achievement—Kielhofner (1985) saw dysfunction as having three corresponding levels—inefficiency, incompetence, and helplessness. He emphasized that both function and dysfunction should be seen as processes, not static states. For occupational dysfunction to exist, Kielhofner explained, the person in his or her social group does not meet expectations for productive and playful participation. Moreover, the person "does not fulfill the urge to explore and master" (p. 64) his or her environment.

Using this model, Kielhofner (1992, 2009) has developed ideas about the optimal use of therapy in treating dysfunction and has worked to fit the model into larger contexts such as the conceptual foundations of occupational therapy. Indeed, the model was initiated with the specific goal of developing resources to guide and enhance practice (Forsyth & Kielhofner, 2003), and Kielhofner's recent collaborations have focused on the model's application to practice. Kielhofner did not engage in the debate regarding terms like *activity* or *occupation* as much as he ignored it altogether. Kielhofner used occupation as his central concept in developing theories regarding occupational therapy, but more fundamentally, he felt that the person's role in the complex process of human occupation defined what people and, following Kielhofner's model, therapists will do to improve human function. Similarly, in Kielhofner's (2007) most recent update to the model, he pointed out that the MOHO has always been a client-centered approach to occupational therapy. Kielhofner's detailed model, with its emphasis on human behavior, goes a long way toward establishing a psychological framework for the human need for occupation in daily life.

Person–Environment–Occupation Model: Mary Law

In conjunction with a variety of different collaborators, Mary Law has focused on the relationship between the practitioner and the person receiving services, or *client,* to develop a client-centered approach to occupational therapy. In developing this approach, Law (1998) and her Canadian colleagues have continued to refine the theories developed in the Person–Environment–Occupation (PEO) Model, which defines the interrelationship of the person to his or her environment and both of these elements in relation to the role of occupation. In defining each element, Law et al. (1994) differentiated among *activity, task,* and *occupation:*

- *Activity* is the basic unit of a task. It is defined as a singular pursuit in which a person engages as part of his or her daily occupational experience. An example of an activity is the act of writing.
- *Task* is defined as a set of purposeful activities in which a person engages. An example of a task is the obligation to write a report.

- *Occupation* is defined as groups of activities in which a person engages over the lifespan. *Occupations* are defined as those clusters of activities and tasks in which the person engages to meet his or her intrinsic needs for self-maintenance, expression, and fulfillment. These are carried out within the context of individual roles and multiple environments.

Using the model, Law and her Canadian team have looked across the literature to validate their approach (Peachey-Hill & Law, 2000) and worked to turn the model into a practical application for occupational therapy (Strong et al., 1999). In its application, the PEO Model becomes a way for the therapist to take into account the multiplicity of factors affecting the client's performance, and a treatment plan is developed that takes into account not only the impact of different activities on the person but also how those activities are appropriate for the environment in which the person will make use of them.

All of this work is informed by the client-centered approach that Law and her team have developed alongside the model. This approach to occupational therapy brings together several strands of observation and research from occupational therapy and other disciplines. As an early basis for the client-centered approach, Law and Mills (1998) cited psychologist Carl Rogers, who emphasized the need for therapists to work with clients in developing solutions to problems rather than to direct the course of therapy. Law and Mills also took into account the views of people with disabilities and their feelings regarding treatment.

The client-centered approach developed in Canada is a series of guidelines for practice produced by the Canadian Association of Occupational Therapists (Gill & Brockett, 1987). Law et al. (1994) produced the Canadian Occupational Performance Measure (COPM), an assessment tool designed to measure "a client's self-perception of occupational performance" (p. 191). Although Law et al. subsequently referred to the pilot testing as covering a "broad spectrum" of clients and environments, the participants were mostly people older than age 60 residing in inpatient geriatric facilities. Thus, their ability to assess their own conditions and treatment needs may have been better facilitated by the client-centered approach than that of a population less able to indicate self-awareness or occupational needs, such as children with developmental disabilities. In fact, contributors to *Client-Centered Occupational Therapy* (Law, 1998) discussed in several chapters the various ways of interpreting the term *client*. The client comes to be seen as not only the person receiving therapy but also as "someone who wishes to make a change through the process of therapy" (Pollock & McColl, 1998, p. 91), that is, possibly the caregiver or parent. A frequent example used in the works of these authors and Law is that of the Alzheimer's patient who may be unable to communicate his or her needs; in such cases, the client is considered to be the caregiving spouse (and the term *spouse* is the one most often used in this example), and as in the client-centered approach, the caregiver's role is that which changes.

In the client-centered approach, then, the client defines the activity and occupation that provide therapeutic benefit, and the client's needs are foremost in the development of interventions created in partnership between the client and the therapist. This approach may seem somewhat reflexive because an assessment model would seem to always require that the client's needs be part of the determination of appropriate therapy. What is important to Law and her colleagues, however, is that the assessment comes from the client and the value of the therapy is always best evaluated by the client; the therapist serves as a facilitator who aids the client in identifying areas of concern and assists in developing a plan to address those areas (and, in theory, those areas alone). One of the central concepts of client-centered practice is that occupational therapy service delivery is flexible and individualized, and the very flexibility and mutability of using occupation and activity makes it difficult to determine a specific approach to using occupation as a means of therapy in the client-centered practice. Law and Mills (1998) acknowledged the lack of specific methodologies in client-centered therapy.

The focus of client-centered occupational therapy is on changing the overall approach to therapy from that of the medical model. In the medical model, therapists are perceived as all-knowing and treatment is evaluated on generalized goals such as "independence at all costs" (Law, 1998, p. 71; see also Baum & Law, 1997). In the client-centered approach, the focus is on the client's finding meaning in everyday occupations and the development of active collaboration between the occupational therapist and client to resolve occupational performance problems (Baum & Law, 1997). Specific assessments and treatment plans are not spelled out because the client-centered approach makes those determinations part of the larger client–therapist process of developing a relationship. As with Fidler (1996), the approach makes scientific and comparative evaluation of treatment methods challenging but refocuses the role of therapy on the benefits to the person.

Since the last edition of this book, Mary Law has begun collaborating with Winnie Dunn (see "Ecology of Human Performance: Winnie Dunn" section) and Carolyn Baum (see next section) on ways to improve outcomes measurement when studying therapeutic interventions and effectiveness (Law, Baum, & Dunn, 2005). As Law et al. explained in the first chapter of *Measuring Occupational Performance: Supporting Best Practice in Occupational Therapy,*

> The health system focuses on outcomes because of the need to be accountable, not only to the clients in need of services, but also to the government and/or the third party who is paying the bill. With a shift in focus toward primary and secondary prevention, it is also important to know if interventions are successful in reducing the impact of secondary problems. Medical outcomes are being defined as well-being and quality of life; improved occupational performance is a critical construct in measuring quality of life regardless of the measure that is used. (p. 10)

Law et al. (2005) went on to discuss the different frameworks—such as Ecology of Human Performance and MOHO—and the different measurement issues with each in an attempt to develop good measurement processes for research and to allow therapists to develop a standard of comparison across frameworks as well. This perspective also reflects a growing sense in U.S. health care that *comparative effectiveness*—the ability to evaluate different treatment options on the basis of the best outcomes for the client—is a key piece of improving health care delivery. Although this work is still in its early stages, developing good measurement tools and focusing on outcomes in a client-centered approach to care is a key step toward taking theories of practice into real-life, practical settings, identifying what works and what works well in improving occupational performance.

Occupation: Charles Christiansen and Carolyn Baum

The Canadian models also informed Charles Christiansen's (Figure 2.2) and Carolyn Baum's (Figure 2.3) attempts to bring together differing theories of activity and occupation to lay a theoretical framework for teaching practice. Although their organizing principle has shifted with each edition, Christiansen and Baum's texts have illustrated the evolving nature of how educators approach theoretical concepts in occupational therapy and the challenges in providing theoretical context to new students. In *Occupational Therapy: Overcoming Human Performance Deficits,* Christiansen and Baum (1991) proposed an Occupational Performance Hierarchy that centers on "*the activity*, which consists of specific goal-oriented behaviors . . . directed toward the performance of a task" (p. 28). The emphasis on activities as related to the performance of tasks creates the theoretical basis for occupational therapy as a way to treat dysfunction or disability.

The work of previous authors serves in this context as a way to take ideas about activity and apply them to the practice of occupational therapy. By contrast, in *Occupational Therapy: Enabling Function and Well-Being,* Christiansen and Baum (1997) focused much more on the development of a definition of *occupation*, moving away from both activity and the notion of disability. The revisions to the text allowed for the incorporation of newer ideas from different theorists but also underscored the difficulty of taking the differing approaches and blending them into a coherent whole. Like Kielhofner, Christiansen and Baum (1997) developed a model that is referred to at the start of each chapter, attempting to encompass all possible facets of human performance in an arrow-shaped form that points to well-being, and each chapter in the text is meant to present a part of this triangular model.

Using the ideas developed by Law and her Canadian colleagues (Gill & Brockett, 1987; Law, 1998; Law et al., 1994; Law & Mills, 1998), Christiansen and Baum (1997) emphasized the client-centered approach, with a resulting deemphasis on specific practice solutions to problems and greater emphasis

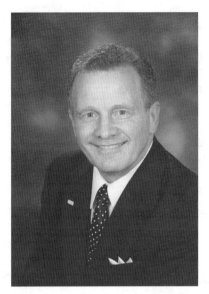

Figure 2.2. Charles Christiansen.

on the client's needs and perceptions. This deemphasis on specific treatments for dysfunction also incorporated the occupational science focus on wellness and healthy occupational performance.

In *Occupational Therapy: Performance, Participation, and Well-Being,* Christiansen, Baum, and Bass-Haugen (2005) moved toward an almost entirely theoretical approach to discussing occupational therapy. Occupational performance now sits at the center of a four-concentric-circle model balancing well-being and quality of life, and the book's essays generally cover different theoretical approaches to various aspects of the field. Although Law's (1998)

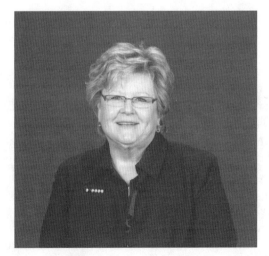

Figure 2.3. Carolyn Baum.

PEO model was still central to the understanding of occupation, Christiansen et al. (2005) examined and discussed a wide range of theoretical concepts in detail, and even when discussing practical concepts, such as interventions, their greater focus is on rationale over specific applications. Although the book is a fascinating compendium of deep thinking about the role of occupational therapy, whether its heavy emphasis on theory is ultimately beneficial to entry-level students remains to be seen. The continual evolution of the text, though, illustrates how a developing theoretical consensus continues to shape the way in which the field is taught.

Activities Health: Simme Cynkin

Simme Cynkin (1979; Cynkin & Robinson, 1990) provided perspective on the fundamental nature of activity as a therapeutic response to dysfunction. In this perspective, the fundamental value of activities to humans is the basis for occupational therapy. Activities are part of people's human existence, and Cynkin (1979) believed the very presence of activity in people's daily lives promotes their physical and mental well-being. This belief is discussed in four assumptions about activities:

- Activities of many kinds are the essence of human existence, based on the interactions of individual and environment. Activities focus on survival, subsistence, and coexistence.
- Activities are a culmination of acceptable norms of behaviors that are defined by a sociocultural system of values and beliefs.
- Acceptable and unacceptable variations exist in individual activities.
- A person's engaging in meaningful activities leads to a satisfying way of life and personal fulfillment (Cynkin, 1979; Cynkin & Robinson, 1990).

Cynkin and Robinson's (1990) assumptions are derived from a historical perspective: Activity has always defined human existence, and activities are basic to human survival. Drawing on the works of psychologist Jean Piaget and Mary Reilly, Cynkin and Robinson centralized human nature and a person's humanity on the performance of a variety of activities, both personal and interpersonal. To this foundation, they added the notion of differing sociocultural norms and differing values placed by various societies on particular activities.

Building on the notion that people can change, Cynkin and Robinson (1990) further argued that behavior related to activity can be changed and that behavioral changes can improve the person's functioning. Moreover, the person can learn to improve function, and this learning process can take place in a variety of ways, both direct and indirect.

The importance of these assumptions, and the framework Cynkin and Robinson (1990) developed from them, laid the foundation for the teaching of ideas behind occupational therapy. "Early occupational therapy was founded on the belief that being engaged in activities promotes mental and physical well-being and that, conversely, absence of activity leads . . . at worst to deterioration or loss of mental and physical functioning" (p. 4). Although theorists such as Fidler (1948) had developed ways of analyzing activity, Cynkin (1979) provided an important additional link: that placing activity in a context of overall human behavior provides greater understanding of its therapeutic importance. Cynkin offered the strongest method possible to give the occupational therapy student not just the tools to assist in restoring function but also the philosophical structure that underlies the importance of activity in everyday life.

Occupational Form and Occupational Performance: David Nelson

David Nelson (1994; Figure 2.4) was particularly interested in the term *occupation* and its meaning for occupational therapists. In his 1996 Eleanor Clarke Slagle Lecture, he related this interest to part of a historical tradition and set of beliefs of occupational therapists: "The human being can attain . . . health and quality of life by actively doing things that are personally meaningful and purposeful, in other words, through occupation" (Nelson, 1997, p. 11). His principal contribution to this perspective has been semantic and includes developing a nomenclature to delimit the use of the term *occupation* by occupational therapists. His terms apply to the therapeutic discipline of occupational therapy.

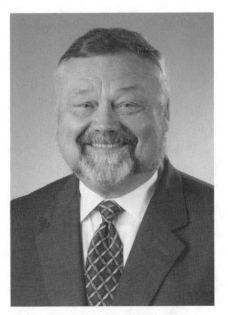

Figure 2.4. David Nelson.

Nelson (1994) divided the term *occupation* into his terms for its essential aspects, *form* and *performance*. *Form* has to do with the objects and circumstances that make the occupation possible. Forms can be a game, a building in which an occupation takes place, a piece of equipment, a piece of music, or another person, to name just a few. Forms are essential to the occupation.

Performance, however, is what the person does to accomplish the occupation. Nelson (1994) stated that performance, in this sense, must be voluntary: "The 'doing' is the occupational performance, and the 'something' to be done is the occupational form" (p. 11). *Performance*, then, is playing the game, constructing the building, lifting the weight for exercise, playing the music, or teaching something to the other person.

Nelson (1994) viewed occupation as the relationship between an occupational form and an occupational performance. Occupations may be as variable as the people who are performing them. If the occupation is eating a meal, the occupational forms, at a simple level, may be breakfast, lunch, or dinner. The occupational performances may be as divergent as a baby eating some oatmeal and "feeding" the rest to the high chair tray and the floor or a diet-conscious 20-year-old woman picking carefully at the low-fat foods on her plate. Some variables that come into play include duration, certainty of outcome, and intricacy.

To Nelson (1994), the term *occupational form* has a physical dimension and a sociocultural dimension. The *physical dimension* is the measurable factors and includes objects, other physical characteristics of the occupation, and the temporal aspects of the occupation. The *sociocultural dimension* includes social and cultural practices, expectations, and settings. For the occupation of playing music, a contemporary, atonal classical piece may be played on an electronic keyboard in a museum in Bucharest, Romania, which might define the piece's sociocultural dimension.

Nelson and Jepson-Thomas (2003) divided the sociocultural dimension into symbols, norms, roles, variations, and language. For the person playing the keyboard, some of the symbols are the notes on the musical score. A norm might be the loudness or softness of the sound itself. The pianist is enacting a role. Variations are present in almost every occupation. In this example, the language, perhaps Romanian in this case, may not be as relevant as the musical sounds. Change and social hierarchies have been incorporated into the system. Occupational form, as Nelson and Jepson-Thomas described it, is a very complex entity.

The person brings all of his or her abilities and characteristics to the occupational performance (Nelson & Jepson-Thomas, 2003). Terms used by occupational therapists, such as *sensorimotor, cognitive,* and *psychosocial,* describe the developmental structure.

Meaning is also brought to the occupation by the person performing it. If the performer in the musical example actually disliked atonal music, his concert might be very different from one for which he had selected his favorite piece.

Any given occupation may have more than one purpose. Not only may a given person have more than one purpose for performing an occupation, but also others may each have different purposes for performing the same occupation. Reading a novel for enjoyment is an example of an *intrinsic motivation*. *Extrinsic motivation,* however, is a purpose found outside of the occupation itself. Reading a textbook for the purpose of passing an exam is an example of an extrinsic purpose. *Conscious* and *unconscious purposes* also exist. An example of an unconscious purpose, according to Nelson (1994), is one involved with a habitual occupation that a person performs routinely with little thought.

One step of an occupation has an impact on those that follow (Nelson, 1994). For example, purchasing fabric and using a pattern to cut out a jacket are steps that have an effect on the actual construction of the jacket. Changes also occur in the person performing an occupation. These are *adaptations*.

Nelson and Jepson-Thomas (2003) defined *activities* as the building blocks of adaptation. They designated these portions of occupations as *suboccupations* or even *sub-suboccupations*.

The occupational therapist, occupational therapy assistant, and occupational therapy student must have a structure and process in which to perceive occupation to move onto therapeutic application. Nelson (1994) termed that process *occupational synthesis*, designating an occupational experience that will have therapeutic impact. The recipient of service is a collaborator in the therapeutic process. Nelson and Jepson-Thomas (2003) stated that occupational synthesis is the job of the occupational therapist.

Nelson (1994) deliberately avoided the word *activity*. In his view and in the view of others, the term is not specific enough because it is sometimes applied to other than human enterprises and because it is not always purposeful. He pointed out that terms such as *molecular activity* and *solar activity* (p. 42) clearly do not refer to human enterprises and that *activity* can refer to any kind of liveliness (see also Darnell & Heater, 1994). Recent writings offer somewhat greater attention to the person performing the occupation but have generally given most attention to the occupation itself.

Ecology of Human Performance: Winnie Dunn

Drawing on the interest in developing a comprehensive framework, Winnie Dunn (Figure 2.5), along with Catana Brown and Ann McGuigan, constructed the Ecology of Human Performance (Dunn, Brown, & McGuigan, 1994). Similar to the Canadian PEO Model (Law, 1998), the central focus of this group from the University of Kansas is on the environment and how the person fits into it. Drawing on Mosey's (1981) notion of frame of reference and Nelson's (1994) occupational forms, the Kansas group developed a framework of context to explain the way in which a person and the tasks the person does fit into an environment.

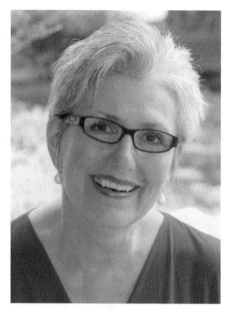

Figure 2.5. Winnie Dunn.

Tasks are defined as objective sets of behaviors necessary to accomplish a goal (Dunn et al., 1994; Dunn, Brown, & Youngstrom, 2003).

Drawing on the work of environmental psychologists, the Ecology of Human Performance thus makes context the center of the therapeutic evaluation and intervention. In this way, it is similar to the notion of lifestyle advanced by Fidler (1996) and the holistic approach envisioned in the Canadian client-centered approach (Law, 1998). A key difference, however, is the change in emphasis to the environment. As with Kielhofner (1985), Dunn et al. (1994, 2003) were less interested in defining *activity* vs. *occupation* and have instead focused more on the external framework into which the person and the therapeutic intervention fit in various situations.

Using the Ecology of Human Performance framework, Dunn et al. (1994) then described five different potential relationships for therapeutic intervention as it relates to the person. Therapeutic intervention can establish or restore (remediate) the person's skills and abilities. Intervention can also alter the context in which a person performs, selecting a context that enables him or her to perform with current skills and abilities. The therapist can also adapt the contextual features and task demands to design a more supportive context for a person's performance. Another alternative is to prevent the occurrence or evolution of maladaptive performance in context. Finally, the therapist can create circumstances that promote more adaptable or complex performance in context. Using these five therapeutic choices, the therapist can evaluate the person in the appropriate context and design an intervention best suited to the person's needs within that context.

By emphasizing the role of context and environment in making therapeutic assessments, the Ecology of Human Performance takes a different look at familiar concepts. In doing so, it exemplifies the value of synthesis within the profession, taking existing ideas and thinking about them in new and different ways. The Ecology of Human Performance takes many things as given: the role of tasks in a person's life and the use of tasks to provide therapeutic benefit. These are ideas that other theorists continue to debate, but clearly the importance of making careful, individualized assessments has become a key part of the theoretical approach to practice, and the Ecology of Human Performance offers yet another way to look at the environmental factors that can affect treatment. As mentioned earlier, Dunn has begun work with Law and Baum to develop an approach to measuring outcomes as a way to establish best practices in the field.

Occupational Adaptation: Janette Schkade and Sally Schultz

Also synthesizing much of the work that came before them, Janette Schkade and Sally Schultz of Texas Woman's University developed the Model of Occupational Adaptation as a holistic approach to contemporary practice (Schkade & Schultz, 1992). This model focuses on the interaction between the person and the occupational environment, which is the context in which occupations occur. *Occupations,* in their approach, are activities characterized by three properties—active participation, meaning to the person, and a product that is the output of a process (Schkade & Schultz, 1992, Part I). In Schkade and Schultz's model, the person's desire for mastery will cause him or her to develop an adaptive response to an occupational challenge. At the same time, a demand for mastery comes from within the occupational environment. In the interaction between the desire and the demand, the person will develop adaptive responses to gain mastery of the occupational challenge.

Schultz and Schkade (1992) then applied this model to occupational therapy practice. In practice, occupational adaptation is focused on *occupational function*—that is, the person's ability to function in the environment—rather than on the acquisition of particular functional skills. In practice, the therapist works in a therapeutic climate with the patient to determine the goal of therapy. The therapist then uses *occupational activities* (discrete activities that can promote occupational adaptation) and *occupational readiness* (skill-based activities and interventions to prepare for occupational activities, e.g. resistive exercise or assistive devices) to allow the patient to develop relative mastery. In many cases, these activities are related to occupations of daily living, the unique patterns of occupations in which the person regularly engages.

In attempting to make the Model of Occupational Adaptation universal, Schkade and Schultz (2003) synthesized many of the prior theoretical notions of activity and occupation to draw together a common perspective. The focus is on synthesizing ideas, not developing new ones altogether, and Occupational Adaptation as a theory adapts the material that has come before to develop a holistic methodology. Although Schkade and Schultz's focus on the adaptive process and the desire for mastery is differentiated from those of others, the notion of activity and occupation (and the client-centered approach) for therapeutic benefit fits comfortably into the theoretical underpinnings of the profession as it continues to develop.

Occupational Science: University of Southern California's Department of Occupational Science and Occupational Therapy

Occupational science is literally the study of occupation and its role in human experience. Florence Clark et al. (1991) defined *occupation* as "chunks of culturally and personally meaningful activity in which humans engage that can be named in the lexicon of culture" (p. 301). The study of occupation is grounded in a Model of Human Subsystems that influences occupation. Similar to Kielhofner's MOHO (Kielhofner & Burke, 1980), it is based on an open systems model that includes feedback, which allows the person to make changes in occupational behavior. We should note that occupational science as a discipline at present encompasses the studies of human and non-human occupation and occupational behavior.

Because of the focus on generalized concepts regarding occupation and not on specific uses of purposeful activities in therapeutic settings, occupational science writings deal with the theoretical issues developed here principally in ways tangential to larger questions. Interest in occupational science as a field of study related to occupational therapy has continued to grow, leading to additional graduate programs around the world, a scholarly journal, and many meetings to share new work. These works range from broad studies of occupations in different societies to looking at occupational roles and their therapeutic benefit.

Yet purposeful activities are embedded within the occupational science definition of *occupation*. A person's participation in meaningful and socially valued activities is emphasized as the core of occupational therapy's moral philosophy (Zemke & Clark, 1996). This belief is generated from the fact that occupational therapists focus on the everyday things that people need to do. Some have felt the need to immerse themselves in the study of these occupations of daily living in which people engage during their lifetime. Henderson (1996) stated that confusion exists between the terms *occupation* and *purposeful activity* because the vocabulary of occupational science has not been agreed on, and the terms are used interchangeably. Similarly to Clark et al. (1991), Henderson (1996) described *occupation* as being chunks or units of culturally and personally meaningful activity within the stream of human behavior, with each level of occupation further subdivided into smaller units. Henderson believed that *occupation* and *purposeful activity* are equated in the field of occupational therapy, and therefore occupational therapists must seek to further understand their interrelationships to distinguish the levels of occupations in which people engage.

Purposeful activities are defined in relation to particular activities and accepted with the notion that adaptations can occur in people's activities. Human beings have a self-reinforcing power to challenge themselves in an array of adaptive strategies to improve quality of life. This power is most relevant after a disability when adaptation is required for people to again participate in occupations in which they previously engaged (Frank, 1996).

An important milestone for human beings that is discussed in occupational science is play. *Play* is a purposeful vehicle for change, one that truly encompasses the traditional definition of *purposeful activity*. The literature on play and purposeful activity go hand in hand and are the root of much of what therapists talk about in the therapeutic process. Play, as a purposeful activity, encompasses much of what occupational science is centered on. Play is an important occupation beginning in childhood and continuing throughout the lifespan. Through childhood play exploration, the child creates the act of doing in the activities that he or she carries out daily. Play has its importance in the ability to interact with our environment; children thus use it to cope with changes when they occur (Burke, 1996).

Occupational science writings often attempt to take theories of occupation and broaden their context to create enhanced possibilities for study and application. Concepts such as *adaptation, work,* and *play* (following theories developed by Reilly [1962]) are all examined for their value as parts of human culture, not as areas of specific application. The very expansiveness of the scope of occupational science suggests a substantial philosophical difference in method and application from occupational therapy as it has come to be understood. Anne Cronin Mosey (1992) has gone so far as to suggest that the field should be "partitioned" from occupational therapy because such a separation would serve to distinguish the role of the discipline from that of the profession. Although the two areas of study may not benefit from a total separation, the ideas of occupational science, developed in the years that have followed its genesis, are clearly far broader than the use of occupation for therapeutic benefit. At the graduate level of study, an occupational therapy student may find a text such as *Occupational Science: The Evolving Discipline* (Zemke & Clark, 1996) useful for contemplating the larger cultural implications of activity and occupation. Because this text contains few practical strategies, however, practitioners may not find these writings directly applicable to practice.

Children and Theories of Learning:
Approaches Out of Australia and Canada

As theories of occupational therapy continue to evolve, new areas of interest come into focus. Many of the theories discussed thus far focus primarily on adults, particularly older adults, but theories of occupation that deal in common adult tasks (activities of daily living, leisure, work) are not necessarily immediately applicable to children. Although it is possible to broaden definitions of *activity* and *occupation* to include nearly everything, the specific role of childhood development, and the process of learning in children, makes for very specific differences in approach and treatment.

Two teams of international therapists—one based in Canada and one in Australia—have begun to examine how theories of learning affect approaches to occupational therapy in children. Both teams have developed new, somewhat different frameworks for approaching childhood developmental issues, but they share a similar learning-based approach to activity and occupational therapy for children, examining how children learn and how the therapeutic experience can be a teaching and learning tool.

Jenny Ziviani, an associate professor at the University of Queensland (Brisbane, Queensland, Australia), along with Sylvia Rodger, head of the Division of Occupational Therapy, has worked to develop a comprehensive view of childhood development and the role occupational therapy can play within it (Rodger & Ziviani, 2006).

> Developing comprehensive knowledge of children's activities demands that we reach beyond an understanding of the age appropriateness of a given object or activity. Likewise, understanding children's activity patterns requires more than decontextualized lists of children's daily activities and pie graphs of children's time use. (Law, Petrenchik, Ziviani, & King, 2006, p. 79)

This view, then, is an adaptation of a client-centered approach, understanding that when a child is the primary recipient of therapeutic intervention, his or her needs are different and the role of parents and community may be very different.

More than with adults, an occupational therapist's role with a child may be very similar to that of a teacher, and thus it becomes important to consider how children learn and what kind of strategies should be used to teach them skills. "Using appropriate instructional strategies may help overcome dependence on the part of the child, while also helping minimize the experience of failure" (Greber, Ziviani, & Rodger, 2007, p. 149).

Out of these considerations of how children approach activity and occupation and how they learn, Anne Poulsen, along with Ziviani and others, developed SCOPE-IT (Poulsen & Ziviani, 2004), a model of occupational performance in time. In this model (which follows from notions developed by Kielhofner [1992, 1995]), environmental and temporal factors are examined to help identify strategies that will engage children in greater physical activity. Although SCOPE-IT, as such, is not a theory, its concerns with how to engage children in activity and strategies that acknowledge the role of both work and play serve as a natural development of the larger considerations about learning and childhood development that are under discussion.

Along with the Australians, a group of Canadian therapists based in Ontario have also been developing a theory of learning that serves as an approach to therapy with children (Rodger & Ziviani, 2006). Led by educators at several universities, these Canadian therapists are drawing on educational theories to provide context for approaches to therapy in children.

> The theories that provide guidance for a cognitive, or problem-solving, orientation arise from the fields of cognitive and educational psychology. In recent years, it has become evident that these theories are also entirely compatible with the evolution of theory that has taken place in the fields of motor learning and motor control. (Missiuna, Mandich, Polatajko, & Malloy-Miller, 2001, p. 71)

In Canada, concerns about developmental coordination disorder and approaches to childhood development have led to the development of Cognitive Orientation to Occupational Performance (CO-OP), which is a practical model of a strategy for learning in children, especially around motor skills. "Through [a] process of guided discovery, the child, in collaboration with the therapist or adult, identifies specific strategies that facilitate performance of the task" (Taylor, Fayed, & Mandich, 2007, p. 125). Here again, the focus on learning in children, and how to break down and teach a task or skill, takes into account how children learn and the therapist's role in facilitating learning of skills. Again, CO-OP is not a theoretical framework, but its practical approaches to teaching skills are grounded in notions of childhood development that serve as an important new theoretical framework.

Legitimate Tool: Anne Cronin Mosey

In 1968, Anne Cronin Mosey (see Figure 2.1) proposed that occupational therapists should develop and use frames of reference to guide their evaluation and interventions. Frames of reference provide therapists with an organized theoretical knowledge base for practice. Occupational therapists use a variety of means to carry out or implement their theoretically based interventions, which Mosey (1981) labeled the profession's *legitimate tools*, or the means that a professional uses to accomplish a goal, including activities, actions, instruments, modalities, methods, and processes. This perspective of a profession's having legitimate tools acknowledges that although many different professions use the same therapeutic modalities, no one profession "owns" them. Professions may share tools, but each profession uses them in unique ways that are authorized by society. This dynamic view of a profession's legitimate tools means that a profession's tools change as the profession evolves. Moreover, this view recognizes that the use of a tool is directed by the theoretical perspective that the therapist has selected to address the client's needs.

Before her classification of legitimate tools, Mosey (1973) had identified the unique therapeutic value of activities in assisting people with mental illness to become part of their communities and to engage in their daily lives. In this text, *Activities Therapy*, Mosey described the power of doing an activity as a means for a person to learn new skills and behaviors. She underscored the potential of learning through doing; purposeful "activities are used to provide familiar life situations in which participants are assisted in identifying faulty patterns of behavior and the ideas, feelings, and values that support these faulty patterns" (p. 2). Activities provide therapists with a means to understand the person and a method to assist him or her in participating in the tasks at hand. Important aspects of using activities therapeutically are, among others, that they involve the here and now, they are action oriented, and they involve learning through doing. Mosey also emphasized the notions of satisfaction and enjoyment of the activity and the therapeutic benefit to the client.

In 1986, Mosey proposed that occupational therapists have six primary legitimate tools: (1) nonhuman environment, (2) conscious use of self, (3) teaching–learning process, (4) purposeful activities, (5) activity groups, and (6) activity analysis and synthesis. In her extensive discussion of purposeful activities as a legitimate tool, Mosey (1986) described the characteristics important for evaluation and intervention in occupational therapy. Therapists develop expertise and skills in using these therapeutic tools as part of their basic professional education and ongoing postprofessional education (Mosey, 1986, 1996).

Mosey (1986) defined *purposeful activities* as a "doing process that requires the use of thought and energy and are directed toward an intended or desired end result" (p. 227). Mosey proposed the characteristics of purposeful activities as follows:

- People who are engaged in purposeful activities are aware of the reason for doing them.
- People participate in purposeful activities of their own free will and are not being coerced.
- Purposeful activities have a planned end result that is not necessarily a material product.
- Purposeful activities have the potential to be symbolic.
- Purposeful activities are universal in that they exist as part of the human experience of interacting with one's environments, and people participate in them throughout their daily lives.
- Purposeful activities are ordinary in nature.
- Purposeful activities are essential to the development of humans in all aspects of their development.
- Purposeful activities are made up of elements that can be identified, holistic, able to be manipulated, promoting differential responses, able to be graded,

facilitating communication, having a focusing organizing effect, emphasizing doing, frequently involving the nonhuman environment, varying on a continuum from conscious to not conscious/unconscious, varying on a continuum from simulated to natural. (p. 241)

Mosey (1986) included purposeful activities as one of occupational therapy's major legitimate tools until 1996 when she proposed a new taxonomy of occupational therapy's legitimate tools. This revised taxonomy of legitimate tools consisted of (1) interpersonal process, (2) activity process, and (3) physical modalities (Mosey, 1996). It did not include purposeful activity itself as a separate legitimate tool, instead including it as a subcomponent of other tools. This categorization may reflect the trend in occupational therapy toward moving away from using specific purposeful activities and instead focusing on the foundation for participation in occupations.

Recently, Mosey (personal communication, 2001) has revised her list of legitimate tools to include seven tools:

1. *Conscious use of self*—preplanned verbal and nonverbal responses to a person
2. *Activities*—tasks or interactions in which people typically engage
3. *Activity groups*—types of primary groups that involve participation in activities or discussion of anticipated or current involvement in activities
4. *Stimulus–response interactions*—specific sensory input with a predictable motor response
5. *Atmospheric elements*—aspects of the physical environment that can be modified
6. *Assistive technology*—devices, equipment, or systems specifically designed or adapted to prevent or remediate dysfunction or to maintain or improve function
7. *Physical agent modalities*—properties of temperature, light, sound, water, and electricity that produce selected effects on soft tissue.

This taxonomy continues to recognize that occupational therapists and occupational therapy assistants may use frames of reference or other theoretically based guidelines for intervention that do not emphasize the importance of purposeful activities. Many guidelines for intervention address a specific component deficit. Other guidelines for intervention may use activities but are less concerned with the purposefulness of the activity to the client. In these situations, the purpose is defined by the therapist who has identified explicit outcomes for the client.

Summary

The nature of *purposeful activities* and *occupation* as concepts for study and theory presents inherent difficulties and always has in that, unlike other treatment modes, the cause and effect in treatment are less easy to quantify and measure. Theories of activity and occupation must take in the broadest possible range of human possibilities and experience but may at the same time be applied in incredibly small and specific ways, always remaining as practical and applicable in real situations as possible. That these theorists have taken on such a daunting task and developed a variety of thoughtful, considered approaches to the questions at the heart of occupational therapy is to be respected and acknowledged. As we said in the introduction, nothing can really substitute for reading these authors' works in their own words.

Some concepts that have been raised are a running thread through the works of theorists whose conclusions can vary widely from one another. Clearly, theorists are moving toward a more personal, individualized approach to therapeutic intervention, one that, in many cases, may be hard to quantify but nevertheless makes paramount the person receiving treatment, respect for the person's environment, and treating the patient with dignity. Although the nomenclature may differ, the role of purposeful activities—be they activities, tasks, or occupations—in therapeutic interventions remains a central focus of the theoretical writings.

At the same time, important unique ideas set these theorists apart from one another. For the practicing therapist, one strategy for processing and incorporating the work of various theorists is to study more than one but to find who best matches the therapist's area of practice. Reilly's focus on pediatrics, Law's focus on gerontological issues, and Kielhofner's focus on mental health all offer ways to take theoretical concepts into specific areas of practice. We think that Fidler, in defining ways to think about activity; Nelson, in deriving a nomenclature; and Cynkin, in developing a notion of how to teach activity theory, stand as important guides to how theorists in occupational therapy approach writing and thinking about these issues.

The terms presented here, and the ways in which they are defined, deal with important theoretical issues, but the questions that are raised are provocative and open to debate. One of the most central is thinking about who is defining these concepts—Who determines what is a meaningful outcome? What constitutes a purposeful activity? Whose purpose should it serve?

Most important, occupational therapy continues to grow and evolve, bringing out new ideas in a rapidly changing field. Room for a variety of perspectives, and a need to constantly reexamine established thought in the face of newly developed concepts and theories, exists. In dealing with the complexities of human occupation and purposeful activities, occupational therapy takes on tremendous challenges and offers substantial rewards. The search for understanding the role of occupation and purposeful activities in human existence is ongoing.

References

Baum, C., & Law, M. (1997). Occupational therapy practice: Focusing on occupational performance. *American Journal of Occupational Therapy, 51,* 277–288.

Burke, J. (1996). Variations in childhood: Play in the presence of chronic disability. In R. Zemke & F. Clark (Eds.), *Occupational science: The evolving discipline* (pp. 413–418). Philadelphia: F. A. Davis.

Christiansen, C., & Baum, C. (Eds.). (1991). *Occupational therapy: Overcoming human performance deficits.* Thorofare, NJ: Slack.

Christiansen, C., & Baum, C. (Eds.). (1997). *Occupational therapy: Enabling function and well-being* (2nd ed.). Thorofare, NJ: Slack.

Christiansen, C., Baum, C. M., & Bass-Haugen, J. (2005). *Occupational therapy: Performance, participation, and well-being* (3rd ed.). Thorofare, NJ: Slack.

Clark, F., Parham, D., Carlson, M., Frank, G., Jackson, J., Pierce, D., et al. (1991). Occupational science: Academic innovation in the service of occupational therapy's future. *American Journal of Occupational Therapy, 45,* 300–310.

Cynkin, S. (1979). *Occupational therapy: Toward health through activities.* Boston: Little, Brown.

Cynkin, S., & Robinson, A. (1990). *Occupational therapy and activities health: Toward health through activities.* Boston: Little, Brown.

Darnell, J. L., & Heater, S. L. (1994). Occupational therapist or activity therapist—Which do you choose to be? *American Journal of Occupational Therapy, 48,* 467–468.

Dunn, W., Brown, C., & McGuigan, A. (1994). The ecology of human performance: A framework for considering the effect of context. *American Journal of Occupational Therapy, 48,* 595–607.

Dunn, W., Brown, C., & Youngstrom, M. J. (2003). Ecological model of occupation. In P. Kramer, J. Hinojosa, & C. B. Royeen (Eds.), *Perspectives in human occupation: Participation in life* (pp. 222–263). Philadelphia: Lippincott Williams & Wilkins.

Fidler, G. S. (1948). Psychological evaluation of occupational therapy activities. *American Journal of Occupational Therapy, 2,* 284–287.

Fidler, G. S. (1969). The task-oriented group as a context for treatment. *American Journal of Occupational Therapy, 23,* 43–48.

Fidler, G. S. (1981). From crafts to competence. *American Journal of Occupational Therapy, 35,* 567–573.

Fidler, G. S. (1996). Lifestyle performance: From profile to conceptual model. *American Journal of Occupational Therapy, 50,* 139–147.

Fidler, G. S., & Fidler, J. W. (1954). *Introduction to psychiatric occupational therapy.* New York: Macmillan.

Fidler, G. S., & Fidler, J. W. (1978). Doing and becoming: Purposeful action and self-actualization. *American Journal of Occupational Therapy, 32,* 305–310.

Fidler, G. S., & Velde, B. (1999). *Activity: Reality and symbol.* Thorofare, NJ: Slack.

Forsyth, K., & Kielhofner, G. (2003). Model of Human Occupation. In P. Kramer, J. Hinojosa, & C. B. Royeen (Eds.), *Perspectives in human occupation: Participation in life* (pp. 45–86). Philadelphia: Lippincott Williams & Wilkins.

Frank, G. (1996). The concept of adaptation as a foundation for occupational science research. In R. Zemke & F. Clark (Eds.), *Occupational science: The evolving discipline* (pp. 47–55). Philadelphia: F. A. Davis.

Gill, T., & Brockett, M. (1987). The guidelines for the client-centered practice of occupational therapy: The basis for practice in Canada. *Canadian Journal of Occupational Therapy, 54*(2), 53–54.

Greber, C., Ziviani, J., & Rodger, S. (2007). The four quadrant model of facilitated learning: A clinically based action research project. *Australian Occupational Therapy Journal, 54,* 149–152.

Henderson, A. (1996). The scope of occupational science. In R. Zemke & F. Clark (Eds.), *Occupational science: The evolving discipline* (pp. 419–424). Philadelphia: F. A. Davis.

Kielhofner, G. (Ed.). (1985). *A Model of Human Occupation: Theory and application.* Baltimore: Lippincott Williams & Wilkins.

Kielhofner, G. (1992). *Conceptual foundations of occupational therapy.* Philadelphia: F. A. Davis.

Kielhofner, G. (Ed.). (1995). *A Model of Human Occupation: Theory and application* (2nd ed.). Baltimore: Lippincott Williams & Wilkins.

Kielhofner, G. (Ed.). (2007). *A Model of Human Occupation: Theory and application* (4th ed.). Baltimore: Lippincott Williams & Wilkins.

Kielhofner, G. (2008). *Model of Human Occupation: Theory and application* (4th ed.). Baltimore: Lippincott Williams & Wilkins.

Kielhofner, G. (2009). *Conceptual foundations of occupational therapy practice* (4th ed.). Philadelphia: F. A. Davis.

Kielhofner, G., & Burke, J. (1980). A Model of Human Occupation, Part one: Conceptual framework and content. *American Journal of Occupational Therapy, 34,* 572–581.

Law, M. (Ed.). (1998). *Client-centered occupational therapy.* Thorofare, NJ: Slack.

Law, M., Baptiste, S., Carswell, A., McColl, M. A., Polatajko, H., & Pollock, N. (1994). *Canadian Occupational Performance Measure* (2nd ed.). Toronto, ON: Canadian Association of Occupational Therapists.

Law, M., Baum, C., & Dunn, W. (2005). *Measuring occupational performance: Supporting best practice in occupational therapy.* Thorofare, NJ: Slack.

Law, M., & Mills, J. (1998). Client-centered occupational therapy. In M. Law (Ed.), *Client-centered occupational therapy* (pp. 1–18). Thorofare, NJ: Slack.

Law, M., Petrenchik, T., Ziviani, J., & King, G. (2006). Participation of children in school and community. In S. Rodger & J. Ziviani (Eds.), *Occupational therapy with children* (pp. 67–90). Oxford, UK: Blackwell.

Missiuna, C., Mandich, A. D., Polatajko, H. J., & Malloy-Miller, T. (2001). Cognitive orientation to daily occupational performance (CO-OP): Part I—Theoretical foundations. In C. Missiuna (Ed.), *Children with developmental coordination disorder: Strategies for success* (pp. 69–81). New York: Haworth.

Mosey, A. C. (1968). Recapitulation of ontogenesis: A theory for practice of occupational therapy. *American Journal of Occupational Therapy, 22,* 426–432.

Mosey, A. C. (1973). *Activities therapy.* New York: Raven Press.

Mosey, A. C. (1981). *Occupational therapy: Configuration of a profession.* New York: Raven Press.

Mosey, A. C. (1986). *Psychosocial components of occupational therapy.* New York: Raven Press.

Mosey, A. C. (1992). Partition of occupational science and occupational therapy. *American Journal of Occupational Therapy, 46*(9), 851–853.

Mosey, A. C. (1996). *Applied scientific inquiry in the health professions: An epistemological orientation* (2nd ed.). Bethesda, MD: American Occupational Therapy Association.

Nelson, D. L. (1994). Occupational form, occupational performance, and therapeutic occupation. In C. B. Royeen (Ed.), *The practice of the future: Putting occupation back into therapy* (AOTA Self-Study Series, Lesson 2, pp. 10–43). Bethesda, MD: American Occupational Therapy Association.

Nelson, D. L. (1997). Why the profession of occupational therapy will flourish in the 21st century [Eleanor Clarke Slagle Lecture]. *American Journal of Occupational Therapy, 51,* 11–24.

Nelson, D. L., & Jepson-Thomas, J. (2003). Occupational form, occupational performance, and a conceptual framework for therapeutic occupation. In P. Kramer, J. Hinojosa, & C. B. Royeen (Eds.), *Perspectives in human occupation: Participation in life* (pp. 87–155). Philadelphia: Lippincott Williams & Wilkins.

Peachey-Hill, C., & Law, M. (2000). Impact of environmental sensitivity on occupational performance. *Canadian Journal of Occupational Therapy–Revue Canadienne d Ergotherapie, 67*(5), 304–313.

Pollock, N., & McColl, M. (1998). Assessment in client-entered occupational therapy. In M. Law (Ed.), *Client-centered occupational therapy* (pp. 89–106). Thorofare, NJ: Slack.

Poulsen, A. A., & Ziviani, J. M. (2004). Health enhancing physical activity: Factors influencing engagement patterns in children. *Australian Occupational Therapy Journal, 51*, 69–79.

Reilly, M. (1960). Research potentiality of occupational therapy. *American Journal of Occupational Therapy, 14*, 206–209.

Reilly, M. (1962). Occupational therapy can be one of the great ideas of 20th-century medicine. *American Journal of Occupational Therapy, 16*, 1–9.

Reilly, M. (1966). A psychiatric occupational therapy program as a teaching model. *American Journal of Occupational Therapy, 22*, 61–67.

Reilly, M. (Ed.). (1974). *Play as exploratory learning*. Beverly Hills, CA: Sage.

Rodger, S., & Ziviani, J. (Eds.). (2006). *Occupational therapy with children: Understanding children's occupations and enabling participation*. Oxford, UK: Blackwell.

Schkade, J. K., & Schultz, S. (1992). Occupational adaptation: Toward a holistic approach to contemporary practice, Part 1. *American Journal of Occupational Therapy, 46*, 829–837.

Schkade, J. K., & Schultz, S. (2003). Occupational adaptation. In P. Kramer, J. Hinojosa, & C. B. Royeen (Eds.), *Perspectives in human occupation: Participation in life* (pp. 181–221). Philadelphia: Lippincott Williams & Wilkins.

Schultz, S., & Schkade, J. K. (1992). Occupational adaptation: Toward a holistic approach to contemporary practice, Part 2. *American Journal of Occupational Therapy, 46*, 917–926.

Strong, S., Rigby, P., Stewart, D., Law, M., Letts, L., & Cooper, B. (1999). Application of the Person–Environment–Occupation Model: A practical tool. *Canadian Journal of Occupational Therapy–Revue Canadienne d Ergotherapie, 66*(3), 122–133.

Taylor, S., Fayed, N., & Mandich, A. (2007). CO-OP intervention for young children with developmental coordination disorder. *OTJR: Occupation, Participation and Health, 27*, 124–130.

Velde, B. P., & Fidler, G. S. (2002). *Lifestyle performance: A model for engaging the power of occupation*. Thorofare, NJ: Slack

Zemke, R., & Clark, F. (Eds.). (1996). *Occupational science: The evolving discipline*. Philadelphia: F. A. Davis.

3

Occupation Across the Lifespan

Ruth Segal, PhD, OTR

Occupations are complex constructs that consist of highly personal yet socioculturally embedded meanings. In Chapter 1, Hinojosa and Blount defined occupations from the person's perspective, writing that *"[o]ccupations* are purposeful activities that are personally meaningful to the person, who engages in them out of personal choice or sociocultural necessity" (p. 2). Clark et al. (1991), however, defined *occupations* from a cultural perspective, as "chunks of activities that are culturally defined" (p. 301). Taken together, these definitions suggest that occupation lies in the transaction between the person and his or her contexts or environments. Thus, the same set of purposeful activities may have different meanings in different situations or contexts. Driving, for example, may be a vocation, a hobby, or a chore, depending on the situation.

The meanings that people assign to occupations occur within "temporal, psychological, social, symbolic, cultural, ethnic, and/or spiritual contexts" (Hinojosa & Kramer, 1997, p. 865). *Meaning* is the sense in which something is understood (*Merriam-Webster's Concise Dictionary of English Usage*, 2002). It is assigned by people who must engage in the act of interpretation to do so (Strauss & Quinn, 1997). Such interpretations are the subject of study of certain academic disciplines such as philosophy, psychology, sociology, and anthropology. None of these disciplines use occupation as the concept guiding their research in the way that occupational therapy does. Yet in occupational therapy and these disciplines, no longitudinal studies

---

EXERCISE 3.1: PURPOSEFUL ACTIVITIES IN YOUR OWN LIFE

Think of a set of purposeful activities in your life, and identify how they may become different occupations when the context in which you perform them changes.

---

have described how occupations evolve and develop across the lifespan. Hence, this chapter represents my attempt to understand the phenomenon of occupation across the lifespan, based on my point of view.

In developing and writing this chapter, I made these five assumptions:

1. The most important aspect of occupation is the meaning attached to it.
2. Meaning is context dependent.
3. The contexts of human life from birth to death are unpredictable, but their number and variety increase from infancy to adulthood and often decline again with old age.
4. Chronic illness and disability often limit a person's life contexts.
5. Poverty limits life contexts.

Building on these assumptions, I take the purposeful activity of eating—getting the nourishment needed for survival and health—and explore its transformation into various occupations in three trajectories: from birth to death, in health and illness, and in affluence and poverty.

Occupations Across the Lifespan

The evolution of meaning is context dependent, and therefore each person's life, in its particular context, will influence but not determine the meaning of activities. This assumption makes it impossible to identify a sequence of occupations that is typical across the lifespan. Indeed, I suggest that at the present state of knowledge, no typical sequence can be identified because social norms and cultural practices limit and afford a person participation in various contexts. These norms and practices are based on age, ethnic background, socioeconomic status, profession, and many other social determinants. Therefore, although a general description of the evolution of occupations and the socially sanctioned activities that are involved in childhood, adolescence, adulthood, and older adulthood can be given, this description is not sufficient because the range of activities within each age category is wide. Therefore, in this chapter, I briefly outline contexts or socially sanctioned activities and elaborate on an example of food in each category. As much as possible, I base these examples on research rather than products of my own construction. I base my discussion of the evolutionary process or development on texts on human development, focusing on its social and psychological aspects.

EVOLUTION OF OCCUPATION

For occupations to become part of one's repertoire of life activities, they must be assigned meanings and must be interpreted in a cultural context. This definition of occupation implies that a child cannot have occupations until he or she can assign meaning to phenomena or activities. Kramer and Hinojosa (1995) described the early emergence of occupations:

> When children are born, they are purely reflexive beings. Their behavior is dominated by sensory responses to their feeling state and their environment, and occupation is not yet evident. However, as children begin to respond to and interact with people and objects within their environment, they begin to develop rudimentary patterns of behavior. Responses to specific people or stimuli become almost predictable, and they develop into patterns. These patterns involve a variety of actions that have meanings to the children; thus, the children are stimulated to engage in selected activities. For example, infants begin to recognize their parents very early. When a parent walks into the room, the infant follows the parent with his or her eyes and begin to wave his or her arms and legs. This indicates that the child expects there to be some interaction. This initial attachment to the person or object is the first phase of object relations (Spitz, 1965).
>
> Often, the infant's responses take the form of motor actions. When repeated, these actions become patterns of behavior. In this sense, behavior is used to mean the emotional responses and reactions of the child. The infant first relates to people in the environment, and then begins to react and respond to objects. These behaviors often become activities. Activity is used in this context to mean constructive action that enhances development and results in a productive outcome, such as when a child learns to reach out for his or her mother when she walks near the crib. The child's repertoire of behaviors and activities expands and forms a multitude of patterns. As these patterns of behaviors and specific activities are repeated over time, they develop more and more meaning to the child and become occupations. Thus, occupations are defined in this context as natural patterns of daily activity that are meaningful to the individual. When observing an infant, one can see a particular child enjoying play with a rattle, while another child may ignore the rattle and spend time with a busy box. Personal preference in activities is evident at a very early age, which can then give rise to varying occupational patterns. (pp. 6–8)

Kramer and Hinojosa's (1995) overview of the evolution of occupations reflects the typical way in which human development is described. That is, the focus is on the increasing abilities and variety of activities and the different meanings assigned to similar activities (i.e., occupations ascribed to people). After the developmental stage described by Kramer and Hinojosa (1995) in the preceding quotation, a different aspect of development begins that is not commonly accounted for, namely, the development of the variety of meanings that each person attaches to similar activities. These meanings, as suggested by Kramer and Hinojosa (1995), Hinojosa and Blount in Chapter 1, and Strauss and Quinn (1997), develop as children's social world enlarges and with it their participation and experiences.

As Kramer and Hinojosa (1995) suggested, occupations in general do not occur during infancy. The significance of food throughout infancy can be discussed only in terms of health and survival. Although attachment is an important aspect of infancy that has been connected with feeding, feeding too can be discussed in terms of survival rather than in terms of infant occupations, consistent with Lowenberg's (1970, as cited in Kittler & Sucher, 2001) application of Maslow's hierarchy of needs to food consumption. The most basic human need is the physical need for survival; infants' motivation to feed is their physical survival. Infants are measured, and these measurements are compared with established growth charts that indicate whether their growth is age appropriate and whether their ratio of length and weight is within normal limits. If either of these measurements is not within normal limits, medical intervention, or at least an investigation into the infant's health and well-being, is needed.

The introduction of eating as a social and cultural phenomenon is important. All humans consume some form of milk at the beginning of life, but by early childhood, the diets of humankind are greatly diverse (Birch, Fisher, & Grimm-Thomas, 1996), suggesting that food is a vehicle for many nonbiological functions and meanings. Food and eating can be viewed as a system of communication (Douglas, 1982). Meals can demonstrate differences in status, social groupings, and relationships. Food also has symbolic social and economic meanings. Finally, giving and receiving food allows people to correctly exercise their roles. For the young, meals are important socialization tools because they teach what is acceptable and unacceptable. Mealtimes are also good for developing self-image and role control. For sociologists, what underlays food and meal preparation, cookery, and consumption hold the most value (Wood, 1995).

CHILDHOOD

Childhood is a socially constructed status (Lee, 2001). That is, social and cultural values, beliefs, and traditions shape what are considered to be the appropriate social interactions for children, including with whom and while

---

EXERCISE 3.2: FOOD

How is food in your life part of a system of communication? What social and economic symbolic meanings does food have for you?

doing what. These have changed with history and still differ among cultures and societies and also within societies (La Fontaine, 1986; Lee, 2001; Shahar, 1990; Wyness, 2000).

Childhood is the period of life in which children are prepared for adulthood by the adults in society. The *social construction of childhood* refers to the patterns of activities and participation that are open to children or in which their participation is required. These activities are constructed on the basis of current scientific knowledge about children's physical, cognitive, psychosocial, and emotional development and are dependent on traditions, beliefs and customs, social status, and ethnic background, to name a few factors. These factors are also time dependent, and they change over time with changes in scientific knowledge and in society (Lee, 2001). The overall structure of childhood in the Western world is one of increasing exposure; as children progress through childhood, they are exposed to a greater variety of environments and activities.

In the modern, middle-class United States, infants tend to be sheltered, and their environment is commonly limited to their own homes, their mothers, and the rest of their nuclear family. Among families with lower incomes or in families in which both parents work, a paid caregiver or a member of the extended family may be retained to care for infants in their home. In both of these scenarios, the infant's environment is limited. To a lesser extent in the United States—and to a greater extent in many other Western countries—infants are cared for in daycare centers. In such cases, an infant's environment is somewhat larger but still very controlled in its nature (Lee, 2001). This sheltering continues until children are considered old enough to join play groups and eventually kindergarten. During this period, young children may attend school and have play dates that include ongoing adult supervision.

In early childhood, usually up to age 7 or so, children's cognitive, physical, emotional, and psychosocial needs are such that their social status does not include any significant social responsibilities for others. During this period, however, their array of social interactions increases in variety, giving ample opportunities for the development of mapping in the brain. Children begin to interact more with other children and adults in a range of contexts. Therefore, similar activities may be performed in a variety of social and cultural contexts and are thus constructed as different occupations. Participating in similar activities in different contexts evokes a variety of experiences that are connected with the occupations. For example, play can take the form of playing alone, with a caregiver, with siblings, with friends, at home, in the park, and at school. The variety of play situations and experiences creates connections in the brain that increase in their versatility and complexity. Participation in play allows children to develop preferences and assert choices (Figure 3.1).

During this period, children begin to eat in a variety of contexts and begin to differentiate between the different meanings of *food* and *eating*. For example, birthday parties are connected with certain foods such as birthday cake and party bags of sweets that are typically considered unhealthy and

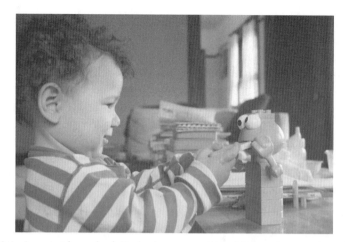

Figure 3.1. A young boy playfully feeds a toy and establishes the meaning of eating.

would not be a part of the child's typical diet. Birthday parties also include savory food such as pizza or hot dogs. The context of eating at a birthday party includes singing a birthday song when the birthday cake is brought in with lighted candles on it and the particular types of room decorations.

At this age, children may be taken to restaurants that serve food appropriate for children and that is consumed in such contexts. These restaurants include self-service fast-food restaurants and full-service family restaurants. Going to school introduces another way of consuming food. School lunches are either brought from home or bought at school, and children socialize while eating their lunches. At this age, lunchtime is supervised closely by educators or other school employees.

During this phase of life, children are exposed to a greater range of foods. Parents provide a variety of food to promote consumption as a means of promoting and maintaining health. The question of what constitutes a *healthy food* is dependent on the dimensions of culture and time. Currently in the United States, particular diets are commonly believed to lead to health and well-being. Therefore, the U.S. government has released a "food pyramid," which can be obtained from a government Web site (www.mypyramid.gov), that delineates the amount and type of foods that make up a healthy diet. The food pyramid is also believed to be based on scientific data, even though these data have been challenged (see Nestle, 2002) as a result of the food industry's influence. Such government publications are not unique to the United States and can be found in many Western countries.

Government policies and recommendations are an example of how social organizations affect individual tastes and construct shared meanings. For example, consider the belief that fresh fruit and vegetables are good for one's health. Such a belief seems obvious to us, but it has not always been that way. In the Middle Ages, for example, cucumbers and melons were considered dangerous to human health (Albala, 2002).

CULTURE AND BELIEFS

Another dimension of food and eating habits that begins in early childhood is the socialization of children into the eating habits identified with the family's particular beliefs, religion, and culture. Many food habits stem from religion; for example, religious groups may use food laws to differentiate themselves from others. These restrictions may come from holy books or from moral attitudes. Often, religious food restrictions are relaxed or ignored. *Cultism* is the word used to describe eating patterns that seem bizarre under conventional wisdom. Cultist food practices satisfy followers' social and psychological needs but are often nutritionally deficient (Fieldhouse, 1986). The following sections summarize some information about food and beliefs that Fieldhouse described in greater detail.

PRESTIGE AND STATUS

Some foods confer high status on those who eat them; others imply status because of the human groups who usually eat them. The differences between the meals of medieval nobles and those of peasants symbolize the power that the nobles held over the food supply and thus over the peasants. Prestige can also be attached to the circumstances and ways in which food is served. Food can make social distinctions, overt or subtle, depending on the situation. The Hindu caste system, which has strict rules regarding who can eat with whom, obviously outlines social distinctions.

STATUS AND FOOD BEHAVIOR

Status through food is conveyed in three principal ways: in the freedom to (1) choose rare and costly items to impress others, (2) select expensive restaurants for personal gratification, and (3) prepare difficult and time-consuming dishes. To be denied any sort of choice in Western society is seen as negative. The ability to choose freely is tied to economic status, which is also tied to social status. When food choices are limited, people feel uncomfortable and are more likely to complain. Lack of choice also decreases self-esteem. Exotic, complex, or expensive dishes convey a higher status. This higher status can derive from several aspects, such as the location, the time or skill necessary to prepare the dishes, or the distance between the person who consumes the food and the person who prepares it. At dinner parties, the food served can be a sign not only of the host's status but also of the status that the host ascribes to his guests.

FOOD AND FASHION

Food may have a high status only because high-status groups consume it. This process is often circular because a food may have a high status but then become widely available to all classes, causing it to lose that status. Preferences for high-status food may develop without any regard to the food's actual taste. Humans are the only group that will shun a nutritional food because of its lower status and replace it with a nutritionally mediocre one of higher status. The importance of prestigious food lies in how much social recognition it will bring.

STATUS AND FOOD OWNERSHIP

In some places in the world, food ownership brings some of the same prestige or status as food consumption. In some parts of Africa, for example, owning cattle conveys tremendous economic status; cows are kept as a sign of wealth and rarely killed for food.

FOOD, FRIENDSHIP, AND COMMUNICATION

The level of intimacy between people can often be gauged by the foods that they share. The act of eating together implies some degree of compatibility. Closeness may be acknowledged with elaborate food. In many places, it is common to keep some sort of food on hand for callers because to not offer food would be to lose social status. One exception is the Bemba people of Africa, who send people food to be consumed in private rather than shared together as a sign of respect.

PEER ACCEPTANCE

Food is also an expression of the human need to belong. The wish to eat what others eat may result in altered food patterns that may not be nutritionally sound. Teenagers are especially susceptible to this. Food choice in specific cases can be limited by social norms dictated by the choices of others.

FOOD AS REWARD AND PUNISHMENT

Children learn what is acceptable and approved of in terms of food consumption through a system of reward and punishment. These may be explicit or implicit and may be accompanied by reinforcing messages.

GIFTS OF FOOD AND SHARING

Shared food is a symbol of social relationships, removed from the food's monetary value. Psychologically, those who were raised in an environment in which food was in abundance tend to develop a predisposition toward sharing, and those who were not raised in such an environment do not develop this trait. As a gift, food can symbolically express a wide range of emotions and sentiments. Three basic types of reciprocity for food exchanges exist: First, *generalized reciprocity* implies that there is no immediate expectation of return, no attempt to determine the gift's value, and no attempt to make gift giving "balance out."

Second, *balanced reciprocity* occurs between social equals who have a personal relationship and takes into account the gift's value and implies some expectation of return. This return may be at a later date. Third, *negative reciprocity* involves immediate exchange and strict accounting of value in an impersonal exchange. Exchanges can also diffuse foods' status. Reciprocity-based food exchanges are common in situations in which environmental resources are limited. If reciprocity is not adopted, then competitive food giving can result.

FEASTS AND FESTIVALS

Feasts and festivals are held for many reasons and for many types of personal, cultural, or religious observances. Feast foods are usually scarce, high quality, expensive, and difficult or time consuming to prepare (Figure 3.2). Festivals are complex, colorful rituals found in nearly every society in some form. The four main types of festival are (1) *ecofests* (astronomical or seasonal events such as May Day), (2) *theofests* (religious events such as Easter), (3) *secular festivals* (national holidays), and (4) *personal festivals* (major life events).

RITUALS AND SACRIFICE

Many pagan and religious rituals involve food. The need for ritualistic food may have contributed to the spread of some religions. In rituals, food offerings were usually animal. In many societies, animal sacrifices have fallen out of favor; instead, they have been replaced by a recommendation for a moral sacrifice, such as one involving prayer or money. Sacrifices may be made for a variety of reasons, but they always imply an asymmetrical status relationship. The following motivations are the most common: to provide food for the gods, to propitiate an affronted deity, to effect communication with a deity through the

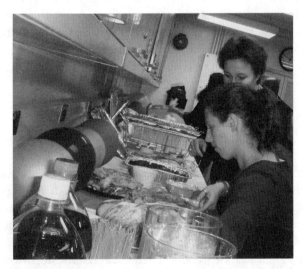

Figure 3.2. Food is an essential part of a feast or festival.

EXERCISE 3.3: MEANING OF FOOD

What meaning does food have in your life? Examine the categories listed in this section and identify how they relate to your life. How do they relate to your family? How do they relate to others with whom you socialize?

---

eating of a victim, for maintenance or renewal of life, for purposes of divination, to confirm a covenant, to ward off evil, and in exchange for favors.

SACRAMENTS

Many cultures, especially ancient ones, have sacred foods that are often embodiments of the gods. Therefore, sacramental killing and eating of these animals implies that they are too sacred to be eaten and should be spared (Fieldhouse, 1986).

CHILDHOOD SOCIAL SITUATIONS

In early childhood, children begin to be exposed to a greater variety of social situations in which food is consumed. In addition, with their increased ability to perceive and interpret the world, they begin to observe and experience different types of foods and their social and cultural meanings. With these changes and developments, children begin to differentiate between different occupations that involve eating; they know the difference between a birthday party and a daily school lunch and between an ordinary family dinner and a holiday dinner. These differences are not only in the type of food consumed but also embedded in interactions with others and the accompanying experiences. This variety of experiences, in turn, helps the development of a multiplicity of connections in the brain that are related to eating and linked to the related experiences and meanings that are unique to each child (Figure 3.3). These meanings are shared with other children and family members because they participate in the same events.

MIDDLE CHILDHOOD (7–11 YEARS OF AGE)

During middle childhood, children gain greater exposure to social contexts and experience decreasing levels of supervision. The interactions among children during lunch time at school are less closely monitored. Peer groups become increasingly important, and empathy and other prosocial behaviors are learned. During this time, children become more aware of themselves and others. They learn to control the expression of their feelings and become more selective in choosing friends. Their self-awareness increases, and self-esteem tends to decrease. Children's peer groups become sensitive to customs and principles of society.

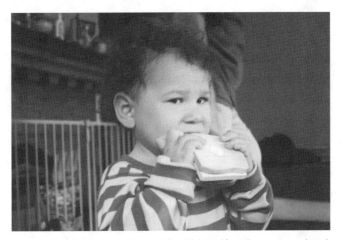

Figure 3.3. Child pretending to feed himself with a toy sandwich.

Children become more aware of their own familial situation in comparison to that of others. Children's well-being continues to depend on the quality of parenting and the social setting rather than on the family's constitution (whether the parents are of the same or different gender, whether single-parent or two-parent family, and whether or not the parents are the biological parents).

School-age children are considered more capable and independent, so they are allowed to venture out into the world more. A key part of their development is social cognition—in other words, understanding other people and groups. During the school years, children gain a better understanding of human behavior, which makes this process complex. Children can see the origins and future implications of an action, and their understanding of personality traits increases. School-age children begin to learn about society's customs and principles.

In terms of food consumption, family dinners, if they occur, become a greater social and educational affair because the child's ability to participate in conversations improves. At home, family dinners are an important means of socialization. Dinner conversations are used to convey rules of conversation, to resolve conflicts, and to establish and challenge social roles (Grieshaber, 1997; Ochs, Taylor, Rudolph, & Smith, 1992; Segal, 1999; Vuchinich, 1987). Although the family dinner is considered an important occupation, even to the point of becoming the space and time in which family members become a family (DeVault, 1991), the nature of interactions during these family dinners may evoke unpleasant experiences when conflicts occur. These different experiences may lead people to attach very different meanings to this particular occupation. In the following sections, I summarize the depiction of family dinners in films and discuss the alternatives presented.

DINING SPACE

The act of eating together shows the quality of relationships and social interactions. Until the 1950s, the site of this act was almost always the home.

Family dining represented family unity. Modern life has seen a shift from dining in the home to dining in restaurants, as reflected in many U.S. films. The bonding once experienced at home can now be experienced at these fast-food establishments and restaurants, whereas dining in the home is shown to be a source of conflict and distress. Eating in a restaurant now shows the sense of wholeness that once belonged to home dining. These films redefine social order and the boundaries between order (purity) and disorder (pollution) in dining. Technology, advertising, changing family structure, and various other factors have led to the rise of fast food and its central place in U.S. society. The films discussed in this section reveal this new place in U.S. society and illustrate the shift of dining from the private to the public domain.

FILMS

MYSTIC PIZZA (PETRIE, 1988)

This film follows three young women, sisters Kat and Daisy and their friend Jojo who work together at Mystic Pizza, as they prepare for adulthood. The pizzeria is depicted as the place where the girls bond over meals. The owner of the pizzeria, Leona, is a motherly figure to them. No meals are ever shown being eaten at home, except for one tense meal at the home of Daisy's boyfriend, Charlie. The characters seem to eat most of their meals at Mystic Pizza. All bonding between characters in the movie takes place inside the restaurant: The restaurant is where Jojo holds her wedding reception; where Kat finds out that Leona has agreed to help with her Yale tuition; and where Daisy reconciles her difficult relationship with her mother.

ORDINARY PEOPLE (REDFORD, 1980)

In this film, home dining is the source of conflict, whereas McDonald's is the only place where the main character can find any nurturing. The film is about the lives of Beth and Calvin and their son Conrad after the death of their other son Buck. Buck died in a boating accident while out with Conrad, and the guilt drove Conrad to attempt suicide. Beth finds herself unable to deal with the disorder in her family and responds by behaving coldly toward Conrad. This behavior is often evidenced in dining scenes. When Conrad reunites at McDonald's with a girl he met in the hospital, and later when he takes another girl there on a date, the viewer sees scenes of peaceful, communal dining.

BETTER OFF DEAD (HOLLAND, 1985)

The family dining scenes in this movie satirize the concept of family mealtime bonding. The mother of the family, Jenny, prepares horrible food that her family does not want to eat. The father, Al, spends meals complaining to or about his teenage son, Lane. The other son, Badger, spends mealtimes cutting coupons from cereal boxes or sitting in his bedroom playing with a

Laser Blaster toy. Lane eats alone, leaves meals early, or is forced into eating with the family by his mother. The film also satirizes the "polluted reality" of fast-food restaurants while also showing them as the only place where Lane can dine with someone and make a connection.

CONSIDERATIONS OF BOUNDARIES AND POLLUTION

The lack of successful family dining in these movies indicates a notion of alienation and pollution when it comes to the act of family dining. According to the anthropologist Mary Douglas, the rules of pollution use elements of environment to support social reality. The activity of eating is based on what society classifies as edible (clean) and nonedible (unclean), and the location of eating is often determined by order and disorder. In the three films, home is shown as a place of disorder, whereas alternative restaurants provide order and a sense of unity of experience. These eating scenes reproduce old ideals and update them for modern times.

CONSIDERATIONS OF STRUCTURAL CHANGES AND LANDSCAPE OF POWER

Changes in societal structure may be the cause of the changes in dining because they shape habits and the meaning of food. Families integrate the power of these changes into daily life. Capitalism, marketing, giant food conglomerates, fast-food chains, and technological advances have all led to the rise of the fast-food restaurant rather than family dining at home.

CONSIDERATIONS OF FAMILY STRUCTURE

Along with social structure, family structure and daily meaning have also changed. With more mothers working, school-age children involved in after-school activities, and teenagers working part-time or playing sports, family dining is harder to coordinate. The cultural importance of family dining has decreased. These films are visual representations of these changes (Ferry, 2003).

ADOLESCENCE (12–18 YEARS OF AGE)

People typically think of adolescence as the time for developing self-identity. This process is related to interactions with family members and friends. It is a time when those relationships evolve into their adult forms. By late

---

EXERCISE 3.4: FILM

Select a television show or movie that you have seen with a storyline that involves a family's daily life. Reflect on how family dining was represented. How have films influenced your thoughts about dining?

adolescence, adolescents are comfortable with relationships with the other sex, their sexual identity has developed, and their communication with same-sex friends and parents has developed. Adolescent children struggle for independence from their parents in term of values, behaviors, and life in general.

One of the issues around food that may begin at this phase of human development is that of eating disorders. These disorders have many psychological explanations. When one talks about an eating disorder as an occupation whose meaning lies within the person (i.e., psychological explanations), one needs to address the social and cultural environments that contribute to the meaning of thinness and the ways to achieve it.

THINNESS IN SOCIOLOGICAL AND HISTORICAL CONTEXT

Whether eating disorders are a modern development or whether they came about over the past 100 years or so is not known. The increased awareness of eating disorders in recent decades signals an increase in both medical knowledge and their incidence. Mennell, Murcott, and van Otterloo (1992) suggested that this increased awareness is the result of long-term changes in society, civilization, and attitudes toward appetites. In the Middle Ages, nutrition was not distributed evenly among social classes and having an abundance of food was a way for the upper class to show its importance. As time went by, the abundance of food reached the lower classes as well, and the quality of the food became what set the higher classes apart from the lower ones. In addition, during the 19th century, the concept of moderation became popular and imposed some restrictions on diets. The 20th century brought an expectation of dietary self-control that stressed the person's control over food.

Anorexia nervosa was first diagnosed in the 19th century. Much of the research on eating disorders has focused on the medical and psychological factors rather than the social factors. The fact, however, that it affects particular demographic groups (most typically young, White, affluent women) cannot be ignored. Throughout the 20th century, the ideal body type for a woman has become thinner and thinner. The pressure to be thin and the importance attached to thinness are rooted in the behavior and personality traits associated with a thin physique, such as success and power, whereas being overweight carries a negative stigma. The fact that the lower and working classes only acquired the means and abilities to afford enough food to become overweight in the past 100 years may be why the upper classes, who had typically been plump, now find themselves stressing slimness. In light of this, it is not surprising that women are more obsessed than ever with food and calorie intake, with most women reporting that they would like to be thinner. Correlations between eating habits that are deemed socially acceptable and those of eating disorders suggest that eating disorders are extreme manifestations of eating habits that are deemed acceptable. Research has also noted that the pressure to be thin is widely felt among women but not nearly as much among men. This difference seems to fit into the pattern of female socialization. Modern women are placed in a tough situation, faced with opportunities for success and power but often raised with traditional female values of compliance and passivity. Women born in the late 20th century were the first to feel this pressure (Mennell et al., 1992).

Women have historically tried to change their bodies to meet the cultural standards of beauty. Wiseman, Gray, Mosimann, and Ahrens (1992) analyzed the measurements of *Playboy* magazine centerfolds (1979–1988) and Miss America contestants (1979–1985) and the number of weight loss, diet, and exercise articles in *Harper's Bazaar, Vogue, Ladies' Home Journal, Good Housekeeping, Woman's Day* and *McCall's* during the years 1959–1988. During the period of analysis, Miss America contestants got smaller, in both size and weight, and showed a significant decrease in hip size, whereas Playboy centerfold models remained at a steady small size throughout this time frame. During these 10 years, 69% of Playboy models and 60% of Miss America candidates were 15% or more below the expected weight for their respective age and height categories, one of the major symptoms of anorexia, suggesting that the cultural standard has stayed thin and grown even thinner. In the Wiseman et al. study, the body sizes may begin to level off at a certain low number because going any lower than that would prove to be dangerous or fatal. The survey of articles shows an increased emphasis on weight loss over the past 30 years. In recent years, the number of exercise articles has outnumbered that of diet articles, suggesting a new trend based on health and fitness for weight loss instead of just dieting, although it must be carefully observed because overexercising can be a sign of bulimia nervosa.

In relation to other aspects of food and eating, adolescents may begin eating in separate social contexts, such as, for example, going on dates or going out in groups. Typically, considering their budgets, fast-food chains at the mall or food at movie theatres might be the popular choice. Adolescents are also left alone at home and may engage in cooking for themselves and younger siblings. That is, at this stage, in addition to refining those skills whose development began in middle childhood around eating and eating appropriately, cooking food and providing for one's own nourishment and that of younger siblings may begin.

ADULTHOOD

Adulthood is different from childhood not only because the adult becomes a legally independent member of society but also because society does not establish a single path for transitioning from early adulthood to older adulthood. In fact, from the late 20th century, adulthood is marked by decreased predictability about the way life will evolve (Lee, 2001). Most texts on human development identify three general foci of adult life: having (1) a family, (2) a career, and (3) intimacy. The way in which adults attend to these foci is determined by social and cultural forces. During adulthood, issues such as gender, socioeconomic status, race, ethnicity, religion, and sexual orientation become more apparent in the options open to people and the choices they make. Although these issues affect children and adolescents as well, the way in which they encounter and address these issues is largely dependent on how their parents construct their exposures to them.

FAMILY

For adults, having a family typically means raising children. The family constitution and legal status may vary from marriage to cohabitation to single parenthood. Parents may be of different sexes or the same sex and may be either biological or nonbiological parents of the children. In each case, the role of parenting is an important aspect of the lives of many adults. As parents, adults are responsible for the physical, psychological, and social well-being and development of their children. One of these responsibilities is to socialize their children to the different occupations of eating in context. They are responsible for introducing culturally relevant foods to their children as a way to socialize them into that culture. These may be fairly simple things such as the kind of breakfast being served. Choices can be to follow the shared meaning of *breakfast* in terms of the types of food served (see Food for Breakfast section) or to break with these traditions by following new scientific information about foods that are good or bad for one's health (e.g., consumption of eggs).

FOOD FOR BREAKFAST

> The most flexible versions of breakfast are probably the Central and North European buffets of breads, pastries, cheeses, and cold meats, or their Middle Eastern equivalents of bread, yoghurt, fruit, and preserves. Really substantial breakfasts include the modern British fry-up, and the North American subspecies of this, with numerous variations on the theme of eggs, plus options of waffles with maple syrup. . . . Traditional Indian breakfasts include dal, rice, breads, samosas, and fruit. Comforting bowls of hot cereal mixtures are popular, from the Scottish oatmeal porridge to the rice porridges eaten across much of Asia, of which congee is the best known. Minimal approaches to breakfast include croissants and café au lait in France, chocolate and churros in Spain, and many variations of the bowl of muesli theme for those who think that cereal, nuts, and dried fruit are key to good health. (Davidson, 1999, p. 104)

The type of food consumed imparts information and signifies meaning. For example, a television advertisement showing a frying pan with two eggs and bacon while the announcer says "breakfast for dinner" suggests that eating eggs in the United States is related to breakfast. In Israel, however, eggs are commonly eaten for the evening meal, which is supper rather than dinner. Even within the United States, a great variety of foods is consumed by different ethnic groups in different geographic locations and according to many other delineations. The variety is so great that Kittler and Sucher (2001) devoted a whole book to describing it.

To make healthy food choices, parents must be knowledgeable about what foods are considered healthy. The health-contributing qualities of food are a good example of how meaning is time dependent, as suggested by Hinojosa and Blount in Chapter 2. For example, the food pyramid published by the U.S. Department of Agriculture is updated on a regular basis because knowledge about the healthfulness of food and diets keeps changing.

In the following sections, I summarize beliefs about healthy foods from the time of the Middle Ages to the present to demonstrate how beliefs have changed.

FOOD AND THE FAMILY

Issues of food and family are closely related to those of nutrition and responsibility, and different cultures can have different working understandings of what is healthy. Women often take on the task of balancing diet and health for themselves and their families. Although knowledge of nutrition among women is high, application of this knowledge is not always consistent. A woman's food choices are primarily affected by her desire to be a good spouse and mother, available time, available money, and influences from her environment and her upbringing.

Research has shown that mass media messages can also serve to influence dietary patterns and decisions, such as those about salmonella, mad cow disease, listeria, and botulism. Informal nutritional education can be just as influential and important as formal nutritional education. In catering to the tastes of everyone else, women often ignore their own tastes and participate less in the domestic dining experience. In times of financial hardship, women are those most likely to go without food. Thus, women are constantly trying to balance the tension between their personal tastes and educational knowledge and those of their families (Wood, 1995).

The role of the middle-age adult as a member of the middle generation of his or her extended family is easier to underestimate. Family ties are strong at this time, and those between the middle-age adults and their elderly parents often improve greatly. When adult children have children of their own, a new link between generations is formed. During this stage of life, women tend to be kin keepers—those who keep in touch with family members who no longer live at home, celebrate achievements, and get the family together. These increased family ties can sometimes be burdensome for middle-age people because they experience obligations to help both the younger and the older members—the so-called "sandwich generation."

FAMILY MEAL

One way of keeping the extended family together is through a holiday get-together such as Thanksgiving or Christmas (Figure 3.4). The preparation of holiday meals may consist of following old traditions and bringing in new ones. For example, parents who did not like certain foods as children may introduce new dishes to make the experience of a festive dinner a better one for their own children. Engaging in festive family meals is an important feature of the construction of a family out of its individual members. Without getting together, regardless of the quality of experiences, interactions and attachments would not occur (DeVault, 1991; Gillis, 1996; Hasselkus, 2002; Kantor & Lehr, 1975).

Another context of eating mentioned earlier is the socialization of children into dining out. Dining out is an experience that has become much more common in the United States and other places with the emergence of fast-food and other affordable restaurants. Dining out as a context for eating is large and diversified in every aspect of that context: The cost of a meal can be close to a dollar or up to a few hundred dollars; the type of food served may represent varied tastes and cultural, social, and religious aspects as well as combinations of those; the nature of service can range from self-service to a restaurant that has servers who specialize in different aspects and stages of the service. With all these variations come different behavioral expectations, experiences, and meanings.

Parents are responsible for socializing their children into the dining-out contexts that are relevant to their social and cultural backgrounds. For example, some cultures whose food is spicy begin introducing spicy food to children around ages 10 or 11 (Davidson, 1999). This introduction may not

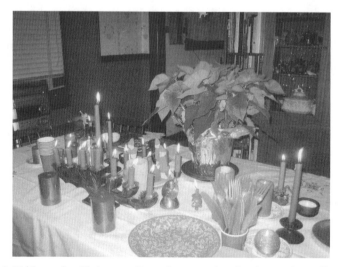

Figure 3.4. Table set for Christmas dinner has meaning for those who will participate.

be a socializing aspect of eating in cultures whose food is not spicy, so people may acquire the taste for it only in later life.

Another aspect of dining out is etiquette or manners. The appropriate way to behave in a self-service restaurant such as a fast-food chain differs from that in a self-service restaurant that presents food buffet style. Eating utensils and their use are also related to the type of restaurant one goes to: chopsticks or knife and fork, one set of utensils or several sets. These observable things can give information about the possible ethnic foods served and how expensive they might be. Observing a person holding and using a knife and a fork can give a broad idea of his or her country of origin: People in the United States do not tend to hold the knife in their right hand and the fork in their left hand while eating, whereas people from Europe do. These are the habits and pieces of information that parents impart to their children to support them in their adult life.

Career

Career is another important aspect of adult life. Career can be a source of income and can be used as a social ladder because of this generation of income and the development of social connections. A career often necessitates special forms of eating. The daily lunch at work can take the form of eating a lunch brought from home, buying a meal and eating it in the office, or going out to a restaurant to eat lunch. The variety of restaurants open for lunch affords a choice that signals differentiation among the levels of employees or business people. The type and price of food consumed can serve as a good indicator of the socioeconomic level of the person eating.

Another type of eating in the context of a career can be eating at workplace parties and special occasions. These parties may be associated with holidays; office events; and personal events such as birthdays, marriages, and childbirth. Each one of these events may occur in the office with food either catered or potluck, in a restaurant, or perhaps in someone's home. Each event and location is attached to unique behaviors and manners as a unique set of experiences and meanings.

Finally, *career* can also include business meals. These can be breakfast, lunch, or dinner, and once again the type of food and location may vary greatly. On these occasions, the focus of the conversation is business rather than social, and the food and location may serve to impress the invited party.

Friendships and Intimacy

Adults take on many roles to fulfill their need for intimacy, each of which demands a type of personal sacrifice. Young adults, free of overriding commitments, find it easy to create broad networks of friends in various settings and among various groups where they can find advice and companionship.

Once marriage occurs, the wide friendship network shrinks because of the time needed to establish a marriage and a home on top of other obligations. Focus on raising a family, however, does not exclude an important occupation that is related to maintaining intimacy and friendships, namely, dining out. Dining out may not be as simple as merely eating at a different location. The experience of dining out can include that of moving into a different world that may help in maintaining and developing relationships.

SOCIAL ASPECTS OF DINING OUT

Dining out is not only about the food consumed but also about the experience of dining out (Campbell-Smith, 1967). Finkelstein (1989) applied a more sociological, structuralist view to this concept and wrote of her findings in her book *Dining Out: A Sociology of Modern Manners*. She wrote that dining out today has much to do with self-presentation and social relationships.

Restaurants have a cultural reputation as being a site of well-being, excitement, and pleasure, which is why things other than the food are important. For example, the restaurant's décor and the cost and nature of the service may serve as indications of its patrons' socioeconomic status. Finkelstein (1989), moreover, suggested that things such as cost and status are more important than the nature and quality of the food because cost and status are objective factors that are easier for people to agree on than food.

The objective factors of dining out allow for standardization of meal experiences. By making these objective factors part of restaurants, the patrons who frequent such restaurants know what the experience should be like and therefore go to the particular restaurant for the particular experience they are looking for at that particular time (Finkelstein, 1989). For example, when taking children out to dine in the United States, the typically appropriate restaurant (other than fast-food chains) would be inexpensive and relatively casual and have a children's menu. In France, however, it is not uncommon to see children in upscale restaurants that may also have a children's menu. Another example could be the parents' decision to dine at an expensive restaurant on their anniversary with the hope of having an experience that is different from their family's typical dining-out experience.

OLDER ADULTHOOD

Older adulthood is sometimes described in terms of increased frailty and health concerns. In sociological terms, *older adulthood* is often defined by the changes in older people's roles and occupations. Some of these changes occur as a result of the biological and physiological changes that occur with aging. Some are the result of life circumstances, such as grown children. Some arise from the organization of society. In general, the way people change their lives with aging greatly depends on their previous lifestyle and their social, cultural, and economic situation. In terms of eating, changes would similarly depend on social status, economic situation, cultural background, and established eating habits. The need to control some aspect of diet may increase as people get older, according to the belief that what people consume affects their health. Most of these changes in food intake occur before one reaches older adulthood and depend on one's personal health considerations, which may include conditions such as diabetes, high blood pressure, or heart disease. Such changes in diet are dominated by scientific findings and common beliefs about the healthful qualities of different foods.

Occupations That Involve Eating

The earlier description of and discussion about the different occupations that involve eating was not meant to be exhaustive but illustrative. My purpose was to demonstrate that the basic human need for food leads all humans to engage in the basic activity of eating. This activity consists of placing food into one's mouth, chewing, swallowing, and digesting. Humans, however, are animals who construct social meanings, and the activity of eating can be performed and experienced in different contexts and in different forms, thus amounting to the creation of multiple occupations that involve eating. Occupations are phenomena that lie within the person because only the person can interpret and assign meaning to activities and events. Humans are social animals, and the interpretations and meanings that they assign to occupations are closely related to their life experiences (Figure 3.5). These life experiences are greatly shaped by temporal, psychological, social, symbolic, cultural, ethnic, or spiritual meanings.

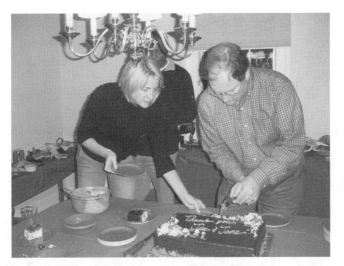

Figure 3.5. As part of a celebration, cakes have important meanings.

EXERCISE 3.5: FOOD STUDY

In the preceding description, the terms *social* and *cultural* were used because these are the main areas of academic study that study food in relation to context. Explore the literature about food to assess the influence of context on food.

In addition to parents, both society and culture shape children's experiences by sanctioning what environments are appropriate for children and at what ages. As children get older and gain increasing experience with the same activity in different contexts, their understanding becomes richer. That is, eating in various contexts teaches children that hunger can be satisfied with different kinds of food and in different situations. They also learn that there are foods other than those served at home and that they will like some of these foods better than those regularly served at home. In addition, they learn that different contexts correspond to different experiences and meanings (e.g., birthday parties, holiday meals).

As children grow up, not only do the environments they frequent become more numerous, but they also spend more of their time with peers in environments away from their families. At this point, activities that are carried out with peers acquire meanings without parental influence shaping the experiences. Such experiences and meanings, translated into connections in the brain, contribute to people's uniqueness. Each child or adolescent has a life context fairly similar to that of his or her parents, yet each participates in new and different contexts that are shared with peers. All of these lead to shared experiences across generations (with parents) and across cohorts (with peers), allowing the social scientist to study the similarities and differences among such groups.

As adults, people are more consciously aware of their contexts, their limitations, and how these relate to lifestyle and experiences. Adults have the power, as sanctioned by society, to raise and socialize their children as long as they do not violate certain boundaries as defined by law (e.g., child abuse and neglect, avoiding schooling, child labor). Parents can shape their children's contexts, thus constructing experiences and meanings for various childhood activities. Examples of such shaping include embracing one's cultural heritage through the types of food served at home and thus supporting the development of tastes for ethnic food. Parents may also decide that they want to do just the opposite, serving nonethnic food with the hope of assimilating their children into the larger society. Alternatively, parents may serve food that is not related to a particular culture but that is deemed at that time to be healthy and most appropriate for the child's development and well-being. In this case, children are socialized into the concept of food as a means of maintaining health rather than a means of cultural identification.

In either case, these experiences are mapped in children's brains as they learn to identify the foods with meanings presented at home. These different meanings associated with eating present different occupations, for example, eating as a marker of cultural identity in which the taste of food is essential in contrast to eating as a means of maintaining health in which the taste of food is not essential.

The sources of parents' decisions about how to socialize their children, although coming from within themselves, are influenced by their life experiences. For example, if parents' social life involves participation in occupations with great cultural emphasis, then they would very likely emphasize food in its cultural forms.

Summary

This chapter is about the commonality and uniqueness of occupations or the meanings that people assign to activities. These meanings are typically shared by one's reference group, which could be based on ethnic and cultural contexts. That is, meaning schemas are a general phenomenon that is shared among a group of people with similar life experiences. Occupations have meaning attached to them by the person who engages in them. Using the purposeful activities associated with eating, I explored the importance of this occupation across the life span. Eating is a social and cultural phenomenon that evolves and changes as the person grows and matures. Culture and life experiences determine its form and significance to the person. The family and social environment influence the life experiences that a person has around food, and meanings are assigned to the occupation of eating that are closely related to life experiences and shaped by temporal, psychosocial, social, symbolic, culture, time, ethics, and spiritual meanings.

Acknowledgment

A special thanks is extended to Kaitlin R. Jessing-Butz, who assisted in the preparation of the manuscript of this chapter.

References

Albala, K. (2002). *Eating right in the Renaissance*. Berkeley: University of California Press.

Birch, L. L., Fisher, J. O., & Grimm-Thomas, K. (1996). The development of children's eating habits. In H. L. Meiselman & H. J. H. MacFie (Eds.), *Food choice acceptance and consumption* (pp. 161–206). London: Blackie Academic & Professional.

Campbell-Smith, G. (1967). *The marketing of the meal experience*. London: Surrey University Press.

Clark, F. A., Parham, D., Carlson, M. E., Frank, G., Jackson, J., Pierce, D., et al. (1991). Occupational science: Academic innovation in the service of occupational therapy's future. *American Journal of Occupational Therapy, 45,* 300–310.

Davidson, A. (1999). *The Oxford companion to food.* New York: Oxford University Press.

DeVault, M. J. (1991). *Feeding the family: The social organization of caring as gendered work.* Chicago: University of Chicago Press.

Douglas, M. (1982). *In the active voice.* Boston: Routledge & Kegan Paul.

Ferry, J. F. (2003). *Food in film: A culinary performance of communication.* New York: Routledge.

Fieldhouse, P. (1986). *Food and nutrition: Customs and culture.* Dover, NH: Croom Helm.

Finkelstein, J. (1989). *Dining out: The sociology of modern manners.* New York: New York University Press.

Gillis, J. (1996). Making time for family: The invention of family time(s) and the reinvention of family history. *Journal of Family History, 21,* 4–21.

Grieshaber, S. (1997). Mealtime rituals: Power and resistance in the construction of mealtime rules. *British Journal of Sociology, 48,* 649–666.

Hasselkus, B. R. (2002). *The meaning of everyday occupation.* Thorofare, NJ: Slack.

Hinojosa, J., & Kramer, P. (1997). Statement—Fundamental concepts of occupational therapy: Occupation, purposeful activity, and function. *American Journal of Occupational Therapy, 51,* 864–866.

Holland, S. S. (Director). (1985). *Better off dead* [Motion picture]. United States: Warner Brothers.

Kantor, D., & Lehr, W. (1975). *Inside the family: Toward a theory of family process.* San Francisco: Jossey-Bass.

Kittler, P. G., & Sucher, K. P. (2001). *Food and culture* (3rd ed.). Belmont, CA: Wadsworth/Thompson Learning.

Kramer, P., & Hinojosa, J. (1995). Epiphany of human occupation. In C. B. Royeen (Ed.), *Human occupation* (AOTA Self-Study Series, p. 5–17). Bethesda, MD: American Occupational Therapy Association.

La Fontaine, J. (1986). An anthropological perspective on children in social worlds. In M. Richards & P. Light (Eds.), *Children in social worlds: Development in social context* (pp. 10–30). Cambridge, MA: Harvard University Press.

Lee, N. (2001). *Childhood and society: Growing up in an age of uncertainty.* Philadelphia: Open University Press.

Mennell, S., Murcott, A., & van Otterloo, A. H. (1992). *The sociology of food: Eating, diet, and culture.* Thousand Oaks, CA: Sage.

Merriam-Webster's concise dictionary of English usage. (2002). Springfield, MA: Merriam-Webster.

Nestle, M. (2002). *Food politics: How the food industry influences nutrition and health.* Berkeley: University of California Press.

Ochs, E., Taylor, C., Rudolph, D., & Smith, R. (1992). Storytelling as a theory-building activity. *Discourse Processes, 15,* 37–72.

Petrie, D. (Director). (1988). *Mystic Pizza* [Motion picture]. United States: Samuel Goldwyn.

Redford, R. (Director). (1980). *Ordinary people* [Motion picture]. United States: Paramount.

Segal, R. (1999). Doing for others: Occupations within families with children with special needs. *Journal of Occupational Science, 6,* 53–60.

Shahar, S. (1990). *Childhood in the middle ages.* New York: Routledge.

Spitz, R. A. (1965). *The first year of life: A psychoanalytic study of normal and deviant development of object relations.* New York: International Universities Press.

Strauss, C., & Quinn, N. (1997). *A cognitive theory of cultural meaning.* New York: Cambridge University Press.

Vuchinich, S. (1987). Starting and stopping spontaneous family conflicts. *Journal of Marriage and the Family, 49,* 591–601.

Wiseman, C. V., Gray, J. J., Mosimann, J. E., & Ahrens, A. H. (1992). Cultural expectations of thinness in women: An update. *International Journal of Eating Disorders, 11,* 85–89.

Wood, R. C. (1995). *The sociology of the meal.* Edinburgh, UK: Edinburgh University Press.

Wyness, M. G. (2000). *Contesting childhood.* New York: Falmer Press.

4

Activity Analysis

Karen A. Buckley, MA, OT/L
Sally E. Poole, MA, OT, CHT

The concept that humans must use both mind and body to maintain health and well-being was documented as early as 2600 B.C. The ancient Chinese, Persians, and Greeks understood that a mutually dependent relationship existed between physical and mental health and well-being. Egyptians and Greeks saw diversion and recreation as treatment for the sick. Later, the Romans recommended activity for those with mental illness (Hopkins & Smith, 1978).

Many centuries later in Europe and the United States, the use of activity and occupation was described as a treatment modality for people with mental and physical illness. In 1798, Benjamin Rush, the first American psychiatrist, advocated the use of domestic occupations for their therapeutic value. Weaving, spinning, and sewing were occupations that he considered to be therapeutic because of their personal interest to the patients of the era and because of their social and cultural relevance (Dunton & Licht, 1957). In the 18th and 19th centuries in the United States, the use of occupations was accepted in the care of people with mental illness. In 1892, Edward N. Bush, superintendent of a psychiatric hospital in Maryland, wrote, "The benefits of occupation are manifold. Primarily, even the most simple and routine tasks keep the mind occupied, awaken new trains of thought and interests, and divert the patient from the delusions or hallucinations which harass and annoy him" (as cited in Dunton & Licht, 1957, p. 9).

In addition to the use of occupations in psychiatric treatment in the 18th and 19th centuries, early documentation has shown that occupations were used to build muscles and improve joint range. In 1780 in France, Clément-Joseph Tissot, a physician in the French cavalry, described the beneficial use of arts and crafts and recreational activities to mediate the physical effects of chronic illness (Dunton & Licht, 1957). Tissot named "shuttlecock, tennis, football, and dancing" (as cited in Dunton & Licht, 1957, p. 9) as activities to promote range of motion for all joints of the upper and lower extremities. In this early literature about the use of occupations or activities, little description is available about the precise methodology used to select activities that addressed specific problems. Instead, activities appear to have been selected for their cultural, social, recreational, and diversional characteristics.

In the early 1900s, occupational therapists embraced the Arts and Crafts Movement that was a backlash against the social ills perceived to have resulted from the Industrial Revolution (Reed, 1986). The Arts and Crafts Movement promoted a simpler life in which activities were performed at a slower pace than required by factory production, where the process was as important as the end product, where the creative spirit was valued, and where manual learning was valued rather than intellectual learning alone (Reed, 1986). Before World War II, little literature indicated that therapists selected activities on the basis of anything other than intuition (Creighton, 1992; Reed, 1986).

At the end of World War I, two factors had a strong influence on occupational therapists' use of activities and related occupations. First, the end of the Arts and Crafts Movement in the United States and Europe meant that many activities were not valued in the same way. Second, therapists found themselves treating patients who were exhibiting both physical and psychological trauma. Therapists began selecting activities on the basis of the patient's particular deficits and needs. They first carefully analyzed each patient's deficits and, using a problem-solving approach, determined which specific activity would be appropriate to address the deficit. Therapists used activities because of their characteristics, but no formal analysis was part of the therapist's treatment routine. Therapists and physicians, however, began to look beyond the profession of occupational therapy to gain knowledge about *activity analysis*.

In this early development of the occupational therapy profession, activity selection and subsequent intervention were influenced by at least two men outside the profession: Frank Gilbreth and Jules Amar (Creighton, 1992). Gilbreth, an engineer by training, studied jobs to identify the most productive and least fatiguing methods of job performance. His work, which was well accepted by industry, examined the worker, environment, and motion. While visiting hospitals in Europe to study physicians and how they worked, he became acquainted with the research of Amar, a French physiologist. Amar had been commissioned by the French government to study how to prepare wounded soldiers for reentry into the workforce, which he did by measuring the physiological requirements of many jobs. His work influenced Gilbreth by making him aware of the possibilities of applying motion studies to the reeducation of returning wounded veterans. Gilbreth presented his work at the 1917 annual meeting of the National Society for the Promotion of Occupational Therapy, which led to the eventual inclusion of this concept of activity analysis into the field of occupational therapy. Activity analysis was incorporated into occupational therapy textbooks as early as 1919 (Creighton, 1992).

The years between World War I and World War II saw the establishment of the American Occupational Therapy Association (AOTA), formerly the National Society for the Promotion of Occupational Therapy, and further development of the profession in general. AOTA encouraged therapists to establish departments and to publish papers to help them do so. In addition, papers were published to assist therapists with the appropriate selection of activities. Crafts were the treatment activities of choice, although *crafts* included both work-related and recreational activities (Creighton, 1992). In 1922 and 1928, AOTA published papers promoting the analysis of crafts for psychiatric occupational therapy and for physical restoration.

World War II propelled women out of the home and into the workforce and propelled occupational therapists from traditional roles into new, real-life circumstances. As a result of improvement in medical and surgical care, veterans were surviving severe physical injuries and living with permanent disability. Occupational therapists began to specialize in the practice area of physical disabilities. Again, occupational therapists referred to Gilbreth's work, now being carried on by his wife Lillian, who proposed that engineers and rehabilitation professionals work together to assist soldiers with disabilities (Creighton, 1992). At the same time, the U.S. Army developed its own manual of therapeutic activities (U.S. Department of War, 1944) that detailed activities to use to improve joint range of motion and strengthening of all extremities. The military, in fact, "divided" the body so that occupational therapists worked with the upper body and physical therapists worked with the lower body (Hinojosa, 1996). Many policies and procedures laid down by the military were, and still are, followed by the profession.

Soon after World War II, Sidney Licht, who at the time was president of the American Congress of Rehabilitation Medicine and the editor of *Physical Medicine Library,* published an article in 1947 advocating the use of a more precise method for analyzing activity for those occupational therapists working in the area of physical disabilities. He believed that *craft analysis* looked at "psychomotor values, economic factors, tempo, or other inherent characteristics" (p. 75). He coined the term *kinetic analysis,* however, to refer to when the tools or activities were to be analyzed for the motions involved. Many of Licht's ideas continue to influence practice in the area of physical disabilities. Contemporary occupational therapists who are concerned about muscle contractions, joint range of motion, precision and accuracy of intervention, ergonomics of body mechanics, and control variants continue to use the criteria for examining motion that Licht originally proposed for kinetic analysis.

Occupational therapists working in physical medicine appear to have become interested in activity analysis before those working in mental health. In 1948, Gail Fidler proposed that occupational therapists working in psychiatric occupational therapy use scientific analysis of activities:

> While the functioning of a personality is certainly not as quantifiable as a muscle, the use of activity for the psychiatric patient should be

more scientifically allied with the principles of dynamic psychiatry
and treatment objectives than it is at the present. (p. 284)

Fidler also proposed an outline for activity analysis to help occupational
therapists meet the goals or aims of treatment so that occupational therapy in
psychiatry could, in fact, be elevated from diversion to the level of therapy.

Activity analysis remained rudimentary in occupational therapy and
focused almost exclusively on the product rather than the process of analysis.
Gradually, the process of analysis has become more important than the end
product. For example, Mosey (1986) proposed that activity analysis is the
process of closely examining an activity to distinguish its component parts.
A careful examination allows a skilled occupational therapist to select the
most therapeutic and appropriate activity from those activities available.
A careful examination ensures that the activities selected are relevant and
correspond to the client's needs.

Activity analysis also plays an important part of deductive reasoning
in whatever frame of reference or approach practitioners use with clients.
Mosey (1986) suggested two goals for using an activity analysis that would
serve to firmly establish the process as a legitimate tool of the profession.
The first purpose enables the student or therapist to learn more about the
activity's inherent properties and the range of skills the person needs to
perform it. After the therapist has an understanding of the person and his
or her personal goals and present performance skills, he or she needs to
select an appropriate frame of reference to initiate intervention. Under these
conditions, the occupational therapist can do a restricted activity analysis,
that is, focus on the function–dysfunction continuum of the specific frame of
reference. This is an alternative purpose for activity analysis. The intent is to
identify whether the activity is well suited to be used to promote change in
the underlying skills or abilities deemed to be the focus of intervention. This
approach to activity analysis is directly related to the postulates regarding
change that were identified in the selected frame of reference.

Activity analysis enables occupational therapists to determine an activity's
therapeutic properties so that they can make an appropriate match between
the client's interests and abilities and the activity that will meet the client's
health needs (Mosey, 1986) and established intervention goals.

Activity analysis can be approached from many perspectives, depending on
the reason for the analysis and the specific focus of interest. Trombly and Scott
(1977) proposed that performance areas be analyzed first. Cynkin and Robinson
(1990) proposed that occupational therapists begin an activity analysis with the
performance context. In Chapter 6, Kramer and Hinojosa stated that activity
analysis assesses the person, activity, and context. For example, a therapist who
works in a hand therapy practice would begin with an analysis of the activity-
based motor and sensory skills; hence, activities used in the clinic would be
selected on the basis of how they address specific deficits. An activity analysis
should consider the person's present, past, and future occupations.

In 2003, Crepeau described three levels of activity analysis: (1) activity analysis, (2) theory-based activity analysis, and (3) occupation-based activity analysis. An *activity analysis* investigates the demands of the activity and its context and personal meaning. *Theory-based activity analysis,* not unlike Mosey's (1986) restricted analysis, asks the occupational therapist to determine the therapeutic use of an activity on the basis of practice theory. Crepeau (2003) stated that activity analysis and theory-based activity analysis are done in the abstract. Only *occupation-based activity analysis* studies the person "engaging in occupations within [that person's] unique physical, cultural, and social environment" (p. 192). We believe that the activity analysis outline, as presented in this chapter, can be used for any of these three purposes. When all three parts of our activity analysis are completed, they will satisfy the description of an occupation-based activity analysis.

Occupational Therapy Perspectives on Activity Analysis

Occupational therapists have an organized conceptual approach to activity analysis. The activity is first viewed as a whole, then an analysis is done to break it down into its component parts. In this section, we outline one method of completing an activity analysis, drawn from various sources within the occupational therapy literature. Many of the ideas presented have become common knowledge within occupational therapy. Hence, it is impossible to determine with whom the idea or concept originated (Allen, 1987; Ayres, 1983; Kremer, Nelson, & Duncombe, 1984; Llorens, 1973, 1986; Neistadt, McAuley, Zecha, & Shannon, 1993; Nelson, 1996; Pedretti & Wade, 1996).

In occupational therapy professional education, much time is spent on activity analysis, that is, learning how to do it and learning the aspects of dividing an activity into its component parts. Traditionally, occupational therapy students learn to analyze an activity by focusing on performance that makes up the individual task. This process of microanalysis often leads the student not to consider the whole activity, the context in which it is usually performed, or the important occupation with which the activity is associated. Students learning how to do activity analysis need to be able to identify more than just the fact that the skill is present; they need to know to what degree this skill is used in the context of the activity being performed. In this section, we outline such a process, with a focus on an analysis that examines activities within the context in which they are performed.

An activity analysis begins with a description of the activity and each of its fundamental tasks, that is, the steps necessary to complete the activity. The occupational therapist describes the activity and how people perform it under usual circumstances. What follows is a suggested outline for occupational therapy students and practitioners to follow when analyzing the component aspects of activities. We present it in three parts: (1) an introduction and description of the activity, (2) the activity analysis outline itself, and (3) a final summary that relates the activity to the person. Like many other activity analysis forms, this form is based on several documents, including the *Uniform Terminology for Occupational Therapy—Third Edition* (AOTA, 1994); the *Occupational Therapy Practice Framework: Domain and Process* (2nd ed.; *Framework–II*; AOTA, 2008); and the *International Classification of Functioning, Disability and Health* (ICF; World Health Organization, 2001).

Part 1: Introduction

In this section, we describe the activity and the factors that influence the person's ability to perform it, including both internal and external characteristics.

ACTIVITY

The occupational therapist describes the activity and how a person performs it under usual circumstances. When the analysis is used as part of an intervention, the practitioner should keep the whole person in mind, that is, how and why the activity is relevant to the person. The practitioner also appraises the activity relative to the context in which the client will perform it and the activity's associated performance areas.

In this section (see Appendix 4.A), the activity is named and the specific sequence of performance (steps) required to perform it is described. Each step is identified in the order in which it is performed to complete the full activity and described in detail. The needed materials, tools, and equipment; space demands; and safety precautions and contraindications are then listed. In this section, the practitioner considers the following:

- Is this an activity that must be completed in one session?
- Is this an activity that can be performed over time?
- Can the activity naturally be divided so that it can be performed over time?
- Do the tasks (steps) in the activity require that it be performed over a period of time?

The practitioner is then asked to consider the influence of social, contextual, and time elements on the activity.

SOCIAL ENVIRONMENT

In this section, the practitioner considers the following:

- Is the activity performed alone or with others?
- Do others place expectations on the person to perform?

PERSONAL CONTEXT AND CLIENT FACTORS

The activity is done by a person. Thus, in the activity analysis, the practitioner must consider the person, including his or her values, beliefs, and spirituality. This section of the analysis form includes demographics.

VALUES, BELIEFS, AND SPIRITUALITY

The practitioner identifies ideas or beliefs that are important to the person. Which of the following features potentially influence the person's participation or engagement in the activity?

- The person's inferred personal value for the activity
- The person's underlying meaning associated with the activity
- The person's perceived purpose of the activity
- The activity's ability to meet a desired need
- The activity's ability to promote independence or self-reliance
- Whether the activity presents a personal challenge or facilitates desired change
- Whether the activity has the potential to facilitate exploration of life's meaning.

INTERESTS

The practitioner identifies mental or physical activities that create pleasure and maintain attention.

- How does the activity stimulate the person?
- Is it repetitive?
- Does it offer an appropriate degree of challenge (e.g., cognitive, motor)?
- Is there variety in the activity?
- What are possible attractions to participating in the activity?
- What are the positive feelings associated with the activity (e.g., physical challenge, fellowship with others, intellectual challenge, demonstration of capacity or creativity)?

The practitioner begins by identifying the roles that might be associated with the activity and determines their relevance and meaningfulness to past, present, and future roles. The analysis can be used to identify whether the activity incorporates skills that can be associated with a desired role. The practitioner also appraises the activity relative to the context in which the client will perform it, considering physical, social, and temporal aspects.

Part 2: Activity Analysis Outline

In this section, we describe the activity analysis's multiple components, including physical signs that influence the performance of the activity.

REQUIRED ACTIONS AND PERFORMANCE SKILLS

The *ICF* is concerned about people's ability to participate in activities and society. Its taxonomy is divided into two broad categories: (1) functioning and disability and (2) contextual factors. According to the *ICF*, functioning and disability themselves include two components: (1) body function and structures and (2) activities and participation. *Contextual factors* include personal factors and environmental factors that influence performance of the activity and the level of participation. The broad categories of required action and performance skills or components (AOTA, 2008; WHO, 2001) serve as a framework for the activity analysis presented in this chapter. We do not use the *ICF* taxonomy in its entirety; rather, we limit its use to categories that we determined were most relevant to the process of activity analysis.

The *ICF* taxonomy provides a broad structure for the analysis and the basis for identifying basic requirements of the activity. The occupational therapist or occupational therapy assistant identifies whether a specific skill is necessary during the performance of the activity (yes or no). A *yes* response indicates that the performance skill will need to be focused on in the subsequent sections of the analysis form. On the basis of the performance (AOTA, 1994), the practitioner assesses the *level of influence* that each element has on the client's ability to do the activity. Eventually, the practitioner must understand how impairment affects or challenges the client's performance of the activity.

Another reason for analyzing an activity is to identify its potential for providing stimulation or opportunities to use specific skills as part of intervention. A 5-point scale is used to rate the level of influence of each element:

- 0 = *The component has no effect or influence on the ability to do the activity.*
- 1 = *The component has only a minimal effect or influence on the ability to do the activity.* The activity would not substantially stimulate or address the performance component element.
- 2 = *The component has a moderate effect or influence on the ability to complete the activity.* If a client has a deficit, compensation may have to be made for the client to perform the activity. The activity would present a challenge to the performance component element.
- 3 = *The component has a significant effect or influence on the ability to complete the activity.* The activity would be extremely difficult to complete if the client has a deficit in this performance component. The activity would present a significant stimulation or opportunity to address the performance component element.
- 4 = *The component has a major effect or influence on the completion of the activity.* A performance component deficit in this area would seriously influence the person's ability to do the activity. Such a person would be very likely not to be able to complete the activity. The activity would

present a major stimulation or opportunity to address this performance component element.

The observation section is used to describe special circumstances or concerns and provides space to include any other comments a practitioner has relative to performance.

In the next section, we define each skill, and several questions are provided to help practitioners assess the role the skill plays in completing the activity. The questions should not be considered definitive but rather as a jump-start when considering each skill or action. After considering each question, the practitioner rates the skill or action's influence and writes observational notes (Figure 4.1).

LEARNING AND APPLYING KNOWLEDGE

Knowledge is what is learned. *Learning* is based on thinking, solving problems, and making decisions. Learning is also influenced by sensory experiences. Activities are about applying knowledge for a meaningful outcome. The first step to examining this aspect of the activity is to consider what the activity requires the person to do. This screening gives the practitioner guidance about which components need to be analyzed further. Answering the following questions guides practitioners to the next step of the analysis:

- Does the activity require watching (using the sense of seeing intentionally to experience visual stimuli, such as watching a sporting event or children playing)? Visual reception is the underlying prerequisite.
- Does the activity require listening (using the sense of hearing intentionally to experience auditory stimuli, such as listening to music or a lecture)?
- Does the activity require other purposeful sensing (using the body's other basic senses intentionally to experience stimuli, such as touching and feeling textures, tasting sweets, or smelling flowers)? Tactile, proprioceptive, vestibular, olfactory, and gustatory senses may need to be examined.

Occupational therapists also analyze activities in relation to their sensory-processing demands. A person's central nervous system processes sensory

Skill	
Level of Influence: ☐ 0 ☐ 1 ☐ 2 ☐ 3 ☐ 4	Observations:

Figure 4.1. Observational notes.

information and integrates this information so that the person can make an adaptive response. *Sensory processing* is the internal mechanism a person uses to process and respond to sensory input. It may influence the client's ability to reach a calm state of alertness and, thus, his or her ability to engage in and complete the activity. Each activity presents unique sensory-processing requirements. Thus, the ability to organize and integrate multiple sensory processes during performance of an activity is critical (adequate response).

SENSORY PROCESSING

- Does the activity require the person to make changes on the basis of sensory input?
- Does continuity of performance depend on the ability to proceed on the basis of sensory input?
- Is the ability to end performance based on sensory processing (e.g., physical discomfort, a problem with the activity)?
- What degree of sensory modulation is required?
- Will an adverse response influence performance (e.g., defensiveness)?
- Will a diminished response influence the activity?

VISUAL RECEPTION

Visual reception involves interpreting stimuli through the eyes, including peripheral vision, acuity, and awareness of color and pattern.

- Does the activity require the person to fixate on a stationary object (visual fixation)?
- Does the activity require slow, smooth movements of the eyes to maintain fixation on a moving object (visual tracking)?
- Must the person rapidly change fixation from one object in the visual field to another (scanning; e.g., locating a misplaced utensil during cooking, locating a dropped object while performing a sport)?
- What degree of discrimination of fine detail is required to do the activity?
- Does the activity require changes in focus such as from near to far?

AUDITORY PROCESSING

Auditory processing involves interpreting and localizing sounds and discriminating among background sounds.

- Does the activity require the person to listen to sounds and interpret their meaning (e.g., musical notes, verbal instructions, verbal communication, warning sounds [e.g., alarm buzzers])? Are there functional sounds that assist the person with monitoring the environment (e.g., water running, frying, opening sounds, traffic, closing sounds)?

- Does the activity produce loud or harsh sounds during its performance (e.g., hammering, power tools)? Could these sounds be stressful to the person?
- Does the activity environment require the person to discriminate or suppress background sounds?
- Does the person use or rely on sound while moving (e.g., search for a source of sound and move toward it)?

TACTILE PROCESSING

Tactile processing involves interpreting light touch, pressure, temperature, pain, and vibration though skin contact and receptors.

- Does the activity require the person to hold objects gently, or is a degree of pressure important?
- Are the materials used at room temperature, or do they require heat or cooling?
- Does the activity require the person to appreciate or tolerate vibration (e.g., electric tools)?
- Does the activity require tactile discrimination?
- Are body parts always within the visual field? When must a person rely on tactile input?
- Could the tactile properties of the activity be perceived as noxious (e.g., defensiveness)?
- Is the ability to localize tactile input part of the task?

PROPRIOCEPTIVE PROCESSING

Proprioceptive processing involves interpreting stimuli originating in muscles, joints, and other internal tissues that give information about the position of one body part in relation to another.

- Does the activity distract or compress joints and tissues?
- Is weight bearing part of the activity (e.g., lower extremities or upper extremities)?
- What is the degree of pushing, pulling, or lifting that occurs during the activity?
- Do movements and position of the extremities occur outside the visual field (e.g., reaching in or out)?

VESTIBULAR INPUT—INTERPRETING STIMULI FROM THE INNER EAR RECEPTORS
REGARDING HEAD POSITION

Vestibular input contributes to appropriate righting and equilibrium reactions, automatic postural responses, and maintaining posture and movement during activity performance.

- Does the activity require quick movements of the head or body?
- Does the activity require postural maintenance or change in relation to gravity or acceleration and deceleration forces (e.g., sit to stand, sudden change in forward movement, vertical or horizontal changes)?
- Does the activity require muscular co-contraction?
- Does the activity require coordinated eye movements?
- Does the activity require postural background movements (e.g., adequate extension; ability to dissociate head, neck, and arm movements)?

OLFACTORY PROCESSING

Olfactory processing involves interpreting odors.

- Does the activity contain odors that might be interpreted as noxious?
- Does the activity involve odors that might be alerting (e.g., burning) or calming?
- How might the scents affect one who is overresponsive to odors?

GUSTATORY PROCESSING

Gustatory processing involves interpreting tastes.

- Does the person need to interpret taste to enhance or contribute to performance?
- Does the taste or texture elicit an overresponsive reaction?

BASIC LEARNING

Basic learning encompasses the skill areas of copying and rehearsing. Answering the following questions guides practitioners to the next step of the analysis:

- Does the activity require copying (e.g., imitating or mimicking as a basic component of learning, such as copying a gesture, a sound, or the letters of an alphabet)? Prerequisites to be examined are recognition, form constancy, spatial relations, and position in space.
- Does the activity require rehearsing (e.g., repeating a sequence of events or symbols as a basic component of learning, such as counting by 10s or practicing the recitation of a poem)? Sequencing is the prerequisite skill.

RECOGNITION

Recognition involves identifying familiar faces, objects, and other previously presented material.

- Does the person have to recognize people, body parts, and objects to engage in the activity?

FORM CONSTANCY

Form constancy involves recognizing forms and objects as being the same in various environments, positions, and sizes.

- Does the activity occur in two dimensions or three?
- Does the activity require the person to respond to changing representations of objects?
- Do the materials change form (e.g., laundry hanging on a line or folded)?
- Does the size of the tools, utensils, or letters change?

SPATIAL RELATIONS

Spatial changes involve determining the position of objects relative to one another.

- Does the activity require the use of spatial concepts (e.g., manipulation, take apart, put together)?
- Does the activity require that the person estimate sizes?
- Does the activity require that the person judge distances or estimate size?
- Does the activity require orientation of shapes, sizes, or designs?
- Does the activity require attention to detail in positioning?

POSITION IN SPACE

Position in space refers to determining the spatial relationship of figures and objects to the self and other forms and objects.

- Does the activity require the person to determine front, back, top, bottom, beside, behind, under, or over?
- Does the activity require that the person understand the relationship between action and his or her body?

SEQUENCING

Sequencing involves placing information, concepts, and actions in order.

- Does the activity require the person to arrange items or perform steps in a serial order?
- Does the activity require an understanding of before and after?
- Does the activity require the person to reverse a sequence (backward; e.g., put on clothing or take it off, put a toy together or take it apart)?
- Does the activity allow the person to have personal choice in the manner of sequencing (e.g., morning care, dressing, showering)?

ACQUIRING SKILLS

Engaging in an activity creates situations in which people gain skills. Skills are the sets of actions that a person has learned and is able to apply in given situations. Skills are often divided into basic and complex skills. *Basic skills* are elementary and purposeful actions, such as learning to manipulate eating utensils, a pencil, or a simple tool. *Complex skills* are integrated sets of actions to follow rules and to sequence and coordinate movements, such as learning to play games like football or use a building tool. Answering these questions guides practitioners to the next step of the analysis:

- Occupational therapists and occupational therapy assistants must often assess a person's cognitive abilities before determining his or her capacity to learn or apply knowledge. Does the activity require the participant to focus intentionally on specific stimuli, such as filtering out distracting noises? Level of arousal, orientation, and attention span must be considered.
- Does the person have adequate skills to support the efficient completion of the activity? Consider motor control, praxis, body scheme, fine motor coordination and dexterity, crossing the midline, right–left discrimination, laterality, bilateral integration, and visual–motor integration.
- When engaged in the activity, what thinking processes does the activity require the person to use (formulating and manipulating ideas, concepts, and images, whether goal oriented or not, either alone or with others, such as creating fiction, providing a theorem, playing with ideas, brainstorming, meditating, pondering, speculating, reflecting)? Consider memory, categorization, spatial operations, generalization, and concept formation.
- Solving problems requires that a person find solutions to problems or challenges to complete the activity. Simple problems involve a single issue or question. Solving complex problems requires the person doing the activity to consider multiple and interrelated issues or several related problems. To solve problems related to activities, a person must identify and analyze issues, develop solutions, evaluate potential effects of the solutions, and execute the chosen solution. Therefore, learning and memory must be examined.
- Making decisions requires choosing among options, implementing the choice, and evaluating the effects of that choice. Consider memory, concept formation, categorization, and generalization.

LEVEL OF AROUSAL

Level of arousal includes demonstrating alertness and responsiveness to environmental stimuli.

- Does the time of day influence the person's arousal level?
- What arousal level is needed to provide an adequate length of time to complete the activity?

- Do fatigue and pain factors affect arousal level and the ability to attend to the task?

ORIENTATION

Orientation includes identifying person, place, time, and situation.

Orientation to Person

- Does the activity relate to the person's lifestyle?
- Is the activity associated with a role that is meaningful to the person?
- Could the activity be influenced by the person's routines (e.g., clean the bathroom on Tuesday, clean the bathroom when it needs cleaning)?

Orientation to Place

- Does the activity require the person to know where he or she is?

Orientation to Time

- Does the person need to know the exact time, date, or time of year to engage in the activity?

Orientation to Situation

- What is the relationship between the activity and the person's environment and roles?
- Does the person need to understand the circumstances in which the activity is performed?
- Does the person understand time restrictions or demands placed on performance?

SENSORY MODULATION

Sensory modulation involves the ability to respond appropriately to incoming stimuli.

- Does the person overrespond to sensory stimuli (e.g., sensory defensiveness, becoming overly stressed by stimuli)?
- Does the person underrespond to sensory stimuli (e.g., does not appear to register stimuli, slow to respond)?
- Does the person seek out sensory stimuli (e.g., rocking, excessive mouthing of objects, spinning)?

ATTENTION SPAN

Attention span refers to the ability to focus on a task over time.

- How long must the person attend?
- Will the person be required to selectively attend (e.g., focus on specific stimuli) or disregard irrelevant stimuli?
- Does the activity demand sustained attention?
- Does the activity require the person to shift attention (e.g., frying eggs, making toast, pouring coffee while cooking)?

MOTOR CONTROL

Motor control involves using functional and versatile movement patterns.

- Does the activity require repetition? If so, what kind (e.g., putting a puzzle together, catching a ball)?
- Do numerous joints need to be controlled during a complex activity?
- Does the activity require the person to inhibit movements to be most efficient (e.g., using scissors)?
- Does the activity require constant or variable changes in speed, tempo, or rhythm (e.g., dealing cards, playing jacks)?
- Is the pace of the activity externally or internally controlled?
- Does the activity require manipulation and control of tools or utensils (e.g., the person must control the tool and the limb)?

PRAXIS

Praxis involves conceiving and planning a motor act in response to an environmental demand.

- Does the activity require the person to assume a novel position (postural praxis; e.g., yoga, martial arts, dance routines for the novice)?
- Does the activity require the person to plan movements that are not habitual?
- Does the activity involve the use of new tools or utensils?
- Does engagement require the person to have a plan?
- Is the activity new and unusual for the person?

BODY SCHEME

Body scheme refers to having an internal awareness of the body and the relationship of body parts to each other. This component is closely related to kinesthesia and proprioception because it requires integration of sensation from muscles and joints.

- Does the activity require that the person have an appreciation for his or her body and be able to sense how the different parts work together (e.g., playing basketball)?

- Does the activity require the person to have an internal awareness of body actions that must happen in a specific sequence (e.g., ballroom dancing)?

OCULAR MOTOR CONTROL

Ocular motor control refers to the ability to move the eyes to focus on and follow objects.

- Is the person able to fixate on a stationary object and follow (track) a moving object with smooth pursuits?

ORAL MOTOR CONTROL

Oral motor refers to use of muscles in and around the mouth.

- Is the person able to coordinate tongue, lips, and jaw for the purposes of clear speech or feeding?

FINE MOTOR COORDINATION AND DEXTERITY

Fine motor coordination and dexterity involves using small muscle groups for controlled movements, particularly in-hand object manipulation.

- What degree of isolated finger use is required?
- Which grasp patterns are used during different functions (e.g., hook, cylindrical, spherical, three-jaw tripod, lateral pinch, tip-to-tip pinch, tripod)?
- Is speed a necessary element of the activity?

VISUAL–MOTOR INTEGRATION

Visual–motor integration refers to the ability to coordinate the interaction of information from the eyes and body movement.

- What degree of eye–hand or eye–foot coordination is required (e.g., tracing, copying, pencil tasks, balance beam)?

CROSSING THE MIDLINE

Crossing the midline involves moving the limbs and eyes across the midline sagittal plane of the body.

- Does the activity require the person to scan the environment to find tools and utensils? If so, how frequently?
- Does the activity require that the person cross the midline of the body with his or her arms or legs (e.g., dressing)?

RIGHT–LEFT DISCRIMINATION

Right–left discrimination refers to differentiating one side from the other.

- What degree of bilateral coordination is required to do the activity?
- Does the person need to be able to use or apply right–left concepts?
- Does the activity require that the person be able to follow verbal or written directions that require actions to the left, right, or both sides of the body?
- Does the activity involve tools that require bilateral coordination, such as the use of one hand as a stabilizer or assist while the other hand operates the tool?
- Does the activity require the person to differentiate right and left on another person (e.g., demonstrated instruction as in Aikido, karate, dancing)?

LATERALITY

Laterality refers to using a preferred or dominant hand or foot.

- Does the activity require a high degree of skill in which the person needs to use a preferred hand or foot (e.g., cooking, sewing, writing)?
- Does hand or foot preference influence how smoothly or effortlessly the person performs the activity?

BILATERAL INTEGRATION

Bilateral integration refers to coordinating both sides of the body. Bilateral integration is considered a prerequisite for gross and fine motor coordination and affects acquisition of skills.

- How frequently do both sides of the body have to cooperate during the activity?
- Does one side of the body need to stabilize while the other side acts?
- Does the activity require crossing the midline in a rotatory, asymmetrical pattern (e.g., golf, baseball swing)?
- Does the activity require that the person use both sides of the body in the same manner (symmetrical performance; e.g., pushing, pulling)?
- Does the activity require reciprocal patterns (e.g., bike riding, swimming, running, martial arts)?

MEMORY

Memory entails recoding information after a brief or long period.

- What are the activity's memory requirements, for example, immediate (1 minute), short term (longer than 1 minute, less than 1 hour), or long term (more than 1 hour)?

- If the activity requires long-term memory, what elements are required?
- What information related to personal experience (episodic) is needed?
- What factual knowledge of the world (semantic) is needed?
- What knowledge of the world or how to do something (procedural) is needed?
- Is the long-term memory modality specific (visual, auditory, verbal)?

CATEGORIZATION

Categorization refers to identifying similarities and differences among pieces of environmental information.

- Does the activity require the person to group objects or information according to characteristics (e.g., visual features, tactile features, similarities, differences)?
- Does the activity require mental grouping (e.g., playing cards, different name brands to be purchased, price differences, nutritional contents)?
- Does the activity require construction in which the person must understand how parts relate to a whole or how to break the whole down into its parts?

CONCEPT FORMATION

Concept formation refers to organizing a variety of information to form thoughts and ideas. This component is related to the ability to categorize.

- Does the activity require synthesis of ideas (e.g., formulation of a hypothesis about the how or why)?
- Does the activity require abstract thought processes?
- Does the activity require symbolic thinking?
- Does the activity require the person to question himself or herself or evaluate performance?

SPATIAL OPERATIONS

Spatial operations involve mentally manipulating the position of objects in various relationships.

- Does the activity require the person to mentally visualize different perspectives (e.g., two-dimensional diagrams, three-dimensional objects)?
- Does the activity involve mental visualization of performance?
- Does the activity require that the person visualize how the object or activity should look on completion (e.g., clothing on a hanger or self, how a table will be set for a dinner party, how a cake will look after baking)?

LEARNING

Learning refers to acquiring new concepts and behaviors.

- Does the activity provide a structured or unstructured learning experience?
- Does the activity provide feedback about performance?
- What type of learning is expected (e.g., motor, verbal, feelings, attitudinal)?

GENERALIZATION

Generalization refers to applying previously learned concepts and behaviors to a variety of new situations.

- Can the activity be performed in different contexts (e.g., bathing at bedside, sponge bathing at sink, tub bathing)?
- Does the activity provide opportunities to apply learned skills to a new situation?

GENERAL ACTIVITY DEMANDS

Completing an activity requires that people carry out simple or complex and coordinated actions. These actions are related to the mental, physical, and social components. Some actions produce a single simple activity that is clearly defined or time limited, such as initiating or terminating the activity. Single complex tasks need to be carried out in sequence or simultaneously, such as arranging the furniture in one's home or completing an assignment for school. Moreover, activities are influenced by the people who participate in them. Consideration of the following guides practitioners to the next step of the analysis:

- A person's mental and physical status influence how he or she carries out simple or complex activities. Prerequisite components to be examined are initiation of activity, time management, termination of activity, coping skills, and self-control.
- Some activities are composed of multiple tasks that need to be carried out in sequence or simultaneously, such as preparing a multicourse meal, with each course requiring initiation and management of time. Space to prepare a salad, main course, and side dishes must be organized, and several tasks may occur together or sequentially. The salad ingredients and vegetables are washed together, and a sequence of peeling and chopping vegetables and salad ingredients must occur to complete the activity. Prerequisite components to be examined are initiation of activity, time management, termination of activity, coping skills, and self-control.
- Simple, complex and multiple activities may be carried out independently or within a group setting. When they occur independently, prerequisite

components to be examined are initiation of activity, time management, termination of activity, coping skills, and self-control. When tasks occur in a group, examine social conduct and interpersonal skills as well.

INITIATION OF ACTIVITY

Initiation of activity refers to starting a physical or mental activity.

- Does the activity require the person to self-start?
- Does the person have to plan the start (e.g., alarm clock)?
- Is the activity motivated by personal meaning and relevance?
- How would the person's mental health status affect the performance of this activity?

TIME MANAGEMENT

Time management involves anticipating, planning, and using parcels of time as they relate to completion of activities.

- Is the activity performed in one session or multiple sessions?
- Are there set time restraints for portions of the activity (e.g., bake at 350°F for 30 minutes)?
- Is the activity part of a personal routine that has self-imposed time restrictions (e.g., morning care consisting of 10 minutes for shower, 10 minutes for dressing, and 10 minutes for grooming)?
- Does the activity allow for choices about the use of time (e.g., a craft project in which the detailing could require additional time because of increased interest or skill level)?
- Does the activity require organization and setting realistic priorities to complete it?

TERMINATION OF ACTIVITY

Termination of activity refers to stopping an activity at an appropriate time.

- What is the person's control over engaging in and disengaging from the activity?
- Is the activity time limited?
- Is the activity rote or repetitive?

COPING SKILLS

Coping skills involve identifying and managing stress and related factors.

- Is this activity new for the person, or is it part of an established personal routine?
- Are parts of the activity automatic and therefore less stressful (e.g., habitual)?
- Does the activity environment influence the perceived stress?
- Does the activity provide an appropriate level of challenge without promoting undue stress?
- Does the activity require exactness, or is there a range of acceptable performance?
- Is performance of the activity externally or internally controlled?

SELF-CONTROL

Self-control involves modifying one's own behavior in response to environmental needs, demands, constraints, personal aspirations, and feedback from others.

- Should mishaps in the activity or environment be expected?
- Does the outcome of the activity lead to attainment of goals?
- Do the activity demands require the person to modify performance in response to changes in the environment?
- Will the person be required to respond to feedback about performance (e.g., criticism or praise)?
- To what degree does the activity challenge physical, social, or cognitive ability?

SOCIAL CONDUCT

Social skills involve interacting while using manners, personal space, eye contact, gestures, active listening, and self-expression appropriate to one's environment and satisfying to oneself and others.

- In what type of social environment does the activity occur?
- Does the activity require cooperative behavior?
- What are the accepted personal boundaries of the activity (e.g., sport, card table)?
- Does the social environment present expectations concerning appropriate interaction and communication (e.g., authority figures)?
- Does the activity require the person to initiate and sustain appropriate communication?
- Does the activity require the person to initiate or answer questions or make suggestions?

INTERPERSONAL SKILLS

Interpersonal skills involve using verbal and nonverbal communication to interact in a variety of settings.

- Does the activity require independence, cooperation, or competition?
- What degree of verbal interaction or casual conversation is required?
- Does the activity require active verbal and nonverbal participation?
- Does the activity require expression of emotions?
- Does the activity require specific nonverbal behavior (e.g., appropriate sitting posture, signs of active listening, changes in facial expression, use of appropriate gestures)?
- Does the activity require the person to assume an unfamiliar interaction style?
- Does the activity require the person to recognize and respond to others' nonverbal behavior?

MOBILITY

Mobility involves changing body positions or location by transferring from one place to another; by carrying, moving, or manipulating objects; by walking, running, or climbing; and by using various forms of transportation. Changing and maintaining body position may occur during performance of the activity. Prerequisite performance components to be examined are postural alignment, muscle tone, postural control, depth perception, and body strength. Answering the following questions guides practitioners to the next step of the analysis:

- Does the activity require changes in body positions?
- When completing specific tasks, must one get into or out of a particular body position?
- Does the activity require moving from one location to another, such as getting up from a chair to lie down on a bed and getting into and out of kneeling or squatting positions?
- Does the activity require the person to transfer from one surface to another?
- What degree of control does the person need to move from one surface to another?

POSTURAL ALIGNMENT

Postural alignment refers to maintaining the biomechanical integrity among body parts.

- What degree of axial alignment does the activity require?
- Does the pelvic position change during performance of the activity (e.g., taking off shoes)?
- Does the activity require frequent changes in alignment (e.g., reading while seated, playing racquetball)?
- What postures are needed to optimally perform the activity?

POSTURAL CONTROL

Postural control involves using righting and equilibrium reactions to maintain balance during functional movements.

- Does the activity have the potential for a sudden displacement of the center of gravity?
- Do changes in the base of support occur while engaging in the activity?
- Does head position change frequently?
- Must the person stabilize against the forces of gravity when engaged in the activity (e.g., lean forward, lean back, lean to the side)?
- Does the activity require the person to anticipate postural adjustments?

DEPTH PERCEPTION

Depth perception involves determining the relative distance between objects, figures, or landmarks and the observer and changes in planes and surfaces.

- Does the person have to reach distances to acquire objects or complete the activity?
- Does the person need to place body parts in relation to changing elements of the environment (e.g., step up or down)?

BODY STRENGTH

Body strength refers to the degree of muscle strength required to complete the activity.

- How does gravity influence the performance of the activity?
- Does the activity provide resistance to movement of the body?
- Does the activity require concentric, eccentric, or isometric muscle contraction?

CARRYING, MOVING, AND HANDLING OBJECTS

Completing many activities requires that a person be able to handle, move, and manipulate objects with his or her upper extremities and hands. Movements may be gross or fine or a combination of both. Sometimes, the actions demand intricate, coordinated finger movements. Other actions require lower-extremity strength and control. Answering the following questions guides practitioners to the next step of the analysis:

- Are any of the following upper-extremity movements done while performing the activity: pulling, pushing, reaching, throwing, or catching?

Prerequisite components to be examined are range of motion, strength, and endurance.

- Must the person move and manipulate objects with his or her upper extremities? Prerequisite skills for upper-extremity control are range of motion, strength, endurance, stereognosis, kinesthesia, and figure–ground perception.
- Must the person carry or transport objects while walking? Prerequisite skills are range of motion, postural control, strength, endurance, and topographical orientation.

RANGE OF MOTION

Range of motion refers to actively moving body parts through an arc of motion.

- What movements are required of the head, neck, and trunk during the activity?
- What degree of range of motion is required of the extremities during the activity (most critical to performance)?
- Which joints are positioned statically, and which joints are active?
- Does the activity require the person to control movements at multiple joints?
- Where are rotational movements required?
- Are there any soft-tissue conditions that would affect range of motion (e.g., hyper- or hypomobility)?

EXTREMITY STRENGTH

Extremity strength refers to the grade of muscle strength required in the extremities to complete the activity.

- How does gravity influence the performance of the activity?
- Does the activity require concentric, eccentric, or isometric muscle contraction?

ENDURANCE

Endurance involves sustained cardiac, pulmonary, and musculoskeletal exertion over time.

- What is the duration of the activity (time)?
- How repetitive is the activity?
- Are portions of the activity resistive?
- Does fatigue occur as a result of the activity?

STEREOGNOSIS

Sterognosis involves identifying objects through proprioception, cognition, and the sense of touch.

- Does the activity require the hands or feet to identify or manipulate objects without reliance on vision (e.g., reaching into a pocket to find a coin, reaching into a drawer)?
- Do aspects of the activity require visual vigilance that may require the person to find, manipulate, or reach for objects outside the visual field (e.g., sewing on a machine, use of machinery)?

KINESTHESIA

Kinesthesia involves identifying the excursion and direction of movement.

- Does the activity require movements to be coordinated over multiple joints?
- Does the activity require visual attention so that the person must rely on the ability to move without the aid of vision (e.g., swinging a bat at a baseball, playing tennis, playing basketball)?
- Does the activity require the person to change directions of movements (e.g., fingers during typing)?

GRASP PATTERNS

The practitioner assesses the types of grasp patterns required to perform the activity.

- What specific grasp patterns are used to complete the activity?
- Does the person demonstrate age-appropriate grasp patterns?

PREHENSION PATTERNS

The practitioner assesses the types of prehension (pinch) required to perform the activity.

- What specific pinch patterns are required to complete the activity?
- Does the person demonstrate an age-appropriate pinch pattern?

FINE MOTOR

Fine motor refers to the ability to use small hand muscles and joints to perform refined actions.

- What kind of fine motor actions does the activity require?
- Does the activity require in-hand manipulation of small objects or small tool use?
- Does the activity require small, joint-isolated movements?

Figure–ground perception involves differentiating between foreground and background forms and objects.

- Does the activity require the person to distinguish an object or image from a complex background (e.g., word-search games, finding hidden objects)?
- Does the activity require the person to discriminate among two-dimensional or three-dimensional figures to complete tasks?
- Does the activity require the person to locate objects from a cluster of objects (e.g., food in a refrigerator, clothes in a closet, an object in a junk drawer)?

TOPOGRAPHICAL ORIENTATION

Topographical orientation refers to determining the location of objects and settings and the route to the location.

- Does the activity require the person to follow a familiar route or negotiate unfamiliar surroundings?
- Does the activity require the person to retrace routes from spatial memory?
- Does the activity rely on the person's ability to identify visual landmarks?

EXERCISE 4.1: EXAMPLE OF ACTIVITY ANALYSIS

Review Appendix 4.B. How does the activity analysis document the activity of getting on a bus and finding a seat? How would an occupational therapist use this information?

EXERCISE 4.2: ANALYSIS OF A DAILY LIFE ACTIVITY

Consider the activity of frying an egg for breakfast or folding clothes. Think about the way in which you normally do the activity. Follow the process outlined in this section. The purpose of this assignment is to appreciate that everything you do is potentially a therapeutic activity. Through the analysis you learn the component pieces outside the context of the real world of activities. In practice, occupational therapists and occupational therapy assistants perform activity analysis with consideration of the client's real activities, the context in which they are performed, and the meanings that the activities have for the client.

Activity Analysis Within the Context of a Frame of Reference

Activity analysis is a tool that occupational therapists use to determine an activity's therapeutic potential. As such, activity analyses provide the means for understanding the client and his or her ability to perform specific purposeful activities. Up to this point, activity analysis has been described as a process to examine or analyze specific activities. When activity analyses, however, are used within the context of a frame of reference, a guideline for practice, or a conceptual framework, the framework provides the guidelines for the activity analysis. For example, if the occupational therapist is going to treat a client with left hemiparesis, the client will most likely have intact language skills. After screening the client, the therapist determines that the client's standing balance, postural control, and sitting balance are fair and that he has problems with upper-extremity motor control. On the basis of this information, the therapist determines that the neurodevelopmental treatment approach is most appropriate to restore performance skills. Given that the client wants to dress himself, the therapist evaluates the client's performance of upper-body dressing, which is best done by having the client attempt to dress. The therapist then does an activity analysis of the way the client performs the activity, with special attention given to the client's neuromotor functioning.

Before observing the client's attempting various activities, the therapist does an activity analysis of the typical performance of the various purposeful activities involved in upper-body dressing, which involves knowing the skills necessary for upper-body dressing. For example, putting on a button-down shirt presents different challenges than putting on a pullover shirt. In the case of the client with left hemiparesis for whom the neurodevelopmental treatment approach has been selected to guide intervention, the therapist attends to the motor and sensory demands of the trunk and upper extremities during dressing. The therapist uses the frame of reference to guide the focus needed as the client attempts to complete the activity.

Summary

The ability to analyze an activity competently is a critical piece of an occupational therapist's repertoire. Without the ability to analyze activities, the therapist is left to use trial and error to plan and carry out interventions with clients. In this chapter, we described the development of activity analysis over the years. No doubt there will be further developments as the profession evolves. The ability, however, to analyze an activity in the context of the person and his or her life enables both the client and the therapist to reach agreement on goals for the client.

This chapter includes a comprehensive outline to approach activity analysis for the occupational therapy student and practitioner. Although the activity analysis may seem tedious and difficult to the beginning student, it is a process that gradually becomes integrated into clinical reasoning as therapists consider activities as therapeutic interventions. Experienced clinicians integrate activity analysis into the evaluation and treatment process so smoothly that it may not be obvious to the novice therapist.

Acknowledgment

We thank Alison S. Robinson, a graduate student at New York University, class of 2011, for providing the activity analysis of her personal experience of getting on a bus and finding a seat.

References

Allen, C. A. (1987). Activity: Occupational therapy's treatment method [Eleanor Clark Slagle Lecture]. *American Journal of Occupational Therapy, 41,* 563–575.

American Occupational Therapy Association. (1994). Uniform terminology for occupational therapy—Third edition. *American Journal of Occupational Therapy, 48,* 1047–1054.

American Occupational Therapy Association. (2008). Occupational therapy practice framework: Domain and process (2nd edition). *American Journal of Occupational Therapy, 62,* 625–683.

Ayres, A. J. (1983). *Sensory integration and the child.* Los Angeles: Western Psychological Services.

Creighton, C. (1992). The origin and evolution of activity analysis. *American Journal of Occupational Therapy, 46,* 45–48.

Crepeau, E. B. (2003). Analyzing occupation and activity: A way of thinking about occupational performance. In E. B. Crepeau, E. S. Cohen, & B. A. Boyt Schell (Eds.), *Willard and Spackman's occupational therapy* (11th ed., pp. 189–198). Philadelphia: Lippincott Williams & Wilkins.

Cynkin, S., & Robinson, A. M. (1990). *Occupational therapy and activities health: Toward health through activity.* Boston: Little, Brown.

Dunton, W. R., & Licht, S. (1957). *Occupational therapy principles and practice.* Springfield, IL: Charles C Thomas.

Fidler, G. S. (1948). Psychological evaluation of occupational therapy activities. *American Journal of Occupational Therapy, 2,* 284–287.

Hinojosa, J. (1996). Practice makes perfect. *OT Practice, 1*(1), 34–38.

Hopkins, H. L., & Smith, H. D. (1978). *Willard and Spackman's occupational therapy* (5th ed.). Philadelphia: Lippincott.

Kremer, A. R., Nelson, D., & Duncombe, L. W. (1984). Effects of selected activities on affective meaning in psychiatric patients. *American Journal of Occupational Therapy, 38,* 522–528.

Licht, S. (1947). Kinetic analysis of crafts and occupations. *Occupational Therapy and Rehabilitation, 26,* 75–78.

Llorens, L. (1973). Activity analysis for cognitive perceptual motor dysfunction. *American Journal of Occupational Therapy, 27,* 453–456.

Llorens, L. (1986). Activity analysis: Agreement among factors in a sensory processing model. *American Journal of Occupational Therapy, 40,* 103–110.

Mosey, A. C. (1986). *Psychosocial components of occupational therapy*. New York: Raven.

Neistadt, M. E., McAuley, D., Zecha, D., & Shannon, R. (1993). An analysis of a board game as a treatment activity. *American Journal of Occupational Therapy, 47,* 154–160.

Nelson, D. (1996). Therapeutic occupation: A definition. *American Journal of Occupational Therapy, 50,* 775–782.

Pedretti, L. W., & Wade, I. (1996). Therapeutic modalities. In L. W. Pedretti (Ed.), *Occupational therapy practice skills for physical dysfunction* (pp. 293–317). St. Louis, MO: Mosby.

Reed, K. L. (1986). Tools of practice: Heritage or baggage. *American Journal of Occupational Therapy, 40,* 597–605.

Trombly, C. A., & Scott, A. D. (1977). *Occupational therapy for physical dysfunction*. Baltimore: Williams & Wilkins.

U.S. Department of War. (1944). *Occupational therapy*. Washington, DC: U.S. Government Printing Office.

World Health Organization. (2001). *International classification of functioning, disability and health, short version*. Geneva, Switzerland: Author.

Appendix 4.A

Activity Analysis Form

Part 1: Introduction

Description of the activity:

Sequence (steps) of activity:

1.
2.
3.
etc.

Timing needed to complete or perform individual steps:

Objects, materials, and their properties:

Physical environment (space demands):

Safety precautions and contraindications:

Social environment:

Personal contextual and client factors:

- Personal (age, gender, socioeconomic, education)
- Client factors (values, beliefs, spirituality)

Note. This form was created by the authors and Jim Hinojosa.

Consider the relevance and meaningfulness of the activity that influence performance:

• Current

• Past

• Future

Cultural, temporal, and virtual conditions within and around the client that influence performance:

• Cultural

• Temporal (time):

• Virtual

Part 2: Activity Analysis Outline

REQUIRED ACTIONS AND PERFORMANCE SKILLS

LEARNING AND APPLYING KNOWLEDGE (SENSORY–PERCEPTUAL SKILLS)

ACTIVITY REQUIRES	YES	NO	FOCUS ON
Watching			Visual reception, sensory processing
Listening			Auditory, sensory processing
Other purposeful sensing			Tactile, proprioceptive, vestibular, olfactory, gustatory, sensory processing

Sensory processing—Internal mechanism used by the person to process and respond to sensory input	
Level of Influence ☐ 0 ☐ 1. ☐ 2. ☐ 3. ☐ 4.	Observations:

Note. Refer to the "Levels of Influence" definitions on page 82 of this text.

Visual reception—Interpreting stimuli through the eyes, including peripheral vision, acuity, and awareness of color and pattern

Level of Influence	Observations:
☐ 0	
☐ 1.	
☐ 2.	
☐ 3.	
☐ 4.	

Auditory—Interpreting and localizing sounds and discriminating among background sounds

Level of Influence	Observations:
☐ 0	
☐ 1.	
☐ 2.	
☐ 3.	
☐ 4.	

Tactile—Interpreting light touch, pressure, temperature, pain, and vibration through skin contact or receptor

Level of Influence	Observations:
☐ 0	
☐ 1.	
☐ 2.	
☐ 3.	
☐ 4.	

Proprioceptive—Interpreting stimuli originating in muscles, joints, and other internal tissues that give information about the position of one body part in relation to another

Level of Influence	Observations:
☐ 0	
☐ 1.	
☐ 2.	
☐ 3.	
☐ 4.	

Vestibular input—Interpreting stimuli from the inner ear receptor regarding head position	
Level of Influence ☐ 0 ☐ 1. ☐ 2. ☐ 3. ☐ 4.	Observations:

Olfactory—Interpreting odors	
Level of Influence ☐ 0 ☐ 1. ☐ 2. ☐ 3. ☐ 4.	Observations:

Gustatory—Interpreting tastes	
Level of Influence ☐ 0 ☐ 1. ☐ 2. ☐ 3. ☐ 4.	Observations:

BASIC LEARNING

ACTIVITY REQUIRES	YES	NO	FOCUS ON
Copying			Recognition, form constancy, spatial relations, position in space
Rehearsing			Sequencing

Recognition—Ability to identify familiar faces, objects, and other previously presented material	
Level of Influence ☐ 0 ☐ 1. ☐ 2. ☐ 3. ☐ 4.	Observations:

Form constancy—Recognizing forms and objects as the same in various environments, positions, and sizes

Level of Influence	Observations:
☐ 0	
☐ 1.	
☐ 2.	
☐ 3.	
☐ 4.	

Spatial relations—Determining the position of objects relative to each other

Level of Influence	Observations:
☐ 0	
☐ 1.	
☐ 2.	
☐ 3.	
☐ 4.	

Position in space—Determining the spatial relationship of figures and objects to self and other forms and objects

Level of Influence	Observations:
☐ 0	
☐ 1.	
☐ 2.	
☐ 3.	
☐ 4.	

Sequencing—Placing information, concepts, and actions in order

Level of Influence	Observations:
☐ 0	
☐ 1.	
☐ 2.	
☐ 3.	
☐ 4.	

ACQUIRING SKILLS

ACTIVITY REQUIRES	YES	NO	FOCUS ON
Basic skills			Motor control, praxis, body scheme, fine motor, crossing midline, right–left discrimination, laterality, bilateral integration, visual–motor integration
Complex skills			

Applying knowledge			Level of arousal, orientation, attention span
Thinking			Memory, categorization, spatial orientation, generalization, concept formation
Solving problems—simple			Learning, memory
Solving problems—complex			
Making decisions			Memory, concept formation, categorization, generalization

Level of arousal—Demonstrating alertness and responsiveness to environmental stimuli

Level of Influence	Observations:
☐ 0	
☐ 1.	
☐ 2.	
☐ 3.	
☐ 4.	

Orientation—The ability to identify person, place, time, and situation

Level of Influence	Observations:
☐ 0	
☐ 1.	
☐ 2.	
☐ 3.	
☐ 4.	

Sensory modulation—The ability to generate responses that are appropriately graded in relation to incoming sensory stimuli

Level of Influence	Observations:
☐ 0	
☐ 1.	
☐ 2.	
☐ 3.	
☐ 4.	

Attention span—Focusing on a task over time

Level of Influence	Observations:
☐ 0	
☐ 1.	
☐ 2.	
☐ 3.	
☐ 4.	

Motor control—The use of functional and versatile movement patterns

Level of Influence	Observations:
☐ 0	
☐ 1.	
☐ 2.	
☐ 3.	
☐ 4.	

Praxis—Conceiving and planning a new motor act in response to an environmental demand

Level of Influence	Observations:
☐ 0	
☐ 1.	
☐ 2.	
☐ 3.	
☐ 4.	

Body scheme—An internal awareness of the body and the relationship of body parts to each other

Level of Influence	Observations:
☐ 0	
☐ 1.	
☐ 2.	
☐ 3.	
☐ 4.	

Ocular motor—Ability to move eyes to focus and follow objects

Level of Influence	Observations:
☐ 0	
☐ 1.	
☐ 2.	
☐ 3.	
☐ 4.	

Oral motor—Use of muscles in and around the mouth

Level of Influence	Observations:
☐ 0	
☐ 1.	
☐ 2.	
☐ 3.	
☐ 4.	

Fine motor coordination and dexterity—Using small muscle groups for controlled movements, particularly in-hand object manipulation

Level of Influence	Observations:
☐ 0	
☐ 1.	
☐ 2.	
☐ 3.	
☐ 4.	

Visual–motor integration—Coordinating the interaction of information from the eyes and body movement

Level of Influence	Observations:
☐ 0	
☐ 1.	
☐ 2.	
☐ 3.	
☐ 4.	

Crossing the midline—Moving the limbs and eyes across midline sagittal plane of the body

Level of Influence	Observations:
☐ 0	
☐ 1.	
☐ 2.	
☐ 3.	
☐ 4.	

Right–left discrimination—Differentiating one side from the other

Level of Influence	Observations:
☐ 0	
☐ 1.	
☐ 2.	
☐ 3.	
☐ 4.	

Laterality—The use of a preferred or dominant hand or foot

Level of Influence	Observations:
☐ 0	
☐ 1.	
☐ 2.	
☐ 3.	
☐ 4.	

Bilateral integration—Coordinating both sides of the body

Level of Influence	Observations:
☐ 0	
☐ 1.	
☐ 2.	
☐ 3.	
☐ 4.	

Memory—Recoding information after a brief or long period of time

Level of Influence	Observations:
☐ 0	
☐ 1.	
☐ 2.	
☐ 3.	
☐ 4.	

Categorization—Identifying similarities and differences among pieces of environmental information

Level of Influence	Observations:
☐ 0	
☐ 1.	
☐ 2.	
☐ 3.	
☐ 4.	

Concept formation—Involves organizing a variety of information to form thoughts and ideas

Level of Influence	Observations:
☐ 0	
☐ 1.	
☐ 2.	
☐ 3.	
☐ 4.	

Spatial operations—Mentally manipulating the position of objects in various relationships

Level of Influence	Observations:
☐ 0	
☐ 1.	
☐ 2.	
☐ 3.	
☐ 4.	

Learning—Acquiring new concepts and behaviors	
Level of Influence ☐ 0 ☐ 1. ☐ 2. ☐ 3. ☐ 4.	Observations:

Generalization—Applying previously learned concepts and behaviors to a variety of new situations	
Level of Influence ☐ 0 ☐ 1. ☐ 2. ☐ 3. ☐ 4.	Observations:

GENERAL ACTIVITY DEMANDS

ACTIVITY REQUIRES	YES	NO	FOCUS ON
Simple task			Initiation of activity, time management, termination of activity, coping skills, self-control
Complex task			
Multiple tasks			
Independent performance			
Group performance			Social conduct, interpersonal skills

Initiation of activity—Starting a physical or mental activity	
Level of Influence ☐ 0 ☐ 1. ☐ 2. ☐ 3. ☐ 4.	Observations:

Time management—The person's ability to manage parcels of time as they relate to the performance of tasks or activities	
Level of Influence ☐ 0 ☐ 1. ☐ 2. ☐ 3. ☐ 4.	Observations:

Termination of activity—Stopping an activity at an appropriate time

Level of Influence	Observations:
☐ 0	
☐ 1.	
☐ 2.	
☐ 3.	
☐ 4.	

Coping skills—Identifying and managing stress-related factors such as anger, disappointment, or frustration

Level of Influence	Observations:
☐ 0	
☐ 1.	
☐ 2.	
☐ 3.	
☐ 4.	

Self-control—Modifying one's own behavior in response to environmental needs, demands, constraints, personal aspirations, and feedback from others

Level of Influence	Observations:
☐ 0	
☐ 1.	
☐ 2.	
☐ 3.	
☐ 4.	

Social conduct—Involves interacting by using manners, personal space, eye contact, gestures, active listening, and self-expression appropriate to the situation

Level of Influence	Observations:
☐ 0	
☐ 1.	
☐ 2.	
☐ 3.	
☐ 4.	

Interpersonal skills—Involves using verbal and nonverbal communication skills appropriately

Level of Influence	Observations:
☐ 0	
☐ 1.	
☐ 2.	
☐ 3.	
☐ 4.	

MOBILITY

Postural alignment—Maintaining biomechanical integrity among body parts	
Level of Influence ☐ 0 ☐ 1. ☐ 2. ☐ 3. ☐ 4.	Observations:

Postural control—Using righting and equilibrium reactions to maintain balance during functional movements	
Level of Influence ☐ 0 ☐ 1. ☐ 2. ☐ 3. ☐ 4.	Observations:

Depth perception—Involves determining the relative distance between objects, figures, or landmarks and the observer and changes in planes and surfaces	
Level of Influence ☐ 0 ☐ 1. ☐ 2. ☐ 3. ☐ 4.	Observations:

Body strength—Degree of gross muscle power when body movement is resisted or is against gravity	
Level of Influence ☐ 0 ☐ 1. ☐ 2. ☐ 3. ☐ 4.	Observations:

CARRYING, MOVING, AND HANDLING OBJECTS

Range of motion—Moving body parts through an arc of motion	
Level of Influence ☐ 0 ☐ 1. ☐ 2. ☐ 3. ☐ 4.	Observations:

Extremity strength—Grade of muscle strength when body movement is resisted or is against gravity

Level of Influence	Observations:
☐ 0	
☐ 1.	
☐ 2.	
☐ 3.	
☐ 4.	

Endurance—Sustained cardiac, pulmonary, and musculoskeletal exertion over time

Level of Influence	Observations:
☐ 0	
☐ 1.	
☐ 2.	
☐ 3.	
☐ 4.	

Stereognosis—Identifying objects through proprioception, cognition, and sense of touch

Level of Influence	Observations:
☐ 0	
☐ 1.	
☐ 2.	
☐ 3.	
☐ 4.	

Kinesthesia—Identifying the excursion and direction of movement

Level of Influence	Observations:
☐ 0	
☐ 1.	
☐ 2.	
☐ 3.	
☐ 4.	

Grasp patterns—Identifying the type(s) of grasp required to perform the activity

Level of Influence	Observations:
☐ 0	
☐ 1.	
☐ 2.	
☐ 3.	
☐ 4.	

Prehension patterns—Identifying the type(s) of pinch required to perform this activity	
Level of Influence ☐ 0 ☐ 1. ☐ 2. ☐ 3. ☐ 4.	Observations:

Fine motor—Ability to use small hand muscles and joints to perform refined actions	
Level of Influence ☐ 0 ☐ 1. ☐ 2. ☐ 3. ☐ 4.	Observations:

Figure–ground perception—Differentiating between foreground and background forms and objects	
Level of Influence ☐ 0 ☐ 1. ☐ 2. ☐ 3. ☐ 4.	Observations:

Topographical orientation—Determining the location of objects and settings and the route to the location	
Level of Influence ☐ 0 ☐ 1. ☐ 2. ☐ 3. ☐ 4.	Observations:

Part 3: Summary

Once you have completed the activity analyses, consider the following:

1. Is the activity part of the client's habits, routines, or rituals?
   - Habits
   - Routines
   - Rituals

2. How does this activity relate to the client's roles?
   - Past
   - Present
   - Future

3. Does the activity facilitate self-expression or enhance self-concept?

Appendix 4.B

Activity Analysis Example

Part 1: Introduction

DESCRIPTION OF THE ACTIVITY

My activity is getting on a bus and taking a seat. This activity has both functional and personal relevance for me. Completing this analysis allowed me to explore the various roles that getting on a bus and taking a seat play in my life, while stirring my curiosity about the process.

SEQUENCE (STEPS) OF THE ACTIVITY

1. At the bus stop, I check the posted schedule for the time of the next-arriving bus and the map to verify my intended route. *(10 seconds)*
2. I stand next to the bus stop and wait for the bus to arrive. *(0–10 minutes)*
3. As the bus approaches, I raise my arm to signal the driver to stop. *(5 seconds)*
4. When the bus pulls up, I walk toward the bus and join the line of people waiting to board it. *(5 seconds)*
5. At this time, I locate my metrocard from within my pants or jacket pocket. *(5 seconds)*
6. I wait my turn to board the bus and eventually take a large step up onto the platform. *(5 seconds–2 minutes)*
7. I locate the metrocard machine, place my card into the narrow slot of the reader, wait for the machine to beep and return my card, and remove my card from the reader. *(4 seconds)*
8. Next, I turn counterclockwise to face the interior of the bus. *(4 seconds)*
9. I scan the bus to ascertain whether any seats are available. *(5 seconds)*
10. If no seat is immediately available, I hold onto the closest handrail and stabilize myself as I wait. *(0–5 minutes)*
11. Once a seat becomes available, I navigate through the bus toward the seat, grabbing onto handrails as I proceed. *(30 seconds)*

Note. This example of activity analysis was written by Alison S. Robinson, graduate student at New York University, class of 2011. Used with permission.

12. Holding onto the back of the seat with my same-side arm and the hand-rail with my opposite-side arm, I place my inside foot in front of the seat. *(3 seconds)*
13. Using my arms as support and shifting my pelvis first horizontally, I lower myself down into the seat. *(3 seconds)*
14. With my pelvis resting on the seat and my feet flat on the floor in front of me, I release my grip on the seat and rails and relax into my seat. *(3 seconds)*

TIMING NEEDED TO COMPLETE OR PERFORM INDIVIDUAL STEPS

One minute, 22 seconds, is the minimum amount of time it takes me to board the bus and to sit down. Additional time is added for any waiting that occurs throughout the activity, including waiting for the bus to arrive, waiting in line to board, and waiting for a seat.

OBJECTS, MATERIALS, AND THEIR PROPERTIES

The only object I use for this activity is a metrocard, which is a thin, flat, plastic-based card. Its size is approximately 2.5 inches × 1.5 inches. A metrocard also represents a previously selected amount of money. I purchased my card for $81.00, and it is worth an unlimited number of rides for 1 month on the bus, the subway, and other participating New York City transit systems.

PHYSICAL ENVIRONMENT (SPACE DEMANDS)

Getting on a bus and taking a seat requires that I live in an urban area with a bus system or in a rural town with a bus station. Taking a seat on the bus demands that there be a seat available to me and that the space is large enough to accommodate me.

SAFETY PRECAUTIONS AND CONTRAINDICATIONS

While I wait to board the bus, I maintain a safe distance from the curb to avoid oncoming traffic. At this time, I also avoid breathing in any exhaust fumes emitted from the back of the bus. Additionally, adverse weather creates unsafe conditions for this activity. Both rain and snow contribute to a slippery surface on the bus platform and also down the center aisle.

SOCIAL ENVIRONMENT

My social environment includes a close relationship with my family. My brother and sister-in-law live nearby, and I visit with them at least once a week. I also spend time daily with a lively group of coworkers and take some time each week to see my friends. My social sphere recently expanded to include numerous classmates and about 30 members of a neighborhood senior center where I volunteer.

PERSONAL CONTEXTUAL AND CLIENT FACTORS

PERSONAL (AGE, GENDER, SOCIOECONOMIC, EDUCATION)

I am a 29-year-old woman currently enrolled in a full-time master's-level program in occupational therapy. In my spare time, I make a modest income working as a licensed massage therapist at a local West Village, NY, chiropractor's office.

CLIENT FACTORS (VALUES, BELIEFS, SPIRITUALITY)

I value the bus and receive enjoyment from this activity. I do not, though, see it as a necessity. The New York City subway system is extensive, and it allows me to easily reach most of my destinations. I am also an avid biker and could use this mode of transportation to travel locally. Although taking the bus is not absolutely necessary in my daily life, it does have personal value for me. I find it to be at times both stimulating and calming. I enjoy discovering new routes and the calming effect of passing by familiar scenery. Riding the bus also reflects my desire to feel tied to my community. If I could no longer ride the bus, it would be important for me to find this connection in a different way, perhaps by spending more time in nearby Prospect Park.

CONSIDER THE RELEVANCE AND MEANINGFULNESS OF THE ACTIVITY THAT INFLUENCE PERFORMANCE

This activity is of daily relevance in my life. Most often, I view taking the bus as a functional activity that serves the purpose of transporting me to and from locations not easily accessible by the subway. I also, however, enjoy the sense of community I gain from riding the bus. In terms of taking a seat, I am familiar with the need to sit, especially when I am returning home from the supermarket with heavy groceries or after a long day of school followed by work. Conversely, I am not aggressive about taking a seat if none are readily available to me.

As an adult, I started using a bus system when I was living in Paris, France. At that time, I discovered that riding the bus enabled me to enjoy the scenery and to connect the location of neighborhoods in my mind. Eventually, I gained a good topographical understanding of the city.

In the future, I plan to continue to use the bus for traveling. I hope to work in the Brooklyn school system, which would allow me to use the bus as my primary mode of transportation. I enjoy the sense of community I feel when taking the bus and see this activity as a way to better connect with my future work population. I expect that taking a seat will increase in importance for me as I age. In the future, I may become injured or ill and require a seat.

CULTURAL, TEMPORAL, AND VIRTUAL CONDITIONS WITHIN AND AROUND THE CLIENT THAT INFLUENCE PERFORMANCE

CULTURAL

Culture affects the way I ride the bus in a couple of ways. In New York City's busy work environment, I almost always ride the bus alone. My friends and family all have very different schedules and destinations from my own, and our lives rarely intersect in this way. When I was growing up, my parents emphasized the importance of self-sacrifice and of respecting older adults. As a result, I feel bound to give up my seat if someone on the bus needs it more than I do.

TEMPORAL (TIME)

Temporal conditions greatly affect my involvement in this activity. First, I take the bus only if my personal schedule and the bus schedule match. Then, if it is around 3:00 p.m. or rush hour, I will not take the bus because of the lack of comfortable space to either stand or take a seat.

VIRTUAL

Virtual conditions do not affect my decision to take the bus.

Part 2: Activity Analysis Outline

REQUIRED ACTIONS AND PERFORMANCE SKILLS

LEARNING AND APPLYING KNOWLEDGE (SENSORY–PERCEPTUAL SKILLS)

ACTIVITY REQUIRES	YES	NO	FOCUS ON
Watching	X		Visual reception, sensory processing
Listening	X		Auditory, sensory processing
Other purposeful sensing	X		Tactile, proprioceptive, vestibular, olfactory, gustatory, sensory processing

Sensory processing—Internal mechanism used by the person to process and respond to sensory input	
Level of Influence	Observations:
☐ 0	—I am alerted to the bus approaching by the integration
☐ 1.	of several cues such as the sight of the bus, the sound of its
☐ 2.	engine slowing down, and the vibrations on the pavement.
☐ 3.	—The bus will start, stop, and swerve in many directions as
X 4.	I am making my way to my seat. I must be able to integrate
	vestibular, proprioceptive, tactile, and visual systems to stay
	upright and walking.
	—I also integrate each of these systems to successfully take
	a seat.
	—In this noisy and visually stimulating environment, I
	must modulate the incoming stimuli to select the sights and
	sounds that are needed for my task.

Visual reception—Interpreting stimuli through the eyes, including peripheral vision, acuity, and awareness of color and pattern	
Level of Influence	Observations:
☐ 0	—As the bus approaches, I am aware of the colors and
☐ 1.	patterns that indicate that this is a city bus, that it is in
☐ 2.	service, and that my route number is displayed.
X 3.	—This activity requires me to visually track the bus as it
☐ 4.	arrives up until it stops to know where to board it.
	—I use scanning to look around the bus for an empty seat.
	—Peripheral vision aids me in navigating my way around
	people, packages, baby carriages, and handrails as I make
	my way to a seat.
	—My focus shifts from near to far as I look for a seat in the
	front and back of the bus.
	—Acuity aids me in locating both the metrocard reader and
	the small slot into which I place my metrocard.

Auditory—Interpreting and localizing sounds and discriminating among background sounds	
Level of Influence	Observations:
☐ 0	—I recognize the familiar sound of the bus approaching
X 1.	without even looking up.
☐ 2.	—The metrocard reader makes a sound to alert me as to
☐ 3.	whether my card has been accepted.
☐ 4.	—This is at times a noisy environment, and sometimes this
	is irritating to me.

Tactile—Interpreting light touch, pressure, temperature, pain, and vibration through skin contact or receptor	
Level of Influence	Observations:
☐ 0	—I rely on tactile input to locate my metrocard.
☐ 1.	—I use light touch when manipulating my metrocard into
☐ 2.	the metrocard reader.
X 3.	—When the bus is crowded, I often cannot see my hands
☐ 4.	and feet. I must rely on tactile input to grab onto a handrail as opposed to someone's arm and to step onto a flat surface rather than someone's bag.
	—As the bus starts to move, I must remain in control despite the ensuing vibrations.

Proprioceptive—Interpreting stimuli originating in muscles, joints, and other internal tissues that give information about the position of one body part in relation to another	
Level of Influence	Observations:
☐ 0	—I am weight bearing on my lower extremities up until I
☐ 1.	take my seat.
☐ 2.	—My arms are at times outside of my visual field.
☐ 3.	—The joints of my upper extremities are elongating and
X 4.	shortening as I hold onto the handrails and the bus swings me back and forth. Often, I am pulling myself along to oppose the forward motion of the bus as it starts up.
	—I weight bear on my upper extremity as I lower myself into my seat.

Vestibular input—Interpreting stimuli from the inner ear receptor regarding head position	
Level of Influence	Observations:
☐ 0	—Walking down the aisle of the bus requires considerable
☐ 1.	vestibular input. I must react to changes in acceleration and
☐ 2.	direction as the bus pulls away from the stop and to rocking
☐ 3.	motions as the bus moves along uneven roads.
X 4.	—Head righting and equilibrium responses assist me in maintaining an upright orientation against the moving forces of the bus.
	—My protective responses are also active in response to the bus's abrupt jerking.
	—As I sit down, I dissociate my head, arms, and trunk.

Olfactory—Interpreting odors	
Level of Influence	Observations:
☐ 0 X 1. ☐ 2. ☐ 3. ☐ 4.	—Although odor does not affect my ability to get on the bus and take a seat, it does affect my enjoyment of it. —In the summer, when people are hot, sweaty, and smelly, I will remain standing to avoid sitting next to someone with an offensive odor.

Gustatory—Interpreting tastes	
Level of Influence	Observations:
X 0 ☐ 1. ☐ 2. ☐ 3. ☐ 4.	I do not use taste as I am completing this activity.

BASIC LEARNING

ACTIVITY REQUIRES	YES	NO	FOCUS ON
Copying	X		Recognition, form constancy, spatial relations, position in space
Rehearsing	X		Sequencing

Recognition—Ability to identify familiar faces, objects, and other previously presented material	
Level of Influence	Observations:
☐ 0 ☐ 1. X 2. ☐ 3. ☐ 4.	—I recognize my bus route number on the approaching bus. —I need to identify the metrocard reader as I enter the bus to pay my fare.

Form constancy—Recognizing forms and objects as the same in various environments, positions, and sizes	
Level of Influence	Observations:
☐ 0 ☐ 1. X 2. ☐ 3. ☐ 4.	—The top of the bus rises high above the other cars on the road. I recognize it from far away by the familiar pattern of lights that is visible. —I identify an empty seat even if it is partially blocked by other passengers. —The bus route number and schedule information are printed at the bus stop. Later, I distinguish my bus from the other buses by locating this same number as it is displayed in lights on the front of the bus.

Spatial relations—Determining the position of objects relative to each other	
Level of Influence	Observations:
☐ 0	—I must judge the distance between my card and the card
☐ 1.	reader as I attempt to pay my fare.
☐ 2.	—I use spatial relations as I orient my metrocard to line up
X 3.	with the card reader.
☐ 4.	—As I walk toward my seat, I estimate the distances between people and objects. This helps me to plan the most efficient route toward my seat.

Position in space—Position in space involves determining the spatial relationship of figures and objects to self and other forms and objects.	
Level of Influence	Observations:
☐ 0	—I determine the distance between myself and the bus as I
☐ 1.	walk toward the entrance.
☐ 2.	—Position in space is very important as I estimate the
☐ 3.	distance between my feet and the step up into the bus.
X 4.	—As I walk toward my seat, I determine the spatial relationship between myself and all people and objects on the bus. This allows me to avoid bumping into people or tripping over objects.
	—I must be able to gauge the distance between myself and the seat and the position of the seat as I slowly sit down.

Sequencing—Placing information, concepts, and actions in order	
Level of Influence	Observations:
☐ 0	—There are many variations in how I step up onto the
☐ 1.	platform, which hand I use to swipe my card, what path I
X 2.	take toward my seat, and which seat I choose. The sequence
☐ 3.	of these tasks does not affect my ability to get on the bus
☐ 4.	and take a seat.
	—It is important, however, to remember to pay my fare before I walk down the aisle of the bus. Also, I must wait for a seat to be available before I go to sit down.
	—Eventually, I will need to reverse my steps to get off the bus. This is, however, outside of the scope of my activity: "get on the bus and take a seat."

ACQUIRING SKILLS

ACTIVITY REQUIRES	YES	NO	FOCUS ON
Basic skills	X		Motor control, praxis, body scheme,
Complex skills	X		fine motor, crossing midline, right–left discrimination, laterality, bilateral integration, visual–motor integration

Applying knowledge	X		Level of arousal, orientation, attention span
Thinking	X		Memory, categorization, spatial orientation, generalization, concept formation
Solving problems—simple	X		Learning, memory
Solving problems—complex	X		
Making decisions	X		Memory, concept formation, categorization, generalization

Level of arousal—Demonstrating alertness and responsiveness to environmental stimuli

Level of Influence	Observations:
☐ 0 X 1. ☐ 2. ☐ 3. ☐ 4.	—It is important that I stay aroused as I wait for the bus to arrive so that I can signal the bus to stop for me. —The act of boarding the bus and sitting down, however, requires that I be aroused for only a matter of minutes.

Orientation—The ability to identify person, place, time, and situation

Level of Influence	Observations:
☐ 0 ☐ 1. ☐ 2. ☐ 3. X 4.	—I identify personally with my activity and my orientation changes in relation to my roles of worker, family member, friend, and home maintainer. At different times, I take the bus to and from work, school, social visits, and the grocery store. —Time is also very important to this activity. The bus runs on a schedule, and I need to be aware of both the current time and when the next bus is set to arrive. —In terms of place, I choose my bus on the basis of where I am and where I need to go. —It is also important that I understand my situation. If I intend to take the bus to school, I should not instead ride the bus toward the grocery store. —Finally, if I am not oriented to my situation, I will not engage in this activity. For example, if I am somewhere unfamiliar, do not know my destination, or a bus arrives displaying an unfamiliar route, I will not get on the bus.

Sensory modulation—The ability to generate responses that are appropriately graded in relation to incoming sensory stimuli	
Level of Influence ☐ 0 ☐ 1. ☐ 2. X 3. ☐ 4.	Observations: —In this noisy and visually stimulating environment, I must modulate the incoming stimuli to select the sights and sounds that are needed for my task. —I must appropriately grade my responses to the level of proprioceptive and vestibular input to stay on my feet despite the swerving and abrupt start of the bus.

Attention span—Focusing on a task over time	
Level of Influence ☐ 0 X 1. ☐ 2. ☐ 3. ☐ 4.	Observations: —Similar to level of arousal, attention span is an important aspect of waiting for the bus. Getting on the bus and taking a seat, however, is a very brief task that does not require me to attend for a long period of time. —I do pay attention to what street the bus is traveling down to know when to exit the bus. Nonetheless, this step is outside of the scope of my assigned activity.

Motor control—The use of functional and versatile movement patterns	
Level of Influence ☐ 0 ☐ 1. ☐ 2. ☐ 3. X 4.	Observations: —All the joints of my lower extremity are active as I climb the bus step, walk down the aisle, and sit down. Many of the joints of my upper extremity are active, including those of my hands, wrists, arms, and shoulder girdle, as I signal the bus, grab onto handrails, and lower myself into my seat. —I manipulate my metrocard with my fingers and hands to orient it toward the opening in the reader while simultaneously controlling my arm and forearm. —My pace of walking to my seat is affected by external forces such as the pace of the person walking in front of me and the steadiness of the bus as it begins to move.

Praxis—Conceiving and planning a new motor act in response to an environmental demand

Level of Influence	Observations:
☐ 0	—Every bus is different. I must be able to act in response
☐ 1.	to these differences. For example, the orientation of seats
X 2.	differs from bus to bus. Also, some have long overhead
☐ 3.	poles to hold onto, and others have the older loop handles.
☐ 4.	Depending on what I find, I need to plan my route to my
	seat and maneuver myself into sitting.
	—There are numerous, potentially unfamiliar combinations
	of obstacles that I might encounter on my way to my seat.
	For example, I might simultaneously need to step over an
	object, lean my upper body to the right to avoid someone's
	backpack, and duck my head beneath yet another person's
	outstretched arm.

Body scheme—An internal awareness of the body and the relationship of body parts to each other

Level of Influence	Observations:
☐ 0	—My body scheme contributes to the gross motor activity
☐ 1.	of walking toward the bus and down its aisle.
☐ 2.	—I use multiple positions during this activity including
X 3.	standing, stepping, arm reaching, and sitting.
☐ 4.	

Ocular motor—Ability to move eyes to focus and follow objects

Level of Influence	Observations:
☐ 0	—I use a near focus to read the bus schedule.
☐ 1.	—I focus on the bus from a distance to read its route
X 2.	number as it approaches.
☐ 3.	—My focus shifts from near to far as I search for a seat in
☐ 4.	the front and back of the bus.

Oral motor—Use of muscles in and around the mouth

Level of Influence	Observations:
☐ 0	—Although I use the muscles in and around my mouth to
X 1.	speak with the bus driver and other passengers, I do not rely
☐ 2.	on oral motor abilities to complete the activity.
☐ 3.	
☐ 4.	

Fine motor coordination and dexterity—Using small muscle groups for controlled movements, particularly in-hand object manipulation	
Level of Influence	Observations:
☐ 0 ☐ 1. ☐ 2. X 3. ☐ 4.	—I use intrinsic and extrinsic hand muscles to perform in-hand manipulation to orient my metrocard with the reader. —I rely on a true synergy of wrist flexors and extensors to keep my hand steady. —I rely on a pronated forearm to manipulate my metrocard into the reader. —I shift quickly between forearm supination and pronation to reach for a variety of handrails.

Visual–motor integration—Coordinating the interaction of information from the eyes and body movement	
Level of Influence	Observations:
☐ 0 ☐ 1. ☐ 2. X 3. ☐ 4.	—I use eye–hand coordination to draw my metrocard up to the reader and insert it correctly into the small slot of the reader. —Eye–foot coordination is extremely important as I control my movements down the aisle of the bus. Navigating the small obstacle-free path down the aisle sometimes feels like I am walking on a moving balance beam.

Crossing the midline—Moving the limbs and eyes across midline sagittal plane of the body	
Level of Influence	Observations:
☐ 0 X 1. ☐ 2. ☐ 3. ☐ 4.	—I do not often move my limbs across the midline. At times I am carrying a bag and only one of my hands is free. During these instances, if I am abruptly thrown off balance, I might reach or stumble toward the contralateral side. —If my eyes were unable to cross the midline, I might be limited to choosing an empty seat on only one side of the bus or another. It is helpful for me to be able to scan across the entire bus, although it is not absolutely necessary for this task.

Right–left discrimination—Differentiating one side from the other	
Level of Influence	Observations:
☐ 0 X 1. ☐ 2. ☐ 3. ☐ 4.	—Although I use both the right and the left sides of my body, I do not need to differentiate my right from my left to board the bus and take a seat. —I am not required to use either my right or my left exclusively during any part of the activity. For example, I can choose to manipulate my card with either hand, and I can step up onto the bus with either foot. —I do check the bus route before boarding, which involves understanding directions. This only, however, mildly affects my ability to do the activity.

Laterality—The use of a preferred or dominant hand or foot	
Level of Influence	Observations:
☐ 0 X 1. ☐ 2. ☐ 3. ☐ 4.	—I am right hand dominant. —I favor my right hand to manipulate my metrocard. I frequently, however, use my hands interchangeably, especially when I am carrying packages.

Bilateral integration—Coordinating both sides of the body	
Level of Influence	Observations:
☐ 0 ☐ 1. X 2. ☐ 3. ☐ 4.	—I stabilize myself by holding onto a handrail with one hand while I manipulate my metrocard with the other. —I use a reciprocal walking pattern as I make my way to my seat. This is often altered by factors such as the distance I am traveling and the obstacles I meet on the way. —Often, my arms reach out in different directions to grab onto seats and handrails. —I hold onto the seat with one hand and a handrail with the other as I sit down.

Memory—Recoding information after a brief or long period of time	
Level of Influence	Observations:
☐ 0 ☐ 1. X 2. ☐ 3. ☐ 4.	—I use either my immediate memory or my short-term memory, depending on how long I am waiting for the bus, to recall my bus route number. —I must also remember where I am going as I select my intended route. —Procedural memory reminds me to take my metrocard out of my pocket as the bus approaches and how to pay my bus fare.

Categorization—Identifying similarities of and differences among pieces of environmental information	
Level of Influence X 0 ☐ 1. ☐ 2. ☐ 3. ☐ 4.	Observations: —I recognize different objects, including seats and handrails. I do not, however, need to group them, take them apart, or put them back together to complete this activity.

Concept formation—Involves organizing a variety of information to form thoughts and ideas	
Level of Influence X 0 ☐ 1. ☐ 2. ☐ 3. ☐ 4.	Observations: —Getting on the bus does not require me to think abstractly. —Although I need to recognize symbols such as the numbers and colors representing my chosen city bus route, I do not need to think symbolically or represent any steps symbolically to accomplish this activity.

Spatial operations—Mentally manipulating the position of objects in various relationships	
Level of Influence ☐ 0 X 1. ☐ 2. ☐ 3. ☐ 4.	Observations: —When I check the bus map, I sometimes visualize the streets that the bus will turn down to ascertain whether this is the correct route. —This helps in the act of choosing to board the bus. Spatial operations are less necessary as a tool for getting on the bus and taking a seat.

Learning—Acquiring new concepts and behaviors	
Level of Influence ☐ 0 X 1. ☐ 2. ☐ 3. ☐ 4.	Observations: —I am much better at maneuvering myself on city buses now than I was when I first moved to Brooklyn 8 years ago. This is because I have learned how to balance myself on an unsteady, moving bus. —The bus provides an unstructured, sensorimotor learning experience that requires the rider to respond to immediate feedback. This feedback often takes the form of losing balance. —Being a novice bus rider, though, never prevented me from getting on the bus.

<table>
<tr><td colspan="2">Generalization—Applying previously learned concepts and behaviors to a variety of new situations</td></tr>
<tr><td>Level of Influence
☐ 0
☐ 1.
X 2.
☐ 3.
☐ 4.</td><td>Observations:
—Each bus is slightly different. I anticipate, however, that on each bus, there will be a step up onto the platform, some kind of a fare reader, handrails of varied shapes and sizes, and a long aisle with seats along the outside.
—When boarding a new bus, I am able to generalize what I already know about boarding a bus and taking a seat to this new situation.
—I generalize my skills to other forms of mass transportation.</td></tr>
</table>

GENERAL ACTIVITY DEMANDS

ACTIVITY REQUIRES	YES	NO	FOCUS ON
Simple task		X	Initiation of activity, time management, termination of activity, coping skills, self-control
Complex task	X		
Multiple tasks	X		
Independent performance		X	
Group performance	X		Social conduct, interpersonal skills

<table>
<tr><td colspan="2">Initiation of activity—Starting a physical or mental activity</td></tr>
<tr><td>Level of Influence
☐ 0
X 1.
☐ 2.
☐ 3.
☐ 4.</td><td>Observations:
—The arrival of the bus initiates my activity.
—Taking a seat, however, requires that I be motivated to sit down. There are not always seats available, and I must be assertive about taking a seat as soon as someone gets up.
—If I were feeling anxious or depressed, I might not be assertive about taking a seat, especially if it initiates a social interaction.</td></tr>
</table>

<table>
<tr><td colspan="2">Time management—The person's ability to manage parcels of time as they relate to the performance of tasks or activities</td></tr>
<tr><td>Level of Influence
☐ 0
X 1.
☐ 2.
☐ 3.
☐ 4.</td><td>Observations:
—This activity is performed in one session and does not require me to manage separate parcels of time.
—Actually getting on the bus and taking a seat occurs within one parcel of time.
—However, this activity requires that I be on time for the bus and that I plan which bus to take to reach my intended destination on time.</td></tr>
</table>

Termination of activity—Stopping an activity at an appropriate time	
Level of Influence	Observations:
X 0	—This activity is self-limited. On sitting down, the activity
☐ 1.	ends.
☐ 2.	
☐ 3.	
☐ 4.	

Coping skills—Identifying and managing stress-related factors such as anger, disappointment, or frustration	
Level of Influence	Observations:
☐ 0	—This activity does not cause me undue stress. It is part of
X 1.	my daily repertoire.
☐ 2.	—There is the possibility of failure should the bus be late
☐ 3.	or there be no empty seats available to me. I do not mind,
☐ 4.	however, either standing or choosing an alternate form of
	transportation.
	—The activity environment can be stressful if it is crowded.

Self-control—Modifying one's own behavior in response to environmental needs, demands, constraints, personal aspiration, and feedback from others	
Level of Influence	Observations:
☐ 0	—Sometimes other passengers ask me to shift my position
☐ 1.	either to let them pass or to gain access to an inside, window
X 2.	seat.
☐ 3.	—I am disappointed when I am carrying heavy bags
☐ 4.	like groceries and there are no empty seats. I modify my
	behavior by finding an empty surface to rest my bags on.
	—I respond to the verbal and nonverbal feedback I receive
	from others regarding behaviors such as the volume of my
	speaking voice and how closely I stand to them.

Social conduct—Involves interacting by using manners, personal space, eye contact, gestures, active listening, and self-expression appropriate to the situation	
Level of Influence	Observations:
☐ 0 ☐ 1. ☐ 2. ☐ 3. X 4.	—Getting on the bus and taking a seat is largely a parallel activity. Each rider has a unique agenda that is carried out individually, while in the context of everyone else. —The activity requires cooperative behavior. People form a single-file line to board the bus and conform their walking pace to that of the people around them. —Personal boundaries must also be taken into account. Although being close is sometimes unavoidable, it is important to maintain some physical distance. —Self-expression is also limited by the environment. There is an expectation that phone conversations and listening devices will be kept quiet. —I make eye contact or lightly tap people's shoulders to get their attention. —Social conduct determines whether I take a seat. If there is someone in more need, such as an elderly person or a mother with a baby, I will forfeit my seat.

Interpersonal skills—Involve using verbal and nonverbal communication skills appropriately	
Level of Influence	Observations:
☐ 0 ☐ 1. X 2. ☐ 3. ☐ 4.	—I use nonverbal communication frequently during this activity. I gesture to the bus driver that I wish to board the bus, I nod my head hello and smile at the driver, and I communicate with the other passengers if I need to pass them by tapping their shoulders or making eye contact. —I at times make casual conversation with the bus driver and say "excuse me" as I pass other passengers. —If someone is sitting in the aisle seat, I will ask them to let me pass by to sit down in the window seat.

MOBILITY

Postural alignment—Maintaining biomechanical integrity among body parts	
Level of Influence	Observations:
☐ 0 ☐ 1. ☐ 2. ☐ 3. X 4.	—I need to maintain both sitting and standing postures. —My pelvic position changes as I move from standing to sitting. —Some rapid postural adjustments take place as I weave between people and objects.

Postural control—Using righting and equilibrium reactions to maintain balance during functional movements	
Level of Influence	Observations:
□ 0 □ 1. □ 2. □ 3. X 4.	—My head righting and equilibrium reactions help me to maintain balance as the motion of the bus moves me back and forth. —My protective reactions are also activated by my displaced equilibrium. —My base of support changes from standing on two feet as I await the bus to alternating between my two feet as I walk to my pelvis as I sit down. —I lean in all directions against gravity as the bus sways. —There is potential for a sudden displacement of my center of gravity.

Depth perception—Involves determining the relative distance between objects, figures, or landmarks and the observer and changes in planes and surfaces	
Level of Influence	Observations:
□ 0 □ 1. □ 2. X 3. □ 4.	—To enter the bus, I must step up about 1 foot to stand on the platform. —I make precise movements with my upper extremity to insert my metrocard into the metrocard reader. —I reach out to grasp onto various handrails and seat backs. —I need to lower myself precisely down onto my seat. —I move my body through the sagittal, coronal, and transverse planes.

Body strength—Degree of gross muscle power when body movement is resisted or is against gravity	
Level of Influence	Observations:
□ 0 □ 1. X 2. □ 3. □ 4.	—I need moderate strength in each of my extremities and my trunk to perform this activity. —I engage my hand and forearm muscles isometrically as I stabilize myself with a handrail. My leg muscles work together both concentrically and eccentrically to allow me to step onto the bus and walk down the aisle. —I eccentrically contract my latissimus dorsi, triceps, and quadriceps muscles, among others, as I lower myself down into my seat. —Trunk control allows me to stay upright as I wait for the bus and walk.

CARRYING, MOVING, AND HANDLING OBJECTS

Range of motion—Moving body parts through an arc of motion	
Level of Influence ☐ 0 ☐ 1. ☐ 2. ☐ 3. X 4.	Observations: —This activity requires a moderate amount of range of motion. I am listing minimum requirements for the following tasks. —Signaling the bus to stop: 90° shoulder flexion or abduction. —Stepping onto the bus: 70° hip flexion, 75° knee flexion, 20° plantar flexion —Swiping my metrocard: 25° shoulder flexion, 75° elbow flexion, 75°forearm pronation —Grasping onto handrails (including overhead): 75° forearm pronation and supination, 150° shoulder flexion or abduction —Sitting down (including lowering myself down with my arms): 90° hip flexion, 90° knee flexion, 90° shoulder abduction, 135° elbow flexion, 75° forearm pronation

Extremity strength—Grade of muscle strength when body movement is resisted or is against gravity	
Level of Influence ☐ 0 ☐ 1. X 2. ☐ 3. ☐ 4.	Observations: —Most of the actions required for this activity are done against gravity. Therefore, a muscle grade of 3 or *fair* will be needed for most involved muscles. —If I am carrying any bags or wearing a heavy coat, all upper extremity movements will require a muscle grade of 4 or *good*.

Endurance—Sustained cardiac, pulmonary, and musculoskeletal exertion over time	
Level of Influence ☐ 0 X 1. ☐ 2. ☐ 3. ☐ 4.	Observations: —This activity requires minimal endurance, and there are minimal resistive movements. —The entire activity takes only a few minutes.

Stereognosis—Identifying objects through proprioception, cognition, and sense of touch	
Level of Influence	Observations:
☐ 0	—I use stereognosis to locate and identify my metrocard
☐ 1.	from within my pocket.
X 2.	—I reach out for handrails and take steps that are outside of
☐ 3.	my visual field. This happens when the bus is crowded.
☐ 4.	

Kinesthesia—Identifying the excursion and direction of movement	
Level of Influence	Observations:
☐ 0	—I coordinate my thumb, finger, wrist, radioulnar, elbow,
☐ 1.	and shoulder joints as I insert my metrocard into the reader.
☐ 2.	—Sitting down requires me to coordinate my ankles, knees,
X 3.	hips, shoulder, forearm, elbow, wrist, and hand joints.
☐ 4.	—Walking requires me to coordinate the joints of my lower
	extremity.
	—Walking down the aisle requires me to make quick
	changes in movement.

Grasp patterns—Identifying the type(s) of grasp required to perform the activity	
Level of Influence	Observations:
☐ 0	—During the activity, I most frequently use my entire hand
☐ 1.	in a power grasp rather than controlling my fingers in fine
☐ 2.	motor movements.
X 3.	—I use a cylindric grasp to hold onto seat tops and
☐ 4.	handrails.
	—I use a hook grasp at times to hold onto groceries or a
	bag.

Prehension patterns—Identifying the type(s) of pinch required to perform this activity	
Level of Influence	Observations:
☐ 0	—I favor a 3-jaw chuck pinch pattern to hold onto my
☐ 1.	metrocard.
X 2.	—A palmar prehension pattern, or "pad-to-pad," would
☐ 3.	also be appropriate.
☐ 4.	—If I could not perform these patterns, I could compensate
	by using a lateral prehension pattern or an ulnar-sided grip;
	however, these would be awkward and difficult.

Fine motor—Ability to use small hand muscles and joints to perform refined actions	
Level of Influence	Observations:
☐ 0	—There are no excessively refined actions needed to perform
☐ 1.	this activity.
X 2.	—My fingers do assist me to grasp onto handrails and seat
☐ 3.	tops and to manipulate my metrocard both in my hand and
☐ 4.	into the metrocard reader.

Figure–ground perception—Differentiating between foreground and background forms and objects	
Level of Influence	Observations:
☐ 0	—I use figure–ground perception to distinguish the empty
☐ 1.	seats from among all of the filled seats.
X 2.	—I distinguish between the bus and all the other cars as it
☐ 3.	approaches the bus stop.
☐ 4.	

Topographical orientation—Determining the location of objects and settings and the route to the location	
Level of Influence	Observations:
☐ 0	—I use the bus stop map to determine whether the
X 1.	corresponding bus will satisfy my route. This is how I
☐ 2.	choose to get on a certain bus.
☐ 3.	—I do not, however, use topographical orientation to
☐ 4.	actually get on the bus and take a seat.

Part 3: Summary

Once you have completed the activity analyses consider the following:

1. **Is the activity part of the client's habits, routines, or rituals?**
   I consider this activity to be a regular part of an irregular routine. At the end of each day, I take the subway from Manhattan to my Brooklyn neighborhood. There, I check the schedule to see if a bus is set to arrive. If it is, I wait and take the bus the rest of the way home. If not, I choose to walk. This same mentality governs my choice to take the bus in many circumstances, including going home from the grocery store and to and from my brother's apartment. If it is available when I need it, I choose to take it. If not, then I find an alternative means of transportation.

2. **How does this activity relate to the client's roles?**
   Past:
   In the past, getting on the bus and taking a seat related to my role of a student studying abroad in a foreign country. I took the bus because my schedule was relaxed and to better orient myself to a new city.

   Present:
   Presently, the activity relates to my roles of student, worker, family member, and friend. I take the bus to and from school, my job, my brother's apartment, and planned visits with friends.

   Future:
   In the future, I hope that the bus will continue to relate to each of my present roles. In addition, I would like to find employment in my neighborhood, which would increase the frequency with which I take the bus. As an older adult, I will probably attempt to take a seat on the bus each time I ride.

3. **Does the activity facilitate self-expression or enhance self-concept?**
   My choice to take the bus as opposed to the subway reflects my self-expression. When I take the bus, I am attuned to the process of transportation and the enjoyment I get from seeing where I am going. It is not a mode of transportation that I choose when my goal is to arrive at my destination by the fastest and most efficient means possible. Taking the bus is a manifestation of the value I place on a slower pace of life.

   Being able to get on the bus is empowering. I am never worried about being lost or stranded in the city. Knowing how to use the bus system grants me a sense of self-efficacy as I become more and more adept at figuring out bus routes and transporting myself where I need to go. Additionally, it contributes to my ability to live an independent life. I am able to buy my groceries, go to the doctor, and commute home from work without any additional assistance. Taking a seat on the bus is another important aspect of this activity. Looking to the future, I see being able to take a seat on the bus as an essential part of my continued use of the bus as an older adult.

5

The Occupational Profile

Judy Urban Wilson, MA, OTR

What we do, and what we think about what we do, encompasses who we are. We act and we react. Sometimes we take a line of action by choice, and at other times we act because we believe we can do nothing else. These daily actions are the occupations that define us to ourselves and also in the eyes of others.

Health is a notion that assumes access to and participation in these occupations. What cuts us off from these occupations consequently impairs our health, and disconnection from our occupations places our sense of who we are at risk. Many conditions can threaten our full engagement in the occupations that are meaningful to us, such as changes in body structure, paucity of available occupations, or a change in the context in which we must act out our occupations. In such situations, we need to regain a full and meaningful set of occupations to restore our health.

In this chapter, I aim to capture what it means for therapy to be occupational in practice. I endeavor to keep it practical, showing that the long heritage of occupational therapy theory is present in our daily work. I cannot cite references for each idea because my thoughts are rooted in a wealth of occupational therapy literature that has brought me to where I am now. My ideas are not new; rather, they are basic to occupational therapy. What I hope I can offer to readers is a series of reflections on occupation from the clinic floor. Keeping my attention on the occupational profile, the focal point of this chapter, reminds me of who we are professionally and propels me to continue growing as an occupational therapist.

Occupational Profile

The objective of occupational therapy is to ensure that people can "engage in everyday activities or occupations that they want and need to do in a manner that supports health and participation" (American Occupational Therapy Association [AOTA], 2008, p. 626). Because the key feature of an occupation is the meaning it holds for the person, the specifics of occupation vary from person to person. Occupational therapy assists in linking a person to those occupations that define him or her. If the objective of occupational therapy is to engage people in occupations, the occupational therapist's first responsibility is to identify the client's occupations.

The *occupational profile* is a summary of set of activities, routines, and roles that describes a client at any one point in time. In practice, the occupational profile is the imperfect collection of data gathered by the occupational therapist to try to capture the individual client's living occupational profile.

An ongoing discussion in the occupational therapy literature concerns how to define *occupations, roles, activities,* and *lifestyles* (e.g., AOTA, 1997; Kielhofner, 1983, 1985, 1992, 2008; Kramer, Hinojosa, & Royeen, 2003; Nelson, 1996; Trombly, 1995). All these terms are used to express human actions and what they mean in the context of people's lives. In practice, the occupational therapist needs to identify and analyze these actions in relation to each client. AOTA (2008) has defined the *occupational profile* as "information that describes the client's occupational history and experiences, patterns of daily living, interests, values, and needs" (p. 649). This definition encompasses a lot of information. In fact, it describes a whole life.

Biography, however, is not the goal of the occupational therapist. Accordingly, the occupational profile focuses on the mundane aspects of living rather than solely on the big events. The story of an accident or a list of a person's life accomplishments is only relevant to the occupational profile because of the impact it has on the person's daily activities and roles, not because of the events themselves. In the evaluation, the therapist seeks to uncover specific features of the client's story; he or she looks for descriptions of activities performed, patterns of behavior, and where and with whom activities are performed. Furthermore, the therapist identifies what makes these activities meaningful or important to the client, thus identifying the client's occupations.

When a person is going to receive occupational therapy, he or she may have a variety of problems or areas of concern. Not all of the person's occupations, however, would be impaired, changed, or threatened. When the therapist begins to evaluate the client, he or she must focus on identifying the client's specific problems or areas to be addressed during therapy. The therapist uses the occupational profile to clarify the person's needs, values, and priorities.

EXERCISE 5.1: PERSONAL PROFILE

What occupations make up your own profile? Which occupations are the most important to you? Why? Pick one occupation and list all the activities that it includes. Where do you perform these activities? With whom? What is unique about how you do these activities?

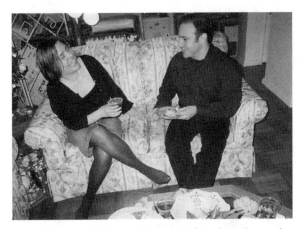

Figure 5.1. Deborah and Jeremy find socializing with friends to be a relevant and important occupation.

Temporal Context

Developing a person's occupational profile requires that the occupational therapist focus on present or recent occupations. These occupations are those most relevant to the client's present sense of self and current circumstances (Figure 5.1). If illness or injury has caused an unfavorable change in occupations, then the occupations just before the change are the most critical part of the profile. These occupations reflect the client's values, goals, ambitions, and aspirations with the most accuracy.

Current occupations are especially critical to explore when the client's current occupations form a negative sense of self, such as in a situation involving an abusive parent or when a person feels like a helpless invalid in his or her present circumstances. If the client is performing activities because of physical, cognitive, psychosocial, or environmental limitations, then the therapist must consider how these limitations influence the client's ability to engage in occupations. If the client desires a change in these occupations, targeting these occupations becomes a central goal of treatment. In sum, when planning treatment it is important to know the client's current occupations because these are the starting points for the creation of any therapeutic change (Figure 5.2).

Even though the occupational profile focuses on present or recent occupations, some understanding of past and future occupations is also important. Past occupations helped shape those of the present and are a source of experience from which the client can continue to draw. It is also important to appreciate the client's vision of future occupations and to understand the importance and value of a particular occupation to the person because such knowledge is essential for planning interventions. In short, past occupations and future aspirations are valuable sources for adjustments or

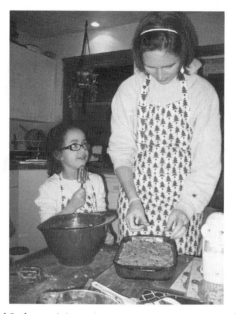

Figure 5.2. Morgan and Judy participate in current co-occupations of daughter and mother.

renewals in a client's occupations as he or she moves forward. One challenge for the occupational therapist is to determine whether current, past, or future potential occupations are the most important and relevant to understanding the person.

Time is a defining dimension of any occupational profile, yet the occupational profile is not simply a resume-like document that builds over time; rather, it is a continually morphing entity. The past, the present, and the future shape a person's roles and routines. People's occupational profiles change both as they mature and in response to life events. A child stops playing with toy trucks and becomes interested in baseball. A student graduates and becomes a worker. A worker retires. A woman gives birth. An aunt becomes ill, and the niece takes her in. These transitions change a person's occupational profiles.

In some cases, the occupational therapist works with a client in response to a particular event that changed the client's occupational profile. The client may have suffered an injury or illness that altered patterns of daily life and daily activities. In other cases, the client comes to the therapist because of an unsatisfying or destructive occupational profile that he or she seeks to change. Whether change is sought because of a sudden event or as a result of longstanding limitations, the therapist needs to learn about the client's previous occupational profile, the client's present occupational profile, and what the client needs and desires for a future occupational profile.

EXERCISE 5.2: TEMPORAL CONTEXT OF PERSONAL PROFILE

Reflect again on your own occupational profile. When has it changed? What are past occupations in which you no longer engage? What impact does this have on your present occupations? What occupations do you aspire to have in the future? Do these aspirations shape any of your present occupations?

CASE SCENARIO 5.1: MARIA, MAUREEN, ALEX, AND DANIEL

For each of the following cases, which time period in their occupational profiles should be the strongest focus of the therapist for treatment planning? Why?

A: Maria is an 11-year-old girl who broke her radius playing soccer in her local league. She is in sixth grade and applying to a specialized science school starting in seventh grade. She has several neighborhood friends with whom she plays on weekends. She lives with her mother and little brother. Her father disappeared 2 years ago.

B: Maureen is an 87-year-old woman referred to a psychiatric day treatment program with a diagnosis of major depression. She has been a widow for 30 years. She retired 2 years ago from her work as a secretary. After retirement, she moved away from the place where she had lived her whole life, leaving friends and her sisters, to move in with her daughter and son-in-law in the next state. She now watches a little TV, knits, and tries to help her daughter around the house. She reports that her relationship with her daughter has become very strained.

C: Alex is a 4-year-old boy with severe developmental delays. He lives with his two parents, 1-year-old brother, and 6-year-old sister. His siblings play with him on the mat in the playroom. He has an adapted highchair in which his parents feed him. They transport him in an adapted stroller. His mother hopes to start him in the town's mainstream school system next year.

D: Daniel is a 65-year-old man who worked as an elementary school janitor for many years. Ten years ago, he was no longer able to manage his work. He was diagnosed with chronic obstructive pulmonary disease. Five years ago, he was placed on oxygen. He is divorced, with an adult son who lives out of state with Daniel's grandchildren. Over the past 10 years, he has stopped his frequent visits to the local pub where he played pool. He is starting to have trouble with his self-care. His clothes are unkempt, and he appears unwashed.

DATA COLLECTION

The process of gathering the information to complete an occupational profile is time consuming and lengthy. It begins at the moment of meeting the client and continues throughout the occupational therapy intervention. The process generally starts with an interview. The client, however, will not share much of the most important data with the therapist until rapport is established. Thus, the intervention plan changes as the intervention progresses.

INTERVIEW

Good interviewing skills are vital for the occupational therapist. The key to good interviewing skills lies not in the questions asked but in effective listening (Figure 5.3). From listening closely to what the client says, the therapist decides on and adapts his or her line of questioning. Once a dialogue has been established, the therapist seeks to clarify details and introduces new topics to explore other areas. The therapist probes for clarification and understanding as he or she listens to what the client says (Figure 5.4).

People are not accustomed to being asked questions about exactly how they do every task in their day. When asked what they do in the morning, many people answer that they get up and go to work. The occupational

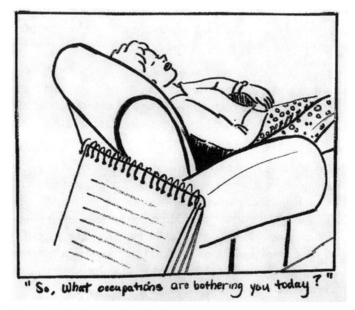

Figure 5.3. Gathering data for the occupational profile is not simple.

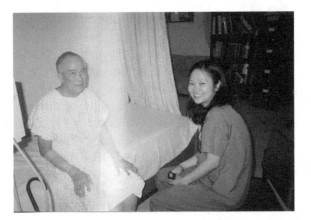

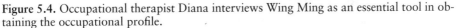

Figure 5.4. Occupational therapist Diana interviews Wing Ming as an essential tool in obtaining the occupational profile.

therapist, however, wants to know when they get up, what kind of bed they slept in, who is in the bed, where they go next, whether they wear slippers, and whether they brush their teeth first or drink their coffee first. The therapist must therefore ask precise and probing questions.

Questions are influenced by the client's particular context. For example, a therapist treating a client with a broken finger will ask more about how the client holds the toothbrush and squeezes the toothpaste and less about what kind of slippers the client wears. For the client with depression, however, the therapist will be less concerned about how the client grips the toothbrush but may focus instead on the time or the regularity of the tooth-brushing routine. The therapist uses clinical judgment and knowledge about the client's condition to shape the interview.

Rarely is the occupational therapist the first health professional in contact with a client. In previous health care environments, clients get used to answering questions about their symptoms; they do not expect to be asked about what they enjoy doing in their free time, what community groups they are involved in, and what responsibilities they have at home. It takes extra effort for the occupational therapist to refocus the conversation, and the therapist must often ask questions in multiple ways to find out about the client's activities and occupations.

EXERCISE 5.3: INTERVIEW A FRIEND OR FAMILY MEMBER

Interview a friend or family member (not an occupational therapist or occupational therapy student). Find out about the person's daily routines, responsibilities, and work and leisure activities.

Sometimes simply asking the client is ineffective. The client may be a young child, may be confused, or may be unable to communicate. In these cases, the therapist can usually turn to family members for information because the family has much more extensive experience with the person and can flesh out the therapist's observations. In some cases, the family may also be considered to be the client, and the therapist may work closely with the family members to develop intervention priorities. For example, a mother may want to be able to fit her daughter into a car seat to ease transportation to school. In another family, the older son may worry about his elderly mother wandering into the kitchen and turning on the stove.

There are times, however, when a client cannot speak for himself or herself, and there are no family members or friends who can speak for the client. This scenario includes both clients who are unable to communicate and those who are resistive to treatment because of confusion or depression. In these cases, a standard interview will be unproductive. The occupational therapist becomes a solver of puzzles who must piece together a hypothesized profile. This profile is constantly updated from the general social data available, from pieces of conversations with the client, and from the client's reactions to activities (Figure 5.5). Success, however, relies on the waning of the client's resistance as rapport builds during the treatment process.

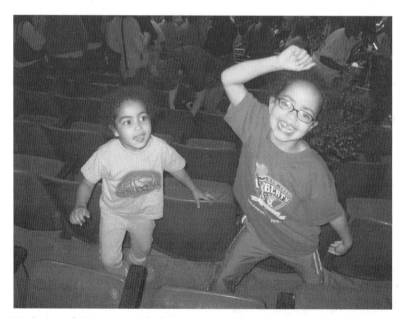

Figure 5.5. Catie and Morgan enrich their co-occupation of sisters as they dance together.

CASE SCENARIO 5.2: LING MEI

Ling Mei is an elderly Chinese woman, found on the streets of San Francisco's Chinatown, who had had a severe stroke. In the inpatient rehabilitation unit, Ling Mei claimed that she was fine and asked that someone take her to the statue of Confucius, where she could sit and panhandle. She told them, "I'll be fine." She had had significant frontal lobe damage impeding awareness and potentially impeding cognitive skills. Her illiteracy and her resistance to formal testing hampered the accuracy of the neuropsychological evaluation. The occupational profile became especially critical when the occupational therapist needed to report to the team whether the client was ready to be discharged safely to the community.

Case questions: Could Ling Mei resume her previous activities adequately without social support? What skills should the therapist consider to be city survival skills? What occupations would you guess recently made up Ling Mei's profile? What activities would you try with her to see how she responds?

PARTICIPANT OBSERVATION

In some sense, the occupational therapist works as an ethnographer. The first ethnographic method he or she uses to learn about the client and his or her life is the interview, as discussed earlier. The second ethnographic method is *participant observation*—a research technique in which the researcher engages in activities with people to learn about them and their lives. In occupational therapy, once rapport is established and the intervention has begun, the occupational therapist learns about the client while engaging in activities with him or her. However, although the ethnographer values not influencing the research participants, the occupational therapist enters the interaction with the purpose of working with the client to create change and gain understanding of the client.

In the *Occupational Therapy Practice Framework: Domain and Process* (2nd ed.; *Framework–II*; AOTA, 2008) Collaborative Process Model (see Figure 5.6), the occupational therapist and the client work together in the process of service delivery. As the therapist and the client jointly engage in the activities within the intervention, they interact, and rapport continues to build. Even when rapport is difficult to develop, interactions between the therapist and the client provide information that broadens the therapist's picture of the client. Therapists use activities pertinent to the client, often within the client's personal context. These interactions are the therapist's "fieldwork" from which observations are made.

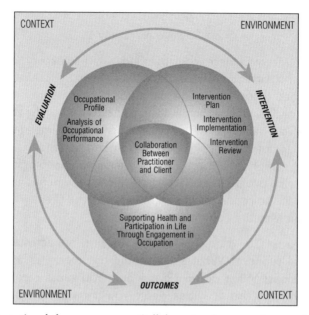

Figure 5.6. Occupational therapy process: Collaboration between the practitioner and client is central to the interactive nature of service delivery.

Note. From "Occupational Therapy Practice Framework: Domain and Practice (2nd Edition)," 2008, *American Journal of Occupational Therapy*, 62, p. 627. Copyright © 2008, by the American Occupational Therapy Association. Reprinted with permission.

Participant observation provides new details about the client's performance in context that support or contrast with what the therapist learned in the interview. As the client chats with the therapist, he or she shares information that triggers new ideas and new questions from the therapist, leading to an increasingly rich occupational profile. A level of intimacy develops between client and therapist, and as this relationship grows, the client may reach a point at which he or she shares sensitive personal information with the therapist.

As the therapist enters the client's world, the client learns about the perspective and principles of occupational therapy through the shared experience of the treatment intervention. In turn, as clients come to a greater understanding of occupational therapy, they themselves become more self-directed in the process. A client may see himself or herself taking part in more activities and may identify which activities he or she wants to work on next in pursuit of a valued occupation (Figure 5.7). The client may bring up an old hobby or a long-held aspiration as he or she perceives that occupational therapy may be able to help him or her achieve such goals. Some clients take on more of a partnership role during intervention and are able to identify occupational issues not previously mentioned as they come to understand the potential of the occupational therapy process. Others need more direction to link the intervention process to their occupations.

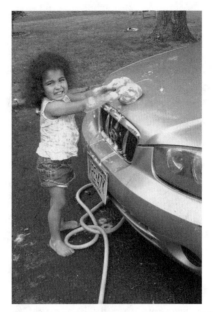

Figure 5.7. Washing a car can be a paid occupation, a chore within the occupation of car owner or driver, or a wet part of the occupation of play.

CASE SCENARIO 5.3: MARTHA

Martha is a 40-year-old woman diagnosed with major depression with borderline personality disorder who was referred to an outpatient psychiatric treatment program. At the initial interview with the occupational therapist (along with the chart review), Martha shared that since her "meltdown" she has been cutting herself, and, as a result, she is on leave from her job as a music teacher in the local school system. Her husband is also a local teacher. She has two daughters, one in college and one doing well in high school. She reported that when she was growing up, her mother had been domineering and emotionally abusive and forced her and her sisters to be performers all their lives. Martha had been sexually assaulted as a child and harbored a lot of anger toward her mother for never stopping or addressing the abuse. She describes herself as shy. Presently, Martha cannot tolerate crowds and is very uncomfortable around other people. The therapist observed that her social interactions were stunted.

The initial treatment plan included practicing relaxation techniques for social situations and to help manage anger in relation to her mother; building self-esteem, beginning with emphasizing her successes, such as her two daughters; using coping strategies for interacting with her mother; and taking

(continued)

CASE SCENARIO: MARTHA (cont.)

on graded resumption of social activities, with the eventual goal of returning to work. Returning to work was especially difficult because in the small town, everyone knew why Martha was on leave. She eventually did return to work. Another big success was attending a concert involving her favorite singer.

After more than 1 year in treatment, small comments from Martha began to emerge when she was talking with the therapist, such as fear in her voice at the mention of bringing financial problems to her husband and complaints about cleaning the mouse cages that her husband brought home from his classroom. At a program family event, the therapist noted that Martha was hyperattentive to her husband and that her husband seemed aloof. Also, others in the program complimented Martha on the townwide children's concerts she once led, about which she seemed proud but reserved and reluctant.

Martha's confidence was growing, which allowed her to answer as the therapist began to question her more about her marriage. Slowly, the therapist learned that Martha's husband was neglectful and emotionally abusive and forced her into an introverted role in relation to his own high achievement. The treatment plan changed to focus on her development of occupations outside the confines of her marriage.

Over time Martha began jogging daily; she resumed playing the organ in church; she made new friends; she took on a caretaker role with her mother, who had had a stroke; she played piano for the town Christmas show; and she restarted the townwide children's concerts. (Case contributed by Kathy Urban, MA, RN. Reprinted with permission.)

Case questions: Why could Martha discuss her marriage later in treatment and not in the beginning? How did this change the treatment plan? How did the revelation about her marriage change the meaning of her past occupation as performer? How might the revelation about her marriage affect her social relationships? What did the therapist observe about Martha's occupations through interaction in activities with Martha?

Data collection for the occupational profile is an ongoing component of the evaluation. As the process moves into the intervention phase, the intervention planning begins to flow more directly from the new data emerging in the profile. The therapist thus uses the occupational profile as an intervention tool. As the therapist learns about the client's occupations, past or future, the therapist recognizes occupations that are still attainable or that are especially self-affirming for the client. The therapist emphasizes the occupations that help the client to see his or her capabilities and encourages the client to actively

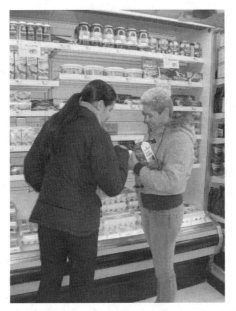

Figure 5.8. In implementing the occupational therapy intervention, Sabrina brings her client Antonia into the community to perform activities in the same physical context that she will use after discharge.

choose which occupations he or she wishes to set as goals. Such a discussion between the client and the therapist is the first step in empowering the client to make changes for a healthier and richer occupational profile (Figure 5.8).

As with all ethnographers, the occupational therapist brings his or her own worldview to the process. Of course, the therapist uses clinical reasoning, understanding of medical and psychological conditions, and a growing understanding of the client to inform his or her decisions about what to ask and how to develop the interventions. The therapist, however, also brings a more personal and subjective perspective to the same process. What questions are asked, what is considered relevant, and what actions are noticed all depend on what the therapist brings to the interaction. The therapist is influenced by the chosen theories and frames of reference, by medical knowledge about the diagnosis and prognosis, by his or her experience with other clients, and by his or her personal experiences and prejudices (Urban 1998a, 1998b). It is important that therapists understand their own worldview and consider how it affects the interaction.

EXERCISE 5.4: MARTHA'S OCCUPATIONAL PROFILE

In the case of Martha, how did the therapist use the occupational profile as a tool? Think about which occupations the therapist reinforced as part of the treatment plan. Which past occupations opened new occupations for Martha?

How Context Affects the Occupational Profile

An activity out of context loses its meaning. Context is the factor that influences a person's performance of activities and occupations, and it can be internal or external to the client. *Internal contexts* include the person's physical, social, and virtual realities, including his or her personal and spiritual beliefs. *External contexts* include the dimensions of time and space. Time dimensions are the time of day or the person's age. Space dimensions are the physical features relevant to the activity, such as the size of the room (AOTA, 2008).

When developing a client's occupational profile, the therapist needs to consider the contexts relevant to each activity and occupation. The context of many occupations is what individualizes them so that they have meaning to the person. The context shapes how the tasks are performed, where they take place, and how important they are. For example, eating is strongly influenced by contextual factors. Having lunch at a restaurant is very different from having a picnic in the park. Likewise, a birthday dinner out is different from dinner at home. Eating is thus heavily influenced by internal and external contextual factors.

Self-care is an occupation found in everyone's profile. Self-care, however, takes different forms for each person. One woman may need to wear nylons to work every day, whereas another may wear them to church on Sundays only. One woman may wear sneakers every day, whereas another may have been raised to believe that sneakers are unfeminine. One may dress in the bedroom, another in the bathroom. One elderly woman may feel that at her age, she has earned the right to have her children help her put on her shoes, whereas another would go barefoot before admitting that she could not do it herself. The elements affecting the single task of dressing are limitless. Understanding the specific contexts relevant to each person provides the critical data that give shape to the occupational profile.

Context also influences the process of obtaining the occupational profile. Issues of class, social norms, and the personal experiences of both the client and the therapist shape and inform the therapeutic relationship and in turn affect what information is shared. As the therapist learns more about the context, the therapist may adjust his or her approach (Figure 5.9). Sometimes a clearer occupational profile will emerge as the therapeutic relationship develops.

Ultimately, the therapist must respect the gaps in the occupational profile and acknowledge that it will never be complete. The therapist needs to identify the occupations, with their contexts, that the person is willing to address with the therapist at that time.

Less obvious is the effect of the occupational profile itself on context. To consider this point of view, one must recognize that people are active forces in their contexts. People's occupations bring them to particular places and

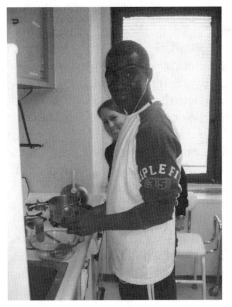

Figure 5.9. Occupational therapist Shannon works with Christopher to change how he performs cooking activities after bodily changes so he can improve his performance of the occupation of living alone.

link them to particular people. Through their occupations, people have the power to change their physical and social environments.

Occupational Therapy Evaluation

The occupational therapy evaluation has two components: (1) the occupational profile and (2) the analysis of occupational performance. Although the occupational profile is the starting point, these two aspects of the evaluation process are not sequential. The process of evaluation is a continuous interplay between the occupational profile and the analysis of occupational performance (AOTA, 2008).

The occupational profile identifies which occupations need to be evaluated for occupational performance. It pinpoints which occupations are priorities for intervention and what configuration of activities currently defines that

---

EXERCISE 5.5: CONTEXT OF PERSONAL PROFILE

Think about one of your occupations, for example, the occupation of student. Reflect on what contexts shape how you perform that occupation. What are the personal meanings of these contexts to you? Include cultural, physical, social, personal, spiritual, temporal, and virtual contexts. How do the details of your occupation differ from those of someone else you know with the same occupation?

occupation for the client. The therapist can then evaluate the client's performance in these activities. As the therapist analyzes the client's actual performance of the specified occupations, he or she observes the individual details of the client's task execution, which further flesh out the profile. People have difficulty describing their habits and routines because these things are so ingrained in their lives that they do not think about them anymore. As the client performs the task, or tries to perform the task, the therapist sees what the client is able to do and how it is completed or attempted.

With the new details observed regarding the client's occupational performance, the therapist can then ask more questions, which further clarify the occupational profile, and in turn refocus the direction of the evaluation of occupational performance. Likewise, as the therapist identifies specific skill deficits through the evaluation analysis, he or she will be able to anticipate what areas of occupations may be problematic and concentrate the questions there. For example, for a client with limited elbow flexion of the nondominant arm, the therapist will delve more deeply into the areas of applying make-up rather than painting fingernails, or golfing rather than reading.

Case Scenario 5.4: Enrique

Enrique is a 22-year-old man with a traumatic brain injury who was recently discharged from an inpatient rehabilitation hospital and referred for outpatient services. In the occupational therapist's initial interview, Enrique says he is having no problems. He lives with his mother, and every morning he gets up and gets his daughter ready for school. He spends his day helping around the house and taking care of his daughter. Enrique is eager to return to work but is concerned that he may not be able to return to construction work because his leg bothers him sometimes.

The therapist's formal testing showed severe disorganization, memory deficits with instructions, and inefficiency and multiple errors in task performance. The therapist decides to ask Enrique's mother about his daily routine. His mother reports that he sleeps late every day. He cannot pick out his own clothes, even though he had always been a meticulous dresser. She takes care of his daughter. She does not let him out alone because he gets lost. She worries when she goes to work because Enrique once left the stove on, and she is afraid that he will wander off.

Case questions: What information for the evaluation do the discrepancies in the reports give us? What suspicions do you think the therapist had that made her ask the mother for the same information she had asked of the client? What occupations does Enrique value? Which occupations are problematic? How does the additional information change the occupational focus of the intervention plan?

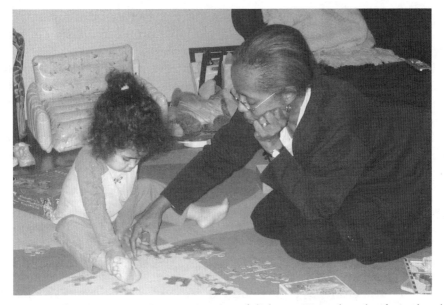

Figure 5.10. Observation is an important aspect of dialogue. Here, the role of grandmother and its value are clear from the activities June engages in with her granddaughter Catie.

Observing a person's occupational performance, particularly in context, is an intimate act. As these activities are shared, the dialogue between the therapist and the client begins to develop. This dialogue is when the therapist learns the most about the client's occupational profile (Figure 5.10).

With a new injury or illness affecting occupational performance, the occupational therapy evaluation may be the first time clients are attempting some of the tasks important to their occupations. This situation makes the clients vulnerable because what they can and cannot do has changed. As they confront familiar tasks with new difficulties, the priorities and values in their occupational profiles shift. Moreover, this shift is emotionally charged. Often, clients struggle down a tumultuous road toward new self-perceptions, which are tied directly to their occupational profile. Clients are struggling to gain a vision of themselves in the future, a vision they use to set their goals and give meaning to the present (Morris, 1994). This metamorphosis spans the evaluation and intervention stages.

Intervention and the Occupational Profile

The constant adjustment of the occupational profile is most extreme with an acute injury or illness. Occupational therapy intervention, however, signifies a point of change for all clients. Even in healthy populations, if a person seeks an occupational therapy consultation, he or she is looking for ways to improve performance or decrease risk factors in occupations. As change occurs, the client's present occupational profile and vision of future occupations also changes.

The occupational profile influences intervention by identifying the client's needs and priorities for intervention. Many clients' articulated goals are too general to use as treatment goals, for example, "I want to go home," "I want to be like I used to be," "I want to walk," and "I want to get better." The occupational profile gives the therapist data with which to interpret these goals and form interventions. In the client's array of occupations, where did the person walk in the past, what activities are necessary to survive at home, and which occupations are presently worse than before?

The occupational profile is also important in choosing types of interventions. It identifies what activities are significant for the client and is also a source of ideas for the purposeful activities implemented in the intervention plan. The therapist seeks purposeful activities that draw on the client's interests to be engaging and motivating for the client. Participating in purposeful activities will build the foundation on which the client's occupations can emerge.

The occupational profile also aids the therapist in choosing a method to approach a goal. Knowing how the client has adapted his or her occupations at previous stages of life can help in the selection of an approach to which the client will be receptive. Where will the client be open to making changes? Would the client rather scale back the performance of an occupation or completely redesign how to fulfill a role?

The intervention process makes a continuous impact on the occupational profile, creating the "dynamic interrelatedness" (AOTA, 2008, p. 626) that entwines evaluation with intervention. The client's awareness of what he or she can and cannot do increases. The therapist exposes the client to new experiences that may open possibilities in the client's eyes. The client travels through different emotional responses to the changes. In addition, the client–therapist relationship is forged, and new revelations and understanding about the occupational profile emerge in the process.

EXERCISE 5.6: LIFESTYLE REDESIGN

Read the story of Penny in Florence Clark's (1993) "Occupation Embedded in a Real Life: Interweaving Occupational Science and Occupational Therapy" (included on CD-ROM). Consider these questions: Which occupations from childhood helped Penny reform her occupations after the "big A"? Which occupations does Penny value most? What occupations did she modify to fulfill her roles? What are new occupations she has taken on to fulfill old roles?

CASE SCENARIO 5.5: GEORGE

George is a 27-year-old who recently experienced a T-4 spinal cord injury and now has a complete paraplegia. He hopes to walk and return to rock climbing and camping. He feels despair at times, convinced that he cannot even shave or feed himself. Sometimes, he just wants to indulge in his role as son and let his mother baby him, bathing him and combing his hair. At other times, he feels empowered, such as during his first time propelling himself in a wheelchair around the hospital unit.

George's occupational profile in relation to the present and the future is like his occupational performance in the evaluation and in ongoing treatment. Sometimes his only goal is to go home as soon as possible, with his mother and sister caring for him. Sometimes he can address his occupations only within the hospital stay, such as his self-care, his exercises, and his leadership role among other patients, but he cannot discuss going home. At other times, he has many questions for the occupational therapist, asking about how accessible public transportation is and for information about wheelchair sports.

Case questions: Which activities will the occupational therapist encourage? How can George's intervention plan capture his changing occupational profile and his changing focus? Which occupations are most urgent in intervention planning as his inpatient stay nears an end? How can his present occupations help build up his ability to support longer term occupations?

Outcomes and the Occupational Profile

Beginning during the evaluation process, the occupational profile is a tool used to set specific outcome measures. The *Framework–II* defines the domain of therapy as "supporting health and participation in life through engagement in occupation" (AOTA, 2008, p. 626). The *Framework–II* divides this statement into three interrelated concepts regarding the desired outcome of therapy interventions: (1) health, (2) participation, and (3) engagement in occupation. The occupational profile identifies which of the client's occupations are desired, valued, and needed. The profile provides details about the occupations in which the client seeks to participate and commits to engage in more fully. In designing the intervention plan, the occupational profile identifies which occupational areas to target. The outcome measures thus flow directly from the occupational issues that surfaced in the profile because the profile identifies the values, roles, personal meanings, and unique contexts of the occupations in the client's life. Successful outcomes represent meaningful change for the client. The direction taken by the outcome measures, however, varies greatly.

The outcome measure can be a resumption of impaired occupations, or it can be a change or redefinition of the occupations themselves. Activities that were health risks or that were unattainable for the client after a bodily change need to undergo alteration. For example, the outcome measures may target a change in leisure skills for a person with a drug addiction or aim to redefine work for a person after a severe brain injury. Because the profile identifies the client's valued roles, it guides the client and therapist in channeling the activity changes to achieve role competence.

The client may identify in the profile certain occupational performances with which he or she is disappointed. The therapist then sets the outcome measure at satisfactory performance of that occupation, such as independence with work skills after a hand injury or resuming independent living at home after a stroke. In other cases in which the client is dissatisfied with his or her occupational engagement, a change in actions is a successful outcome. In this case, the profile identifies the components of the occupational challenge. For example, a client who describes a series of job losses because of fights with his coworkers illustrates a profile that is not satisfactory to the client at present. The adaptation outcome measure is the change in performance that allows the client to maintain a job.

The therapist may choose to look at the occupational profile with the client as a conscientious part of jointly evaluating outcomes. This process allows the client to identify his or her own satisfaction with changes that have occurred. This process may also reveal a change in the client's perceptions and whether there is great or little change in performance. The ultimate goal of occupational therapy is for the client to spontaneously engage in occupations that he or she values. The client's quality of life is determined by the client's perceptions of his or her life and is strongly influenced by his or her ability to engage in meaningful occupations. The occupational profile's temporal context is most critical in setting outcome measures. To determine outcome measures, the occupational therapist considers the client's future, anticipated occupations, and past occupations. During intervention, the therapist also guides a realistic development of that future occupational vision, and outcome measures are reworked throughout the intervention process as the client and the therapist reconfigure the occupational profile. The outcome is therefore both a product of the occupational profile and a transformative factor in the occupational profile.

The outcome measures arise from the occupational profile, and the client and therapist set goals while exploring the occupational profile together. This is not to say, however, that a successful outcome is a return to a set occupational profile. It is important to remember that the occupational profile is a fluid entity. Indeed, throughout the occupational therapy intervention, the profile continues to transform. The client factors may have changed, the interventions may have changed the makeup of the activities, and the intervention may have modified the context or environment of the occupations. Even when body function has returned to normal and the

---

EXERCISE 5.7: OUTCOMES FROM THE OCCUPATIONAL PROFILE

Review several of the cases presented in this chapter (i.e., Maria, Maureen, Alex, Daniel, Ling Mei, Martha, Enrique, Penny, and George). Identify appropriate outcome measures for each.

---

occupations are performed in the same context as they were previously, the meaning of these occupations to the client has changed because of his or her experiences during the occupational therapy intervention. The outcome measures stemmed from the occupational profile; nevertheless, the outcome itself is part of the new occupational profile.

Conclusion

The occupational therapy profile is a useful tool to gain information about a client's occupations, and it is critical for planning and implementing occupational therapy interventions. The occupational profile provides a structured process for obtaining information about a client's set of activities, routines, and roles. Using the information obtained from the occupational profile, a therapist is able to determine meaningful therapeutic goals that reflect the client's values and needs.

References

American Occupational Therapy Association. (1997). Statement—Fundamental concepts of occupational therapy: Occupation, purposeful activity, and function. *American Journal of Occupational Therapy, 51,* 864–866.

American Occupational Therapy Association. (2008). Occupational therapy practice framework: Domain and process (2nd ed.). *American Journal of Occupational Therapy, 62,* 625–683.

Clark, F. (1993). Occupation embedded in a real life: Interweaving occupational science and occupational therapy [Eleanor Clarke Slagle Lecture]. *American Journal of Occupational Therapy, 47,* 1067–1078.

Kielhofner, G. (1983). Occupation. In H. L. Hopkins & H. D. Smith (Eds.), *Willard and Spackman's occupational therapy* (6th ed., pp. 31–41). Philadelphia: J. B. Lippincott.

Kielhofner, G. (Ed.). (1985). *A Model of Human Occupation: Theory and application.* Baltimore: Lippincott Williams & Wilkins.

Kielhofner, G. (1992). *Conceptual foundations of occupational therapy.* Philadelphia: F. A. Davis.

Kielhofner, G. (2008) *Model of Human Occupation: Theory and application* (4th ed.). Philadelphia: F. A. Davis.

Kramer, P., Hinojosa, J., & Royeen, C. B. (Eds.). (2003). *Perspectives in human occupation: Participation in life.* Philadelphia: Lippincott Williams & Wilkins.

Morris, J. (1994). Spinal injury and psychotherapy in treatment philosophy. In G. M. Yarkony (Ed.), *Spinal cord injury: Medical management and rehabilitation* (pp. 223–229). Gaithersburg, MD: Aspen.

Nelson, D. L. (1996). Therapeutic occupation: A definition. *American Journal of Occupational Therapy, 50,* 775–782.

Trombly, C. A. (1995). Occupation: Purposefulness and meaningfulness as therapeutic mechanisms [Eleanor Clarke Slagle Lecture]. *American Journal of Occupational Therapy, 49,* 960–972.

Urban, J. (1998a). *A critical analysis of "cultural sensitivity" in health care practice.* Unpublished master's thesis, Hunter College of the City University of New York, New York.

Urban, J. (1998b, June 3). *Cultural issues in occupational therapy.* Paper presented at the 12th International Congress of the World Federation of Occupational Therapists, Montreal, Quebec, Canada.

6

Activity Synthesis as a Means to Occupation

Paula Kramer, PhD, OTR, FAOTA
Jim Hinojosa, PhD, OT, FAOTA

The magician's sleight of hand is smooth and sinuous, creating the illusion of a reality that is not really there. The audience members watch in awe, trying to reconcile the reality that they know exists with what they think they are seeing. It seems so simple, yet creating the illusion is actually very complex (Hunt, 1997). In many ways, the magician's act mirrors the activity synthesis carried out by an occupational therapist or occupational therapy assistant. Make no mistake, the practitioner does not perform magic. Rather, he or she puts so much thought and skill into developing and creating activities that the client's experience becomes seamless, much akin to observing the misleading simplicity of a magician's illusions.

Activity synthesis occurs in everyday life, yet people generally do not conceptualize the development of activities as synthesis in any special way. Occupational therapists, however, view activities and their synthesis in a complex and theoretical manner while still building activities on what people do on a daily basis. Throughout this chapter, we view activity synthesis as a means to advance a client's ability to participate in occupations. Despite the fact that activity synthesis is thus central to the art and practice of occupational therapy, very little has been written specifically about this aspect of intervention. In this chapter, we delve into the myriad concerns and reasoning processes involved in activity synthesis in occupational therapy, with particular attention to the importance of gaining an understanding of a client's specific occupations.

Activity Synthesis in Everyday Life

All thought, in its early stages, begins as action. The actions which you have been wading through have been ideas . . . but they had to be established as a foundation before we could begin to think in earnest. (White, 1977, p. 11)

Activity synthesis is not unique to occupational therapy. It occurs in everyday life, albeit in a much more simple form. At the most basic level, *synthesis* is simply changing or creating an activity so that a person may engage in it successfully. For example, when an occupational therapist or occupational therapy assistant presents a task to a child and encounters resistance, he or she will often change or modify the task to engage the child and diminish the resistance. Many young children, for instance, do not like to have clothes put on over their heads because it occludes their eyes. When a parent turns this task into a game, for example by saying "Where did Johnny go?" while putting the shirt over the child's head, the child will often laugh rather than be frightened. This parent has just synthesized the activity by modifying it to prompt the child's engagement with the task, leading to a successful outcome. As another example, if a person becomes tired while performing a task standing up, he or she will try to find a way to do the same task sitting down. This could be as simple as pulling up a chair, or it might require moving the activity to a counter or table at a different height so that the task can be done sitting down (Figures 6.1a and 6.1b). In other words, synthesizing activities is something that people take for granted—people often modify, adapt, or alter activities without even thinking.

Activity Synthesis in Occupational Therapy

Although people naturally modify activities in this relatively unconscious manner, they do not generally adapt the activity in an organized fashion. No

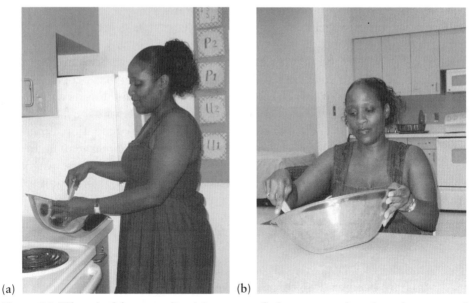

(a)   (b)

Figure 6.1. When tired from standing (**a**), a person finds a way to adapt the task to a seated position (**b**).

theoretical rationale exists for the adaptation of the activity, and the person instead relies on what appears to be common sense. In doing so, people tend to look for a simple change in the activity that will bring about success rather than looking critically at the activity as a whole. Occupational therapists, however, use activity synthesis in an organized manner, often determined by the frame of reference or theoretical perspective they are using to guide their intervention. Therapists provide intervention on the basis of specific theoretical perspectives. Therapists' theoretical perspective directs them in the use of specific tools during the intervention.

Theoretical Perspectives in Activity Synthesis

How do occupational therapists and occupational therapy assistants use activity synthesis as part of their intervention? Where does activity synthesis fit into the overall intervention process? As presented in this chapter, *activity synthesis* involves and encompasses a complex reasoning process that guides practitioners in how activities are used. It is important to use activity synthesis in an intervention within a frame of reference or theoretical context. Occupational therapy intervention is indeed based on theoretical perspectives, frequently referred to by a variety of different names (including *models of practice, theoretical orientations, guidelines for intervention,* or *frames of reference*). In this chapter, we use *frames of reference* to include all interventions that are theoretically based.

Activity synthesis, therefore, is based on the practitioner's skills and abilities, his or her understanding of the client and the client's needs, the context in which the activity will occur, and the frame of reference that the therapist has determined to be the most appropriate for the client. Use of the frame of reference forces the synthesis to take place in the context of theoretical information that guides what is actually done. Thus, activities are used, adapted, modified, or created within the parameters of a chosen frame of reference.

Case Scenario 6.1: Juan

Juan, an 8-year-old boy, was referred to occupational therapy for a handwriting problem. After a comprehensive evaluation, the occupational therapist assigned Juan to an occupational therapy assistant to implement a program to develop hand coordination for writing based on muscle strengthening. Thus, a sensorimotor frame of reference was chosen. The therapist selected this frame of reference because she had determined that Juan had poor muscle strength and limited experience with fine motor activities. The intervention must be carried out within the context of Juan's

(continued)

Case Scenario 6.1: Juan *(cont.)*

class. After meeting Juan, reviewing the recommendations, and discussing the frame of reference with the therapist, the occupational therapy assistant uses activity analysis and synthesis to develop activities for Juan. These activities involve Juan's using an adapted pencil for writing and paper with raised lines that will give him increased sensory feedback. In addition, the assistant observed the computer-based activities used in the classroom. After careful analysis of these computer-based activities, the assistant decided to replace Juan's keyboard with one that provides more resistance. The keyboard was also raised so that Juan must use more shoulder motion while working on the computer.

If a different frame of reference (such as one based on play and theories of psychosocial development outside the classroom environment) had been chosen, then a different approach would have been used. The focus would be on Juan's personal interests, analyzing those purposeful activities, and synthesizing activities in response. For instance, the occupational therapy assistant might observe that Juan enjoys the game Connect Four.® The objective of this game is to pick up small checkers and put them into a vertical form to line up four in a row. An understanding of theories of psychosocial development suggests that an 8-year-old boy would be expected to relate to others in a competitive manner. Therefore, the occupational therapy assistant involves Juan in creating a new competitive game based on Connect Four. Guided by the psychosocial frame of reference, the assistant then competes with Juan in the newly adapted game. To make the game address some of Juan's motor needs, they decide to place the checkers under various heavy objects around the room, forcing Juan to develop his strength. In addition, before putting the checker in the vertical form, Juan and the assistant must attempt to balance themselves prone over a small ball, using the nondominant hand to balance and support their weight. Thus, guided by the psychosocial development frame of reference, the assistant has synthesized an activity that will be both engaging for Juan in terms of his stage of development and therapeutically valuable for his particular motor needs.

In such a way, all occupational therapy practice should be based on theoretical information or rationales. Activity synthesis is no exception. It should be undertaken by the practitioner within the context of the theoretical information; it is not separate or outside of the theoretical framework but is guided by it throughout the process.

Activity analysis and synthesis have long been considered important tools for occupational therapists and occupational therapy assistants (Mosey, 1981). They have been discussed as separate processes that are associated with providing the practitioner with the means to understand and use pur-

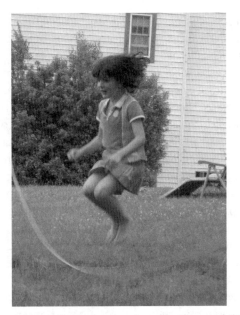

Figure 6.2. Jumping rope is a complex task to analyze. Teaching a child to jump rope involves synthesis.

poseful activities successfully; the two processes (activity analysis and activity synthesis) are used together for the client's benefit. Interestingly, in occupational therapy professional education much time is spent on activity analysis, and very little time is spent on activity synthesis. Hence, students and clinicians get the impression that activity analysis is more important and significant to the intervention process than is activity synthesis (Figure 6.2).

The assumption is that once the clinician understands the step or stage of a task that is problematic to the client, intervention can take place, and the client will then work toward the successful completion of the task. However, the assumption that synthesis is unimportant is not accurate; in fact, a constant interplay exists between analysis and synthesis. Indeed, Nelson (1997) characterized occupational analysis as "what occupational therapists do" (p. 15), thus noting the importance of synthesis as interconnected with analysis rather than separate from it. Synthesis is considered to be an intellectual process and part of the clinical reasoning and decision-making aspects of practice (Mosey, 1996; Nelson & Jepsen-Thomas, 2003).

Perspectives on Occupation and Client Participation

From a therapeutic perspective, activity synthesis begins with conceptualizing the activities the client wants or needs to perform. Responsibility rests with the client and the practitioner to determine the importance of these actions, to think them through carefully, and to use this knowledge as the foundation for activity synthesis.

Let us take a step backward. Before analysis or synthesis can take place, the clinician needs to understand the client and his or her life situation, which involves understanding the client's personal goals, desires, capacities, and limitations. Personal goals and desires may depend on context, and in some cases they may be those of the family or society and may depend on certain life circumstances. Goals and desires then need to be explored within the context of capacities and limitations, for although one may be have desire to achieve something, the capacity for that goal may not be present. Activities can be synthesized effectively only once the practitioner has a clear understanding of the client, his or her life, and all the contextual factors that affect this client (Figure 6.3).

Identifying and defining potential goals for the intervention require negotiation and collaboration between the client and the practitioner. This process goes two ways, and each person involved brings his or her own perspective: The practitioner brings a clinical understanding of the client's condition from a medical and psychosocial perspective and an understanding of the potential sequela of the disease, and the client brings his or her unique sense of self and an understanding of his or her own aspirations, along with the drive to achieve the goal. Together, the practitioner and client develop goals that define the course of treatment and the outcomes of intervention. Ideally, the goals should relate to the occupations that the person currently wants to carry out or will engage in in the future and should be oriented to the ability to participate in life and society.

The next step is to complete an activity analysis to give the occupational therapist or occupational therapy assistant a rudimentary understanding of the tasks that might be adapted or changed. With this information, the therapist can begin to design or create activities that meet the client's needs. The therapist synthesizes an activity that is consistent with the theoretical perspective, model,

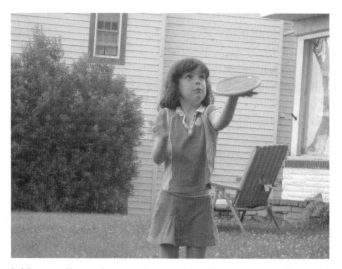

Figure 6.3. A child naturally synthesizes the activity of learning to catch a Frisbee—but it can still be scary!

or frame of reference that has been selected to guide the therapist's interventions with the client. The theoretical perspective determines how and in what ways an activity is synthesized in the therapeutic situation. Putting together the therapist's professional knowledge, the expected outcomes of the therapeutic process, and the client's (or family's) mutually agreed-on goals, the synthesis begins.

Process of Activity Synthesis in Occupational Therapy

When the activity analysis is complete and the theoretical perspective has been considered, the activity synthesis can begin in earnest. This process starts with defining the key elements of the activity because one can adapt an activity only so much until it becomes a different activity. For example, is it still baking if no oven or heat is involved? Is it still baseball without a ball and bat? When these key elements are no longer present, the activity is no longer the same. Once the activities are created and presented to the client, the therapist observes the client's performance and continually reanalyzes it to adapt and resynthesize the activity to meet the client's changing needs and to move toward the end goal. The process is thus ongoing and dynamic: Sometimes the activity needs to be reconstructed or synthesized in a different way to allow the client to be successful. The dynamic nature of this process shows that analyzing the activity is not enough—understanding how one can construct or synthesize and resynthesize an activity is equally important. Therefore, both activity analysis and activity synthesis are important tools for occupational therapists and occupational therapy assistants.

It is important to remember that synthesis involves more than just the activity itself; it involves the personal meaning of the activity. As discussed earlier, practitioners view synthesis in the context of the person as an occupational being. They ask the following questions: Who is the person involved in the intervention process? What occupations are important to this person? How do specific purposeful activities relate to these occupations? Does the accomplishment of a purposeful activity build on or allow this person to engage in meaningful occupations at his or her current stage of life or in the future? The creative process of synthesis requires a thorough understanding of the activity and a visualization of the goal and the desired end product.

As noted at the beginning of this chapter, occupational therapists and occupational therapy assistants have an organized conceptual approach to activity synthesis. The activity is viewed as a whole, and an activity analysis is done to break it down into component parts. The final step in the process is to synthesize or re-create the activity with change, modification, or adaptation to allow the client to achieve success in the task. Traditional activity synthesis requires that the chosen activity be reconstructed, incorporating the client's therapeutic goals, areas of strength and limitations, and the therapeutic relationship. The activity is reconfigured in ways that allow the client to approach it with minimal fear of failure and with greater potential for success. We should also note at this point that activity synthesis can be used for various purposes: as an evaluative tool or within the intervention process. More specifically, activity synthesis can be used to evaluate performance within a context, teach a new skill, refine a skill, or maintain a client's functional status or performance ability. These applications of activity synthesis are discussed later in this chapter.

For occupational therapists and occupational therapy assistants, activity synthesis is a complex process of adapting and grading activities, modifying activities, and creating new activities. In the next section, we discuss the processes involved in activity synthesis: adapting and grading activities, modifying activities, and creating new activities. Although we address each process individually as though it is distinct from the others, in practice one or more processes may be used in combination; they overlap and are not mutually exclusive. As with learning any process, it is important that each component (process) be appreciated and understood in relation to the others. By understanding the components of activity synthesis, one can attain a distinct knowledge of the whole process of synthesis.

ADAPTING AND GRADING ACTIVITIES

Adaptation involves a change to the environment or the activity, not a change to the person. Adaptation of activities, therefore, involves changing the environment in which the activity occurs or the activity itself rather than working to bring about change in the person doing the activity. When a client has difficulty with a task or activity, the activity is adapted for the client. This process begins with an activity analysis that considers the capabilities of the client, the activity, and the context in which it will be done. After analyzing the activity or completing the activity analysis, the therapist uses the theoretical perspective to decide how the activity should be adapted or changed to meet the client's abilities, allowing the client to perform the activity in a specific context. For example, with a rehabilitation frame of reference, the therapist can simply provide the client with a spoon with an adapted handle, have the client change his or her position when engaging in the task, or have the client sit down during the activity for energy conservation. If the therapist selected a different theoretical perspective, the adaptation could also involve a more complicated process in which defining features of the activity itself are changed. Theoretical perspective thus guides the adaptation process.

EXERCISE 6.1: ADAPTATION

Think about an activity that you adapted to make your life easier. Reflect on the adaptation. How did you deduce the appropriate adaptations? Because you knew your capabilities and had a goal in mind, how did that influence the way you approached the adaptation?

EXERCISE 6.2: ADAPTING AN ACTIVITY FROM A BIOMECHANICAL PERSPECTIVE

Observe children playing in a playground or a schoolyard. Select one activity in which they are engaged. Using a biomechanical perspective, how would you adapt the activity so that a child in a wheelchair could participate?

EXERCISE 6.3: ADAPTING AN ACTIVITY USING A SENSORY INTEGRATION FRAME OF REFERENCE

Adapt a playground activity for a child with tactile defensiveness using a sensory integration frame of reference.

Grading is a common way to adapt an activity. Although it is a basic principle in learning theory, occupational therapists and occupational therapy assistants almost universally use grading. For this reason, it is critical to think about grading and how it is used in the context of specific theories that guide intervention. Grading can involve simplifying the activity, making the activity more complex, modifying the sequence or physical nature of the activity, or modifying the amount of time taken to complete the task. Simplifying the activity (also known as *grading the activity down*) entails making the activity easier for the client in some way. For a child who is learning how to undress him or herself (an acquisitional frame of reference), grading might involve having the parent roll down the sock from the heel and then have the child pull it off or open pants fastenings and then have the child remove the pants. In this case, the practitioner does part of the task and allows the child to do the remainder. Once the child has accomplished a certain segment of the task, the task can be made slightly more difficult, thus grading the activity up rather than down. Grading a task down allows the client to feel successful and gain confidence so that he or she becomes willing to try more difficult tasks, develop skills, or build on a previously acquired level of skill.

EXERCISE 6.4: GRADING AN ACTIVITY

Select an activity at which you are very competent but that one of your peers cannot perform. For example, if you are good at playing chess or the piano or at baking, then select a peer who does not know the rules of chess, how to play the piano, or how to bake. Develop and carry out one teaching session with that person. How did you grade the activity so that the other person would have a positive learning experience? How would you have graded the activity for a different person?

Whether adapting or grading, theoretical perspectives often require that the physical nature of an activity be changed by modifying the materials used in a task. From a developmental perspective, for example, if a child has difficulty building with wooden blocks because they are hard for him or her to grasp and lift, then smaller foam blocks could be provided that are lighter and easier to handle. This adaptation allows the child to play with blocks without having adequate grasp or strength for lifting. The adaptation here is grading the activity down so that the child can participate in the block building despite having limited strength and grasping ability.

MODIFYING ACTIVITIES

Activity modification does not involve changing the activity itself, but rather changing the way the activity is done. The purpose and goal of the activity remain the same, but the sequence or time requirements of the tasks encompassed in the activity may be altered. Modifying the sequence of tasks involves changing the order in which tasks are done so that the person can engage in the task more successfully. This approach is frequently used for energy conservation. For example, to avoid energy depletion caused by a client repeatedly walking up and down stairs or back and forth across a room, the client can change the order in which he or she performs activities of daily living (ADLs) tasks. Modifying the activity may also mean moving the venue of the activity from the kitchen counter, where the client has to stand to complete the activity, to the kitchen table, where the client can complete the task while sitting down. Another type of activity modification may involve scaling the activity, like finishing part of a puzzle (e.g., the outer edges of the puzzle or one section) rather than the whole puzzle.

Performance (the actual doing) of tasks involves a time factor. To be functional, tasks have to be done either within a specified amount of time or at a specific time of the day or year. For example, a child's spending a half hour putting on a shirt would not be considered functional. In the therapeutic environment, the timing of a task can be modified or the time requirements of a task or activity can be changed: A client can take longer to complete a task without repercussions, or dressing can be done

---

EXERCISE 6.5: ALTERING THE SEQUENCE OF TASKS

Think about the way in which you accomplish the self-care occupation of getting ready for work in the morning. List the tasks that you do to accomplish each activity (e.g., personal hygiene, selecting clothes, dressing). Select one activity. Consider how you would change the sequence of the task if you had to get ready in a shorter period of time one morning.

EXERCISE 6.6: ALTERING THE TIMING OF TASKS

Select an activity at which you are very skilled. Determine how much time it takes you to do the activity from beginning to end. Divide the time in half and do the activity. How does it affect your performance? Now, double the time that it takes to do the activity. How does this affect your performance?

---

in the middle of the day rather than in the morning. Once a client has mastered an activity within an extended time frame, the time allotted can be decreased. The following example illustrates the use of time to modify an activity: When working with a child who is learning to put on a pullover shirt, the child might be allowed to take as much time as he or she needs. Slowly, a time requirement would be added. After the child has mastered putting on the pullover shirt in a reasonable amount of time, he or she might be asked to put on a button-down shirt in the same amount of time, even though this shirt is more difficult to put on. In this way, the task of putting on a shirt is made more challenging by the use of layered adaptation. Each successive task in this scenario is more complex than the previous one, with time becoming a more important component of the task at each stage.

CREATING NEW ACTIVITIES

The most complex type of activity synthesis is creating new activities. This synthesis occurs after the practitioner evaluates a client and determines the areas that require intervention. In response to the evaluation, the practitioner creates an activity specifically for the client. The therapist can engage in creating new activities in two different ways. First, the creation of an activity may arise from the practitioner's responsibility to present a specific level of challenge to the client and thus promote growth. The other type of creation may be based on the client's occupational needs and desires to move to a certain level. It is important to note that creating an activity is on a different plane from grading and adapting because an entirely new activity will emerge from this process rather than a modification of the previous activity.

Some theoretical perspectives and frames of reference, such as neuro-developmental treatment and sensory integration, almost define the role of the therapist as the creator of activities. This places responsibility on the practitioner; the role of the therapist is based on the client's therapeutic needs, and the goal of the frame of reference is to promote future growth and skills. From this perspective, client collaboration is secondary and derived from engagement in the task: If the client does not engage, the therapist must create new activities to entice the client.

In other theoretical perspectives and frames of reference, such as occupational adaptation and occupational performance, the creation of activities comes from the client and is based on perceived occupational needs rather than therapeutic needs per se. This synthesis requires skill, creativity, and an in-depth understanding of the client. The resultant activity is based on an understanding of the client's interests, problem areas, and goals. It is not based on activity analysis but is client centered and has a "just-right" fit for the client. In this type of synthesis, the nonhuman environment plays a very important role. The practitioner, therefore, must gain an understanding of both the human and the nonhuman environment of the client's occupations to create activities that will engage the client. For example, if the client has a special pet and the practitioner can involve the care of that pet in an aspect of the intervention, then the client will be more likely to engage in that intervention (Figure 6.4).

CASE SCENARIO 6.2: JANET

Janet, a woman with multiple sclerosis, is confined to a wheelchair and resides in a nursing home. Before she came to the nursing home, she raised several dogs who were very important to her. The nursing home has a pet therapy dog, and the occupational therapist found that Janet was much more likely to come to groups when the therapy dog was present. The therapist's understanding of Janet's interest in pets allows him or her to design activities that will fit with Janet's interest.

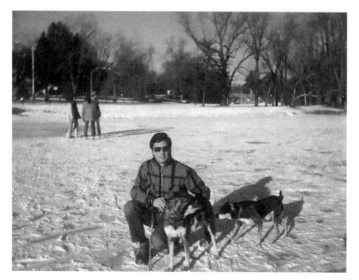

Figure 6.4. Sometimes the presence of a pet can make it easier to engage in an activity.

EXERCISE 6.7: CREATING A NEW ACTIVITY

Identify a skill, such as grasping fork and using it for self-feeding, that needs to be developed. Determine a goal that you have that is related to the development of that skill. After selecting the skill, look around your home and develop an original activity in which you could engage that would develop the skill.

EXERCISE 6.8: CREATING NEW ACTIVITIES WITH DEFINED DEVELOPMENTAL GOALS

You have been hired to work in a new occupational therapy practice with limited space and materials. All that you have in the treatment environment are two chairs and one small table. You also have in the supply closet masking tape, a box of colored 1-in. blocks, and two boxes with 12 (unsharpened) pencils each. You have two children scheduled for the day: Steven, a 19-month-old boy with developmental delays who functions at about a 9-month developmental level, and Shana, a 3-year-old girl with cerebral palsy spastic diplegia. Develop goals for a treatment session for Steven and Shana and develop an activity using only the materials, supplies, and environment described.

EXERCISE 6.9: CREATING NEW ACTIVITIES ON THE BASIS OF THE CLIENT'S NEEDS

Diego is a 12-year-old child with attention deficit hyperactivity disorder. He wants to join the local Little League team but needs to develop basic skills in baseball and self-control. Create an activity that will move Diego toward his goal of playing on the team.

Activity Synthesis in the Context of Occupation

All these activity synthesis scenarios require skill on the part of the occupational therapist or occupational therapy assistant. First, why is this activity important to the client? How does this activity relate to the client's occupations? What role will it play in his or her life? How will it help the client to engage in meaningful occupations? Determining the answers to these questions allows the practitioner to understand the activity and its relationship to the client's occupations. To accomplish this successfully entails engaging the client, developing rapport, and developing an understanding of who the client is as an individual. Then, using the creative process within a theoretical framework, the practitioner devises or synthesizes activities that will meet the client's needs. If the client has no interest in the activity or does not see it as meaningful to his or her life, then he or she will only go through the actions with no personal investment. Moreover, the client may not be self-motivated to participate in the activity at all, and its therapeutic value will thus be minimized. In sum, for the intervention to be successful, the synthesis of activities has to take the client into account. Some theoretical perspectives explicitly address the client's personal motivation, and others address the meaningfulness of the activity to the client. On the basis of the client-centered nature of occupational therapy, the therapist needs to explore the value of the occupation to the client and his or her personal choices in terms of occupations. If the client values the occupation, the chance that he or she will be motivated to engage in that occupation is greater. When motivation is not a major concept in the theoretical framework chosen, other theoretical perspectives may need to be introduced to explore personal motivation. Occupational therapists and occupational therapy assistants should not make assumptions about a client's motivation, nor should they just choose occupations for the client. Context should also be considered when the synthesis of activities is related to intervention because the ultimate goal is for the client to be able to perform the activity in the real world, not just in the simulated environment of the occupational therapy practice setting.

Importance of Activity Synthesis to Intervention

It is often difficult for a person to change or modify the way in which he or she does particular tasks, especially when he or she has engaged in those tasks for many years. Even if completing the task in the usual manner becomes very difficult, change may still be hard to accept. If a person is accustomed to preparing a meal standing at the kitchen counter and then develops limited standing tolerance, he or she can move that meal preparation to the kitchen table to complete the task sitting down. This is likely to be an acceptable modification. Yet it is sometimes difficult for people to make adjustments and modifications to their occupations if the modification alters the value or enjoyment they derive from them. For example, when cleaning one's home becomes too strenuous or difficult, some obvious options include getting assistance from others, cleaning one room each day until all are done, or doing minimal cleaning. Some of these options may be more acceptable than other options. For some people, getting assistance with cleaning is not an acceptable option because cleaning has been one of their life's occupations or a source of enjoyment and pride. For others, doing minimal cleaning may not be acceptable because of their personal beliefs or their desired standard of living. The case scenario of Betty illustrates a person successfully adapting an activity to make it easier, yet in a way that retains the value of the occupation for that person.

CASE SCENARIO *6.3:* BETTY

Betty had collected porcelain figurines over the years, and she liked to clean them periodically. These objects, however, were displayed on high shelves, well out of reach without climbing on a ladder. She did her own analysis of the task: As a senior citizen, she was aware that climbing on a ladder was no longer an acceptable option because she would risk falling and injuring herself. She considered hiring someone to do the task for her, yet her collection was personally valuable to her and she did not like the thought of other people handling the objects. Betty thus hired someone to help her but was very clear in defining this person's role in the task. The helper was to climb the ladder to retrieve the objects from the shelf, and Betty would then wash them and direct how they were to be put back in place. This modification of the activity allowed Betty to have control over the task and to handle the things that were precious to her while avoiding the aspects of the activity that were difficult and potentially dangerous. Betty synthesized the revised activity in a way that is acceptable to and safe for her.

Other Uses of Activity Synthesis in Intervention

Up to this point, we have discussed activity synthesis as an intervention process used to bring about change in the client. We have stressed the use of theoretical grounding in this process. Indeed, occupational therapists and occupational therapy assistants typically think about activity synthesis as a tool for treating a client. It is generally a medium that is used to improve function once a deficit has been identified. Activity synthesis can, however, be used creatively in many more ways. As discussed previously, it can be used as a tool with which to evaluate client performance. We also noted earlier in the chapter that activity synthesis may be used to teach a new skill, to refine a skill, and to maintain functional status or performance abilities. The next section presents the use of activity synthesis for these various purposes.

EVALUATION OF PERFORMANCE

Activity synthesis can assist the therapist in evaluating a client's performance within a certain context. The therapist may first see whether a child can close a zipper on a doll or on an ADL board. The therapist may then observe the child's ability to close a zipper on his or her own clothing. It may be easy for a child to close a zipper on an ADL board or on a doll, but it is critical for the child to be able to close a zipper on his or her own coat. The therapist uses the synthesized activity to evaluate the child's performance within two different contexts and by doing so can determine whether intervention is necessary and how to intervene.

CASE SCENARIO 6.4: BOB

A therapist works with Bob on developing social skills. In a group, Bob role-plays purchasing an item in a store. During the role playing, the therapist observes how Bob handles himself, whether his verbalizations are appropriate, and his ability to count out money to pay for the item. On the basis of Bob's ability to perform in the role-playing situation, the therapist can take Bob into an actual store and observe his abilities in a real context rather than a simulated situation. The therapist uses these observations to give feedback to Bob and to develop a plan for intervention. The therapist can also point out to Bob the differences in his performance in the simulated situation and in the real-life activity to help set mutually acceptable goals for performance.

TEACHING NEW SKILLS

Using learning theories, a practitioner can use synthesis to teach new skills. This type of intervention is what an occupational therapist or occupational therapy assistant typically thinks of as activity synthesis. How does one devise a meaningful activity that will assist the client in developing new skills? Expanding on a previous example, when teaching a child to fasten clothes, the practitioner may first work on the skill in isolation with a doll and then make it more complex by applying the skill to the child's own clothes. In this situation, the practitioner is identifying the skills that need to be developed and creating activities that will promote the development of that new skill.

REFINING SKILLS

Similarly, a practitioner can use activity synthesis to refine a skill, again using learning theories. Once the client has attained a basic skill level, the practitioner can enhance and embellish the activity to make the skill level required more complex. When working on developing communication skills with a cli-

---

CASE SCENARIO 6.5: AYISHA

Ayisha has difficulties with money management skills. She does not watch how much money she gives to the store clerk and does not count her change. The therapist uses an acquisitional frame of reference and sets up a simulated store. Ayisha must pay for everything that she wants from the store, and the therapist works with her on money management within this context. Periodically, the therapist takes on the role of consumer and has Ayisha take on the role of cashier. Through this activity, the therapist can begin to teach Ayisha the basic skills necessary for developing the ability to manage her money.

CASE SCENARIO 6.6: SAM

Sam is developing social skills in a group doing role playing. He then tries out the skills he has acquired in a real situation. The therapist works with Sam on refining his behavior in the real-world environment. Is he dressed appropriately to go out shopping? Does he make eye contact with store personnel? Can he ask questions appropriately if he needs to find an item he wants to purchase? Can he handle money responsibly?

---

ent with psychosocial dysfunction, the practitioner might first work on having the client say "Good morning" to others in a protected environment, such as a therapy group, and then work on conducting an entire conversation. Although the activity synthesis might begin in a protected environment, eventually the skills would need to be tested in the real world to determine their viability.

In both the preceding discussion and the case scenario of Sam, the therapist continually resynthesizes the activity to increase the demands on the client and refine the skills necessary for application in the real world. In essence, by grading up the task, the therapist is synthesizing the activity to meet new goals.

MAINTAINING FUNCTIONAL STATUS OR PERFORMANCE ABILITIES

Synthesis can be used to maintain a person's functional status or performance ability. If a client has been working on strengthening her hands and has achieved an acceptable level of strength, then it would be incumbent on the practitioner to work with the client to synthesize activities that would maintain that level of strength after completion of intervention. The therapist would first need to understand the client's meaningful occupations and then within this understanding synthesize activities that would be of sufficient interest to the client so that she would want to continue doing them to maintain her hand strength.

CASE SCENARIO 6.7: OLIVIA

Olivia has had difficulty with range of motion in her shoulder. She has received intervention and has been responsive to therapy. She can now raise her arms to 180° of shoulder flexion. The therapist initially suggested that Olivia do certain exercises to maintain function and ability, but Olivia did not follow through on the exercise program. During a subsequent home visit, the therapist suggested that Olivia place the dishes that she uses most often on the second shelf of her cabinets so that she would have to reach for them. Olivia was willing to do this because it was more meaningful to her than doing specific exercises, even though she understood their value. Thus, the maintenance of her shoulder range became a part of her everyday life (Figures 6.5a and 6.5b).

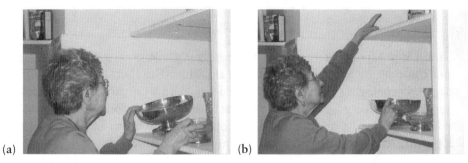

Figure 6.5. Dishes are placed on the second shelf (a) to maintain shoulder range of motion (b).

This case scenario shows that if the activities devised by the occupational therapist or occupational therapy assistant hold no interest for the client, the client subsequently has little incentive to continue with them. Therefore, synthesized activities should incorporate purposeful and meaningful occupations for the client to maximize their success. As another example, squeezing Theraputty may not be a meaningful occupation for a particular individual, but molding clay into animals that could be given as gifts might be more purposeful, enjoyable, and rewarding. In this case, activity synthesis is based on the fundamental assumption of the profession rather than on a theoretical perspective: As occupational therapists, we believe that engagement in occupations keeps people healthy. A fundamental assumption of occupational therapy is that people are more likely to engage in activities that are meaningful to them; in other words, these activities are purposeful. Therefore, primary goals of the occupational therapy process are not only to assist people in finding meaningful occupations but also to help them maintain and restore function so that they can engage in these meaningful occupations and to facilitate the exploration of various means by which people might continue to engage in their chosen occupations.

ACTIVITY SYNTHESIS FOR HEALTH PROMOTION AND PREVENTION

Occupational therapy practitioners have a responsibility that goes beyond intervention to promote health in the client. Activity synthesis is an important tool in this process in which the therapist can take an active role with the client, collaborating on the developing of activities to promote health. Synthesis may be necessary to develop activities that will assist the client to meet goals and optimize their lifestyle. With the knowledge that the occupational therapist gains concerning the client's desires and abilities, he or she can assist in developing specific activities that will maintain physical, mental, and social health. For example, through activity synthesis, the occupational therapist can customize activities that will promote continued engagement in social activities, reinforcing participation. Synthesis may take many forms. For example, the therapist may encourage clients to participate in a community center or may customize a home exercise program to address specific needs and abilities.

Artful Practice and Activity Synthesis

In the synthesis of activities, the practitioner needs to be artful in developing or choosing an activity that suits the client's needs from a functional perspective and the client's interests from a personal perspective. If both needs and interests are not met, then the activity will not be successful in achieving its goal. The occupational therapist or occupational therapy assistant first takes the time to learn about the client, focusing on who he or she is as a person and his or her strengths and limitations. Then the practitioner, with the client's input, identifies goals for the client and the intervention, which may involve analyzing the client's performance in particular activities and identifying performance components that are interfering with successful completion of the task. It may also involve some aspect of client education to increase the client's awareness of how performance can be improved or how performance in a particular area is affecting overall functioning. Activities are then synthesized with the client so that they are meaningful and beneficial to him or her. Gaining the client's input at this stage of the intervention is key.

It is important to remember that synthesis is not concrete: It does not follow a step-by-step process and may be undertaken in many different ways. Several elements, however, should be present for synthesis to be successful. These elements are developing an understanding of the client, including what is important to this person and his or her meaningful occupations; analyzing activities to determine how deficits are interfering with performance; and selecting a frame of reference that will help the client to overcome his or her deficits. Additionally, together with the client, the practitioner identifies or devises activities that will help the client to overcome his or her deficits or develop the skills necessary for successful task performance.

CASE SCENARIO 6.8: JANAY

Janay has a weakness in her hands. When first synthesizing activities for Janay, the therapist considered using modeling clay as a therapeutic intervention, but Janay showed no interest in working with clay. She enjoys baking, however, and has expressed an interest in learning to bake bread. Baking bread requires kneading the dough, which will strengthen Janay's hands. Thus, baking bread has therapeutic value and is also a meaningful and pleasurable activity for Janay. The successful meeting of the therapeutic and personal needs specific to Janay and her situation will potentially lead to a more successful intervention.

EXERCISE 6.10: SYNTHESIZING ACTIVITIES USING A FRAME OF REFERENCE

You have just been assigned to a new client, Malcolm. He has a right hemiplegia secondary to a cerebral vascular hemorrhage. Before this trauma, Malcolm was an engineer in the U.S. Navy. He had a very high-level position designing equipment for ships. His hobbies included building things for his family and home using multiple media (e.g., woodwork, electricity, mechanical devices). Choose a frame of reference or a theoretical perspective and synthesize several activities for this client using the chosen perspective and incorporating Malcolm's personal interests and preferred occupations. Describe the activities and how they reflect both Malcolm's interests and the theoretical perspective you have chosen.

EXERCISE 6.11: ACTIVITY SYNTHESIS IN A CLINICAL ENVIRONMENT

Observe an intervention with a client. Identify the activities that have been synthesized for that client. Try to identify the theoretical perspective or perspectives that provide the foundation for this intervention. Have the activities been synthesized specifically for this particular client? Can you determine the client's investment in the intervention? Are you observing artful practice?

Development of Artful Practice

As discussed earlier, activity synthesis requires artful practice on the part of the occupational therapist or occupational therapy assistant. This is not something that can be taught easily. It is, in part, the product of experience because one does not start out as an artist. One must learn how to use and play with materials; study techniques; develop skill with the materials; and, finally, develop a personal style. These are the prerequisites to becoming an artist. Once a person possesses the basic skills, he or she may be able to develop into an artist, but it will take time, practice, and experience. The same is true of the occupational therapist and occupational therapy assistant. Initially, the practitioner starts out as a novice with a technical or procedural understanding of what is going on with the client. The practitioner develops into an expert with time and experience. He or she learns how to get to know the client quickly and how to use this information to synthesize meaningful occupations for the client. Once the practitioner possesses expert-level skills, he or she can use synthesis as an effective tool and become an artful practitioner.

The clinical reasoning process is part of the art of practice. The practitioner develops reasoning skills in different areas and during different stages of professional development. Some aspects of clinical reasoning include scientific reasoning, narrative reasoning, pragmatic reasoning, and ethical reasoning (Schell, 2003). These different types of reasoning are discussed in depth in Chapter 7, "Clinical Reasoning." Clinical reasoning skills develop as the practitioner matures and reflects on his or her cumulative experiences. Engaging in the practice of synthesis, however, involves more than just reasoning: It involves understanding the client, his or her life, and oneself as a practitioner. Experience contributes to one's ability to be an artful practitioner, enhancing knowledge of different approaches, a range of techniques and responses, and greater interaction skills. Having a multitude of experiences with clients with various disabilities and cultures, and in various settings, expands one's repertoire. The knowledge gathered from experience provides the practitioner with options for intervention and with options for interaction. Such knowledge is not necessarily an expansion of theoretical knowledge but an expansion of practical knowledge and a greater understanding of the self and the human condition—all elements essential to successful and appropriate occupational synthesis. The practitioner needs to be reflective (Schön, 1983) and have a clearer understanding of the role of activity and occupation in the client's life. He or she is then able to creatively match intervention with the client's needs. The art thus comes from within the practitioner, not from a greater understanding of theory (Schell, 2003). It is a personal and professional development, not exclusively an intellectual development.

Although the art of practice does not come from an understanding of theory, it does, however, occur within a theoretical context. The therapist should choose a theoretical framework or frame of reference that will fit the setting, the client's needs, and also the therapist's own knowledge base. The choice of a theoretical approach and, therefore, the choice or synthesis of activities should consider all of these things and not be based on one area alone. Understanding the personal, organizational, and client contexts is critical to effective practice.

Occupational Synthesis

If one practices artfully, then it can be assumed that occupational synthesis will take place. But what exactly is occupational synthesis? Our view of occupational synthesis is that the process takes place within the client: Activity synthesis is performed by the practitioner, whereas occupational synthesis happens internally (and sometimes subconsciously) within the client. At the initiation of occupational therapy services, the client, or his or her significant others, conveys to the therapist those occupations that are meaningful to him or her. The therapist needs to use this knowledge within the intervention process as activity synthesis. Then, once the client has experienced occupational therapy and has engaged in tasks and activities that have improved functional performance, the client develops a sense of which of those activities contribute to personally meaningful occupations. Those occupations become a part of that person—occupations that he or she is willing to continue to take part in to maintain functional performance once occupational therapy is finished. For example, in the case of Olivia, placing the dishes she uses frequently on a higher shelf helped her to maintain the range of motion in her shoulder. If reaching up has become part of her occupational synthesis, then she would keep her dishes on the higher shelf and incorporate this activity into her daily life. The ongoing use of the activity (and its adoption into Olivia's routine) signals that it has been synthesized into her daily life and occupations.

In this view, the occupational therapist or occupational therapy assistant provides activities and options for the client as a means of intervention. The client then incorporates some of these activities into personally meaningful occupations. The occupational synthesis then takes place within the client as the client chooses those occupations to continue as part of everyday life. We should note that the perspective we propose is not consistent with that proposed by Nelson and Jepson-Thomas (2003). They defined *occupational synthesis* as what the practitioner does—they did not use the term *activity* at all. We believe that what the practitioner does is activity synthesis, whereas occupational synthesis occurs within the client.

The artful occupational therapist or occupational therapy assistant creates the circumstances in which occupational synthesis can take place within the client. The practitioner uses his or her knowledge of human occupation integrated with theoretically based guidelines for intervention to provide activities and opportunities that the client then uses for occupational synthesis. The definitive goal of occupational therapy is to provide interventions that will produce the desired changes so that service recipients can participate in occupations that are personally significant to them (Hinojosa, Kramer, Royeen, & Luebben, 2003). They facilitate opportunities for occupational synthesis to occur by providing interventions that are relevant and creative. Again, this synthesis requires a successful interaction between the therapist and the client so that the therapist can gain an understanding of those activities that are meaningful to the client, and the client can give feedback to the therapist on the effectiveness of specific activity syntheses.

Artful practice requires that the practitioner experience the treatment with the client, using his or her own life experience as an active agent of change to design and implement treatments (Weinstein, 1998). As proposed by Schön (1983), the art of professional practice is built on a professional's reflection in action. The practitioner reflects on what is happening during treatment to continually modify, adapt, or change the intervention process or activity. Beyond the theoretical perspective, the practitioner experiences what is happening and is prepared to change strategies spontaneously. This skill does not occur automatically; rather, it is based on both reflection and experience. In some cases, modifying the activity, the environment, or the interaction will help to make the intervention more effective for the client. In other situations when the predicted changes are not happening, the practitioner decides to change the intervention. In these cases, the artful practitioner proposes new hypotheses and implements the revised intervention. These modifications ensure that occupational synthesis takes place and that interventions are also related to the client's future occupations.

When interventions are relevant, the client is able to transpose the tasks or activities easily into his or her real-life occupations. Relevant interventions are judged by two criteria. First, are they appropriate for addressing the client's deficits? Second, are they pertinent to the client's life situation (e.g., goals, values, culture, lifestyle) as defined by the client? Occupational synthesis is more likely to take place when the occupational therapy program is relevant to the client. The practitioner begins this process by considering the following four questions to ensure that the client's life situation is being addressed:

1. Do I understand the client's occupations?
2. Do I respect the client's occupations and personal choices?
3. Do I understand the client's activity patterns, particularly in relation to his or her cultural background, and do I respond to them appropriately?
4. How do my client's occupations influence other people in his or her daily life?

After reflection on this first set of questions, Hinojosa (2003) identified five additional questions that an occupational therapist or occupational therapy assistant might ask to assess the relevance of his or her interventions with regard to the concept of occupation:

1. Are my interventions reflecting an understanding of the client's life situations and his or her culture?
2. Have I developed an understanding of my client's occupations through discussions with him or her?
3. Have I considered clear ethical reasoning when developing my interventions within the context of the client's goals, priorities, and capacities?
4. Are my interventions based on an understanding of how the client defines his or her occupations?
5. Do my interventions result in enabling the client to engage in occupations and increase his or her life satisfaction?

Developing meaningful intervention using synthesis is a complex process. The practitioner usually starts by developing an understanding of activity synthesis. At the same time, he or she is developing sound clinical reasoning skills and, over time, gaining experience to develop the art of practice. With experience, the practitioner comes to understand the client's critical role and his or her unique situation. This process is not necessarily linear, but it is one that takes time and experience to develop. Once this development has occurred, occupational synthesis can be facilitated, and intervention becomes truly meaningful. The ultimate demonstration and most valuable outcome of occupational synthesis can be observed when the client engages in his or her chosen occupations in real life rather than in an artificial clinical situation.

Summary

Activity synthesis is a common phenomenon that occurs in everyday life. People have many occupations and activities that are meaningful to them, and they modify and change activities so that they can perform them successfully. Activity synthesis appears simple precisely because it is so commonplace, yet most people do not synthesize activities in an organized and systematic manner. True activity synthesis is a complex skill, yet very little has been written specifically about it. Occupational therapists and occupational therapy assistants approach activity synthesis from an organized theoretical perspective requiring an understanding of activity analysis, the underlying components, the context, and, of course, the client. Furthermore, activity synthesis is strongly influenced by the frame of reference chosen for intervention and the artfulness of the practitioner. Activity synthesis is a critical function of the occupational therapist and occupational therapy assistant and is used frequently in day-to-day interventions. If used successfully in the intervention process, activity synthesis should result in occupational synthesis within the client. In this chapter, we propose that the practitioner needs to understand the importance of activity synthesis and how to approach it in an organized and systematic manner. Through effective activity synthesis, the therapist will be able to help the client develop true occupational synthesis. Then, through ongoing development, reflection, and experience, the practitioner becomes both skillful and artful in developing interventions that are meaningful for the client.

References

Hinojosa, J. (2003, August 4). Occupation and continuing competence: Part II. *OT Practice, 8,* 11–12.

Hinojosa, J., Kramer, P., Royeen, C. B., & Luebben, A. (2003). The core concept of occupation. In P. Kramer, J. Hinojosa, & C. B. Royeen (Eds.), *Perspectives in human occupation: Participation in life* (pp. 1–17). Philadelphia: Lippincott Williams & Wilkins.

Hunt, D. (1997). *The magician's tale.* New York: Putnam.

Mosey, A. C. (1981). *Occupational therapy: Configuration of a profession.* New York: Raven.

Mosey, A. C. (1996). *Applied scientific inquiry in the health professions: An epistemological orientation* (2nd ed.). Bethesda, MD: American Occupational Therapy Association.

Nelson, D. L. (1997). Why the profession of occupational therapy will flourish in the 21st century [Eleanor Clarke Slagle Lecture]. *American Journal of Occupational Therapy, 51,* 11–24.

Nelson, D. L., & Jepson-Thomas, J. (2003). Occupational form, occupational performance, and a conceptual framework for therapeutic occupation. In P. Kramer, J. Hinojosa, & C. B. Royeen (Eds.), *Perspectives on human occupation: Participation in life* (pp. 87–155). Baltimore: Lippincott Williams & Wilkins.

Schell, B. A. B. (2003). Clinical reasoning: The basis of practice. In. E. B. Crepeau, E. S. Cohn, & B. A. B. Schell (Eds.), *Willard and Spackman's occupational therapy* (10th ed., pp. 131–139). Philadelphia: Lippincott Williams & Wilkins.

Schön, D. A. (1983). *The reflective practitioner: How professionals think in action.* New York: Basic.

Weinstein, E. (1998). *The nature of artful practice in psychosocial occupational therapy.* Unpublished doctoral dissertation, New York University, New York.

White, T. H. (1977). *The book of Merlin.* Austin: University of Texas Press.

7

Clinical Reasoning

Fran Babiss, PhD, OTR/L

Professionals whose work requires collaboration with the people they treat have an enormous responsibility. During an occupational therapy student's fieldwork, an inevitable moment comes at which this enormity becomes very tangible, often in the form of fears about saying or doing the wrong thing with a client. That "what if" is the starting point of clinical reasoning. It is an awareness of the power that each of us has to affect destiny through the choices we make. What we say or do is never guaranteed to have the outcome for which we strive, but we are responsible for taking action, and the practitioner's job is to develop the skill to make such choices.

I have had students ask me, "How did you know what to say to that client?" The attempt to operationalize the decision-making process is complex. Reasoning about activities and occupation is how we make decisions about what course of intervention to pursue with a client. Can we make the best decision? How do we know we have taken the right course, and essentially, how do we go about the process of deciding what purposeful activities to choose in working with others? Moreover, how do we know that we have chosen from viable and validated treatments? We live in a time when consumers are asking, "Does your treatment really work?" In an era in which even the Joint Commission on Accreditation of Healthcare Organizations (2008) is requiring proof of the use of evidence-based practice, it is essential to understand the mechanism of cognitive reasoning.

This chapter assists readers in the process of both becoming more aware of the concept of reasoning about activity and engaging in clinical reasoning. It is filled with examples and exercises designed to give you the opportunity to think about your thinking.

EXERCISE 7.1: MAKING A DECISION

Take a few minutes now to reflect on the way in which you decided to become an occupational therapist or occupational therapy assistant. Think about your age at the time of the decision. What was going on in your life? Did you have other career choices from which you fixed on occupational therapy? Can you tease out the cognitive and emotional mechanisms you used to settle on your chosen course? More important, can you remember what happened immediately after the point at which you made the decision?

Most often, people do not function in a meta-cognitive mode. By this, I mean that it is a rare occurrence to think about one's own thinking in an overarching manner. Therefore, it is a difficult task. Whether it is something you are aware of or something you develop over time, decision making and reasoning about activity and occupation are skills you will need to hone as a professional. You may not always make the right decision, but you can learn to make the best decision.

Definitions

Many years ago, when I was beginning my study of occupational therapy, I was told repeatedly that practitioners worked holistically. This meant that I paid attention not only to a person's physical or mental health concerns but also to the interaction among body, mind, and spirit. I still believe this holistic view to be true, and it contributes to the intricacy of my reasoning about activities and occupations. It also makes defining *clinical reasoning* very difficult. As Hinojosa and Blount stated earlier in Chapter 1, "The labels used [to describe reasoning] are not always the same, and the ideas behind them are not necessarily uniform" (p. 1). Defining this concept is, however, a starting point, and its inherent difficulty supports the argument for looking at the concept of clinical reasoning from a pluralistic standpoint.

Clinical reasoning is complex (Mattingly & Fleming, 1994), and many definitions exist. Consistent with my views on clinical reasoning, Schell (2003b) defined it as a process that is both complex and multifaceted. She went on to define *clinical reasoning* as "the process used by practitioners to plan, direct, perform, and reflect on client care" (p. 131).

Building on Exercise 7.1, think about what happened to you once you decided to become an occupational therapist or occupational therapy assistant. A decision is nothing more than what you think until you begin to take action on the basis of that decision. This is the planning stage of clinical reasoning. At first, deciding to become an occupational therapist or occupational therapy assistant seems no different from deciding to become a black belt in karate. The way in which you or anyone else knows that a decision has been made is by the behavior you engage in after having made the decision. This is the performance stage of clinical reasoning. Imagine deciding to become an occupational therapist or an occupational therapy assistant and finding a sensei on the basis of that decision.

A decision that Mr. Ames will need 120° of forward shoulder flexion to permit him to return to his job stocking shelves in a warehouse determines a clear course of action designed to assist him in a return of range of motion. Complexity enters in the form of deciding just what to do to implement that increase in movement. In addition, how does one know that Mr. Ames really wants to return to work, and can he be provided an environment that closely approximates the conditions of his workplace? A dozen more questions can and should be asked before action can take place.

Clinical Reasoning—A Very Brief History

A close examination of the process of clinical reasoning was a natural development in the maturation of occupational therapy as a profession. Cohn (1991) traced the origin of the inquiry to Joan Rogers's 1983 Eleanor Clarke Slagle lecture devoted to explicating clinical reasoning. In closing, Rogers spoke of the need to examine thinking more systematically for the purpose of making it accessible to the profession. She correctly connected an improvement in one's art of practice with a greater awareness of the ways in which one thinks about that practice.

On the basis of this beginning, Mattingly and Fleming (1994) worked with the American Occupational Therapy Association (AOTA) and American Occupational Therapy Foundation (AOTF) to conduct an ethnographic study to begin to explain the thinking that takes place when occupational therapists solve treatment problems. Today, clinical reasoning has been incorporated into occupational therapy curricula to address the expanding knowledge required of practitioners. The need to move to evidence-based practice models has furthered the necessity of teaching students professional reasoning (Coster, 2008). Christine Peters, director of occupational therapy at Stony Brook University, stated,

> Clinical reasoning and evidenced-based practice [are] integrated throughout the Stony Brook Occupational Therapy curriculum, starting at the foundational courses, when basic concepts and principles are introduced philosophically and historically. As the student advances in various practice areas, clinical reasoning is revisited, using in-classroom case studies and integration of examples from community-based practice and internships. Our goal is for a developing therapist to be able to think in the immediate and tacitly understanding why and how decisions are made that

reflect occupation-based practice. (Personal communication, February 2, 2009)

This addition is based on the following premise: With the ability to perform reasoning about activities and occupation, occupational therapists should be able to solve treatment problems that exist outside of their experience or training, and learning how to think about a profession improves the ability to engage meaningfully in that profession. Throughout their professional careers, practitioners continue to develop their clinical reasoning skills.

Underlying Framework

The catalyst for much of the thinking about thinking in occupational therapy is based on the work of Schön (1983). In addition, Dreyfus and Dreyfus (1986) contributed to our understanding of the movement of the practitioner from novice to expert. In this section, I summarize the work of Schön and of Dreyfus and Dreyfus so that readers can have a better understanding of the development of the categories of clinical reasoning in occupational therapy.

REFLECTIVE PRACTITIONER

Schön's (1983) work is credited as being the starting point for the exploration of the workings of clinical reasoning in the occupational therapy profession. His area of exploration was the development of professions, more specifically, of how professions acquire their particular knowledge. He created this epistemology of practice on the basis of the premise that most practicing professionals know more in practice than they can verbalize. This situation is what I wrote about in the beginning of this chapter, and it represents the strongest argument for participating in the training of occupational therapy students as they keep thinking about choices made in practice. When asked how decisions are made during practice, the occupational therapist is sometimes at a loss to explain the process. This not being able to say what one knows (p. 49) is what Schön explored.

The task for professionals is to develop an art of practice in spite of the multiple frames of reference that exist. Schön (1983) believed that the conflicts and difficulties that exist in solving professional problems are what allows a person to grow in his or her ability to solve these problems artfully, and I agree. Pluralism is healthy for a profession (Mosey, 1985), and the art of practice can be developed regardless of the techniques chosen:

> It is true that there is an irreducible element of art in professional practice; it is also true that gifted engineers, teachers, scientists, architects, and managers sometimes display artistry in their day-to-day practice. If the art is not invariant, known, and teachable, it

appears nonetheless, at least for some individuals, to be learnable. (Schön, 1983, p. 18)

Schön (1983) labeled the simple application of learned techniques of practice as *technical rationality*. The movement to full professional status of an artful practitioner involves moving from what Schön termed *knowing-in-action* to *reflection-in-action*. Knowing-in-action involves the concept of *tacit knowledge*, a term credited to Polanyi (1962/1974) that describes a form of knowing without knowing how one knows. For example, you may have no difficulty knowing that you like or dislike a certain work of art, but you might not be able to say what it is that makes you like or dislike it. In the same way, people often use language without the slightest understanding of its grammatical underpinnings. A sentence may be dissonant to a person's ears, but he or she would be challenged to provide the grammatical rule broken that is the cause of discomfort. Similarly, a practitioner may interact with or choose a purposeful activity with a client without being able to explain why a statement was made or an intervention chosen.

Much knowing-in-action is a function of experience as a practitioner. As the practitioner experiences situation after situation, a database is built. After time and repetition, experience and action become separated, much in the same way that a person can daydream while driving home from work, yet find himself or herself at the front door without any difficulty. While writing this chapter, I asked many therapists to pay attention to their thinking about what they did as they practiced, and some likened the experience to waking up. This is not to say that many occupational therapists and occupational therapy assistants sleep in practice but that certain practices become so automatic that they disappear from our awareness and become tacit knowledge. Hence, the question from a student, "How did you know how to do that?" is an opportunity to explore knowing-in-action and make the tacit explicit. Then, a piece of the art of practice becomes learnable.

Danger lurks, though, in the habituation to tacit ways of applying clinical knowledge, which is addressed by the cliché "When all I have is a hammer, the whole world looks like a nail." In my practice, I have come to specialize in working with people with borderline personality disorder. As a result, I often see the patterns associated with this disorder in many of the clients with whom I work. This perspective creates a tunnel vision that negates the possibility of entertaining other possible explanations for the way in which a client functions, which was made explicit to me by an occupational therapy student who had worked in the school system for many years before pursuing a career in occupational therapy. During an occupational therapy activity, a client got up from the table and took a lap blanket from a chair, reseating herself wrapped in the blanket. After the group, the student and I were reflecting on the group, and I described the client's behavior as a need to direct the group's attention to her because the group was focused on another client. The student opined that perhaps the client's behavior had been an indication of a need for tactile pressure because she was starved for sensory input. I return to this example shortly.

Reflection-in-action is a characteristic of a professional who is practicing at the highest level of expertise. It is the ability to reason about what is going on as it is in process. Schön (1983) saw reflection-in-action as the positive outcome when the professional is confronted by a situation that falls outside of the applied science of technical rationality, the experience of knowing-in-action, and catapulted into a world of problem solving in which he or she must entertain new thinking and actions. Schön said,

> Many practitioners, locked into a view of themselves as technical experts, find nothing in the world of practice to occasion reflection. They have become too skillful at techniques of selective inattention, junk categories, and situational control, techniques that they use to preserve the constancy of their knowledge-in-practice. For them, uncertainty is a threat; its admission is a sign of weakness. Others, more inclined toward and adept at reflection-in-action, nevertheless feel profoundly uneasy because they cannot say what they know how to do, cannot justify its quality or rigor. (p. 69)

At this point, it is helpful to return to the previous anecdote in which I and my student had such different explanations for the behavior of the client who wrapped herself in a blanket. In terms of reasoning about the incident, we each saw it through the lens we had been using, either sensory or psychological. Either conclusion could lead to differences in intervention, even interventions that could be counterproductive for the client. Schön (1983, p. 157) spoke of a virtual world in which the student and supervisor can imagine a situation without being in the situation. Although this strategy works for the architect planning on paper or the psychotherapist analyzing the transference, it is not helpful in this situation because not enough information is available about the client. The answer to the problem of the need for attention versus the need for tactile pressure can be solved by reflection-in-practice, which involves continued observation of and interaction with the client. As it turned out, by asking questions and providing different input, we determined that the client needed both tactile input and others' attention, and the incident provided a learning experience in creating interventions that worked along both axes. Schön likened reflection-in-action to a form of research designed for learning new and different ways of thinking about phenomena. It challenges the practitioner to stretch the limits of his or her knowledge.

Many occupational therapists have used Schön's (1983) work to guide their own practice and to assist students in reflection for the purpose of professional growth. Duncombe (2008) spoke of her own personal journeys in reflection as a path to using reflection with interning occupational therapists.

She made use of a population of 57 students over the course of 115 affiliation experiences to gather material about how the students reflected on their practice. The information gathered by means of questions such as "How have you used occupation-based practice in this fieldwork?" was analyzed by using qualitative methods that allowed the faculty of Boston University to realize that they needed to explain and address occupation-based treatment in greater depth.

Schön (1983) acknowledged the value of experience in passing on the skill of being a reflective practitioner. The movement of a practitioner from novice to professional is another area of professional development that has a strong impact on reasoning about activity.

CLINICAL REASONING AND EXPERIENCE

Suppose you were told that to become an expert practitioner you would have to rely on intuition? In other words, what you could learn by rules, regulations, and experience was not enough. If learning the rules and exceptions were enough, the problem of computer artificial intelligence would have been solved by now. Dreyfus and Dreyfus (1986), brothers who are professors of philosophy and industrial engineering, have explored the progression of people from novice to expert in different careers and skill acquisitions. Their investigations have provided a framework for understanding growth in the ability to reason about activities as a function of time and experience. The five stages that an individual may pass through are (1) novice, (2) advanced beginner, (3) competence, (4) proficient, and (5) expert.

STAGE 1: NOVICE

The beginner who is learning a new skill is taught to recognize certain features and rules that are based on features of the task at hand. For example, when a novice dancer is learning to waltz, the order of the steps is the focus of the activity. The rules about the order of steps in the dance are what Dreyfus and Dreyfus (1986, p. 21) referred to as "context free" because they can be recognized without a need to be aware of anything else that is happening. In fact, the novice dancer might not be able to learn the steps of the dance if she or he had to focus on anything other than the rules for the steps. The novice could not account for the crowd on a dance floor or the dance style of a partner. It would not be possible for the novice to carry on a conversation while waltzing.

Novice occupational therapists beginning school 25 years ago were given rules for behavioral health practice in their introductory classes. At that time in the history of the profession, students were often taught exact prescriptions of activities to be used with clients, much of them based on psychodynamic theories of the meaning of symbols. They were taught that male clients would prefer leatherworking and woodworking, and female clients would be motivated by needlework crafts. When they wrote papers for school, these students followed these rules assiduously.

STAGE 2: ADVANCED BEGINNER

At the advanced beginner stage, the learner of a new skill or profession is continuing to gather more context-free facts. The context the learner perceives is becoming larger because of the experience gained through practicing in concrete situations in the world. He or she is beginning to gather a "database" of past situations with which current experiences can be compared. Thus, the advanced beginner begins to use situational cues for reasoning and practice. The dancer begins to be able to look around the dance floor and negotiate and adjust steps so as not to collide with others. Knowing the steps is not enough. To survive on the dance floor, one must learn to avoid others in the same space.

In the behavioral health clinic, it did not take long to gather a collection of situations in which the "gender" of a craft was often useless. From these experiences, practitioners learned that although preference for activities might still relate to generalizations about gender, asking a client what he or she enjoyed doing had more value and helped the practitioner to establish a rapport with the client. The rules these practitioners had learned as novices did not serve them well in each real-world situation.

STAGE 3: COMPETENCE

At the competence point in learning a skill or profession, the learner has amassed so many context-free rules and situational experiences that he or she can feel overwhelmed. So much is known that extracting the significant from the irrelevant is difficult. The competent professional adopts or is taught a hierarchy of decision making to assist him or her in making a way through the confusion of too much information. At this level, the learner begins to have a sense of responsibility for the outcome of a decision, and this emotional involvement is critical to the move to the level of competence. The dancer is now able to decide that dancing close to the judge of a dancing contest is the most important task and feels confident in doing so while dancing. Other components of the dance no longer require intense focus. The steps of the waltz are second nature, the synchronization with a usual dance partner is established, and the dancer rarely bumps into other couples on the dance floor. Thus, she or he is able to begin to plan and establish goal-directed behavior in the larger environment.

At this level, practitioners working in a behavioral health setting have had experience with hundreds of clients and several dozen activities. Access to all of this information allows them to begin to construct a form of triage in activity selection. A competent practitioner can interact with a client in a way that allows him or her to understand that the client's self-esteem is so damaged that an activity in which a successful outcome is ensured is of primary importance. After that decision, an exploration of the type of activity in which the client might be motivated to engage might follow. In other words, it is a search for an activity that is meaningful to the client. The competent practitioner's task is then to adapt and grade the client's choice to ensure a positive outcome. The practitioner has an emotional stake related to both empathy for the client and a desire to make the right choice in activity with the client. Dreyfus and Dreyfus (1986) stated that many people do not develop beyond this level of skill because to do so would entail moving into intuitive levels of thought and action.

STAGE 4: PROFICIENT

The proficient practitioner functions without a conscious reach for rules, situations, or hierarchies. Intuition, as described by Dreyfus and Dreyfus (1986, p. 109), consists of a "holistic understanding" in which response to patterns occurs without having them deconstructed into component parts. It is knowing the right thing to do without thinking about why it is the right thing to do. It is akin to Csikszentmihalyi's (1990) description of the concept of *flow* as a seamless flow of activity. The proficient practitioner functions effortlessly. The proficient dancer is at one with his or her body, partner, the dance floor, and the entire experience in which they exist.

A proficient behavioral health practitioner senses when a client is ready to tackle a more challenging task, tolerate an intervention about his or her behavior, or take an interpersonal risk. The practitioner does not break down the client's interactions or behavior into units but looks at the entire client moving through the environment. This level is difficult to explain to the novice student because it goes beyond the simple acquisition of thousands of hours of experience. It is a leap into the intuitive realm that many practitioners never make.

STAGE 5: EXPERT

Dreyfus and Dreyfus (1986) said, "When things are proceeding normally, experts don't solve problems and don't make decisions; they do what normally works" (p. 31). Being one with what one does is the essence of expertise. The move from proficiency to expertise mirrors that of the move from advanced beginner to competence. As the advanced beginner accrues more and more situations and rules, he or she groups them together to improve his or her decision-making skills. In the same manner, the proficient learner groups intuitive experiences into larger chunks so that thinking recedes and acting and living become one. As long as things unfold as usual, the expert will not make mistakes. The dancer on the floor will waltz in a way that all can recognize as expert, but to say why would be to break the experience into parts that would render it incomprehensible as a whole. If asked what makes her an expert, the waltzer may not be able to say because at this level, such a question is akin to asking her what makes her who she is.

An expert practitioner in behavioral health practice might be able to sense that a client is in acute distress even if the client is not manifesting symptoms. Many of my peers related experiences of becoming disquieted by the behavior of a client during a group. They could not tell me why, but they knew somehow that increased intervention or even intervention of a more restrictive nature might be necessary. They could not tell the client's psychiatrist why they requested an immediate consult, but in most instances they were correct in their belief. They did not think but acted according to instincts they could not identify.

The five stages from novice to expert, along with the concept of reflective practice, provide a structure around which a discussion of the different types of reasoning occupational therapists use can proceed.

Types of Reasoning About Activity

In this section, I describe ways of looking at the complexities of clinical reasoning as they relate to occupational therapy. This subject is abstract, and readers are advised to equate the perspectives presented with their own thinking, reasoning, and decision-making processes.

THERAPIST WITH THE THREE-TRACK MIND

The concept of the occupational therapist or occupational therapy assistant operating in three spheres of reasoning emerged from the clinical reasoning studies conducted by Mattingly and Fleming (1994) and Mattingly and Gillette (1991), supported by the AOTA and AOTF. This small qualitative study examined the reasoning of a small group of therapists with a specialization in physical disabilities as they provided treatment.

PROCEDURAL REASONING

When in Exercise 7.1 you engaged in thinking about the process of deciding to become an occupational therapist or occupational therapy assistant, you were engaging in procedural reasoning. The practitioner who thinks about the activities he or she might use with a client to improve on the client's functional limitations is engaging in procedural reasoning. The evaluation process, focusing on the relationship between performance in daily life and the barriers to engagement and participation in daily activities, requires the ability to reason in a procedural way. The connection between this evaluation and the creation of an intervention plan is procedural as well.

Mattingly and Fleming (1994) distinguished between the procedural reasoning of an occupational therapist and that of a physician engaging in medical reasoning. The goal of medical reasoning is to postulate a diagnosis. Occupational therapists do not engage in diagnosis, but they work with the functional sequelae of diagnoses (A. C. Mosey, personal communication, 1986).

An experienced practitioner has a great deal of past information to which to refer to identify patterns and offer hypotheses about what might work with a client. Through a form of what I call "cognitive figure–ground," practitioners sort and sift through the information gathered while speaking with and observing a client. The practitioner pushes aside what he or she reasons to be irrelevant and extraneous in the hope of finding what is meaningful and worthy of attention. As Mattingly and Fleming (1994) stated, this type of thinking does not take place without the other two tracks operating in concert.

INTERACTIONAL REASONING

Relationships form the context within which practitioners function. During evaluation, the dialogue in which practitioners engage is part of the intervention. The way in which practitioners interact with a client can determine the efficacy of the entire course of treatment. Interactional reasoning is all of the ways in which one decides how to communicate with and listen to a client. Experienced practitioners develop what they would call an instinct for knowing how to speak with clients.

The most powerful and meaningful intervention is that which allows the client to determine what goals are important to him or her. Collaboration with a client is essential to this process. Beginning practitioners have to juggle so many new ideas, thoughts, frames of reference, and facts that the simple act of listening to the client's story becomes lost. Yet, it is this very act that can lead the practitioner to the point at which the direction to take with a client becomes clear.

In addition, knowing how to speak with a client allows practitioners to provide encouragement and motivation in a positive manner. This is not to say that reasoning about the interaction is to create a positive relationship. Often, the hardest concept for an occupational therapy student to grasp is that the job is rarely about being liked. Practitioners need to be honest and say the things that will move a client to pursue his or her goals. Using interactional reasoning skills, occupational therapists can judge the point at which they can push a client to move beyond the safety of the movements he or she has been trying around the house or the interactions he or she has been risking with his or her spouse.

Interactional reasoning requires that practitioners know themselves well. What practitioners say has to match their personalities and styles, or they will not be taken as genuine. The question becomes "What do I need to communicate with this client, and how shall I express it so that it is coming from me?" If you have a sense of humor, it can be used to connect with a client, as can a very serious nature. A practitioner has to be able to observe the effect of his or her interaction on others and adapt or alter it when needed.

CONDITIONAL REASONING

The joy of working with clients comes from the moment when the narrative they are sharing rings with meaning for them and allows the practitioner a glimpse into their world. For example, Martha, a young woman with borderline personality disorder who refused to sit during her interview, became engrossed in telling me what it was like to be in her head: "It's like in the movies, when those whirling disks are chasing the star, and she just escapes one, when, just like that there's another and another, and she can't keep up. I feel like I'm being chased and captured." Thanks to her eloquent metaphor, I was able to ask her whether she wanted help learning how to control the whirling disks. For the first time during the occupational profile process, she sat down, made eye contact, and seemed to be listening to me. All at the same time, I watched her movements in space, I watched the room in which she sat, and I listened to her words. For a brief moment, I entered her world, and she was ready to begin to do the things she needed to do to decrease her disorganization and emotional pain. I address this type of reasoning further in the section on narrative reasoning.

The holistic roots of the profession of occupational therapy suggest the need for conditional reasoning in that it provides the connection from meaning to action. *Conditional reasoning* is the ability to place thinking in an environmental context at the same time that thinking takes place in a context that is beyond the bonds of strict linear cognition. It is phenomenological, creative, and imaginative. It is the synthesis of all of the other forms of reasoning, some of them beyond what is known explicitly.

The phenomenology of the client is of paramount importance in conditional reasoning. The practitioner's task is to understand how the client makes meaning out of his or her life and the activities of which it consists. As with clinical reasoning, conditional reasoning is difficult to conceptualize.

Mattingly and Fleming (1994) said, "We think that conditional reasoning revolves around the ways that therapists think about which of the actions that the patient takes have potential for meaning-making" (p. 198). They believed that meaning-making connects with activity in three ways, which they labeled *intentionality, habits,* and *symbolic meaning.* This connection is an integral one for practitioners. It is the framework for the jump from meaning to action.

Intentionality implies choice. Consider the thinking involved in collaborating with a client about the choices he or she will make about purposeful activities and occupations. The therapist's goal is to see to it that the client is choosing activities that will allow him or her to move back into his or her life, but the therapist's ideas may not match those of the client. A weak grasp may preclude tooth brushing, but the client may want to be able to pick up a fork first. In a clinic devoid of forks and toothbrushes, we may be working with pencils and pick-up sticks. The idea of doing an activity with many useful applications and outcomes is one of the caveats Mattingly and Fleming (1994) identified. Most people's conception of occupational therapy practice is based on a linear observation of activity provision. They are not aware of the clinical reasoning in the form of conditional reasoning that is the impetus for the choice of purposeful activities. What looks like playing pick-up sticks to an observer may mean independence in feeding to the practitioner and the client. The richness of the many layers of meaning for the client and the practitioner is often misperceived. When the practitioner explains to clients what he or she is doing and why, the practitioner lets clients into his or her phenomenology and provides them with the opportunity for greater understanding of the power of occupational therapy.

Habit is a word that has its origins in the very beginnings of occupational therapy. Habit training harkens back to the earliest days of the profession. Life is made up of a series of routines and rituals that simplify and secure meaning. Practitioners understand the importance of habits to people whose daily routines have been interrupted by disability. The meaning of a morning cup of coffee is far grander than the mechanics of the praxis that brings the coffee to the lips. Although the importance of praxis may not have been apparent when the person did not have to think about how his or her body moved in space, it is of the utmost importance when it prevents the event from happening.

On an even more ephemeral level, the symbolic meaning of *activity* is critical to the practitioner's clinical reasoning skills.

EXERCISE 7.2: THE MACRAMÉ LESSON

Read the following case scenario and identify when the therapist uses instances of procedural, interactive, and conditional reasoning.

CASE SCENARIO 7.1: ROXANNE

Thinking about thinking is not always an exercise that results in the expected outcome. The most glaring example of this that I have experienced came many years ago in working with a young woman, Roxanne, who came to day treatment after a long inpatient stay for depression, several suicide attempts, and severe self-mutilating behavior. Although she was a respiratory therapist and social worker, school had always been difficult because of what she called her learning disabilities, which made it hard to process information and directions. Roxanne had not been able to maintain her employment in respiratory therapy because she could not arrange the equipment correctly when she was under pressure. When stressed, she became unable to tell left from right, a disability that could result in the death of a patient. At the time of our interview, Roxanne had no plans to return to work.

(continued)

CASE SCENARIO 7.1: ROXANNE *(cont.)*

During my interview with Roxanne, she helped me to see how important it was to her to be able to spend some time with her children. She had great difficulty engaging in arts and crafts secondary to her perceptual difficulties, a symptom of her learning difficulties. She asked me whether I could teach her a craft that she could do with her children. She challenged me by letting me know that it would be a difficult undertaking. She suggested that she be taught to do macramé so that she could make the knotted friendship bracelets popular at the time. I agreed and made plans to carry out this activity. As she left for the day, Roxanne turned to me and said, "Get a good night's sleep before we meet again. I want you to have the stamina to make it through." I knew Roxanne well enough at this point that I understood her statement as a way of feeling close to me. Roxanne was extremely bright and liked when those around her spoke in an intellectual way; sarcastic language was very acceptable. In an instant, I had a riposte that may have sounded inappropriate had a student been watching, but was the right thing to say to Roxanne: "Oh, but I shall endeavor to have you in knots tout à fait." The word *endeavor*, the use of French, and the sarcasm and play on words were all chosen to establish a bond and to validate Roxanne for her brightness.

My reasoning after the interview followed this path. First, I believed that macramé was a purposeful activity that the client had identified as meaningful. The chances of Roxanne being motivated to engage would be high. Second, in this case macramé would be a purposeful activity that made up a piece of the occupations of child care, leisure, and social interaction, adding to the client's repertoire. Third, I was familiar enough with the activity to know that I could break it down into component parts that could be taught by rote over and over until the client could perform it in spite of her perceptual difficulties. I believed that I had thought about the most important aspects of the task and had strategies for the intervention, and I was confident that the experience would be a positive one.

In fact, the experience was a very positive one. Although it took a long time for Roxanne to master the basic square knots of macramé, she was able, eventually, to repeat the mantra I used to help her remember the steps involved in making the knot. At one point, Roxanne told me that using the phrase "crossover in front" was confusing. Eventually, we figured out by trial and error that saying "Lay the cord on top of the macramé" allowed her to visually process the act. By the end of the session, Roxanne had begun to make an interlocking strand of knots and said that she would teach her son and daughter how to make the knots using the way in which she had been taught. I knew that written instructions would be unintelligible to her without a reader, but I gave her sheets with instructions and macramé cord to take home anyway.

After Roxanne left, I basked in the self-satisfied glow that is the prize of every therapist who knows the joy of a session that goes well. Roxanne was grateful, and I was fulfilled by having planned a useful intervention. I felt I had provided Roxanne with something that would improve her ability to engage in life in a meaningful way.

The next week, I asked Roxanne how she had fared in her arts-and-crafts session with her children, and she told me that it had gone well. Now that she could master the basic knots, she wanted to go on to do the finer work of making the friendship bracelets. But first, she wanted to tell me why she had adored the activity most of all. I was all set to hear how wonderful it had been to be provided with a means of interacting with her children in a meaningful and "mommy-like" way. Roxanne whispered to me, "I can't tell you what it meant to me that you let me take string home. You know I tried to kill myself three times when I was in the hospital." I was stunned. I believed that I had thought about what the ideal activity would be, why it was ideal, how to present it to Roxanne, and even what the outcome of the activity might be. Yet Roxanne focused on the interaction and relationship between us. I adjusted my response on the basis of this surprise and told Roxanne that I trusted her and would be glad to spend a few more hours teaching her how to make the friendship bracelets. In the end, Roxanne did master the macramé and went on to trying to learn to knit, but could not master this activity successfully.

PRAGMATIC REASONING

Health care has undergone major changes since the inception of managed care, and these changes are those that are taken into account by pragmatic reasoning (Schell & Cervero, 1993; Schell & Schell, 2008). Schell and Cervero (1993) identified pragmatism after they completed a literature review on the topic of clinical reasoning. Pragmatic reasoning is similar to conditional reasoning in its recognition of the integration of environmental and personal factors, but goes farther to embrace the phenomenology of the therapist, the input of the treatment team, and the political–economic factors of present day health care (Schell & Schell, 2008, p. 170). The difference between the 10-page treatment plans done for school assignments and the one-goal plans created for a 2-day length of stay for a patient in a hand surgery clinic are enormous.

ETHICAL REASONING

Within the context of pragmatic reasoning is the thinking that is done with regard to ethics. The mechanics of managed care and caps on reimbursement are often in conflict with both the needs of the client and the desire of the practitioner. How is reasoning affected when a therapist determines that a client requires 6 months of rehabilitation and the reimbursement is for 10 visits? How does one construct a context of improvement under these constraints? The opposite is just as common an occurrence. In my practice, the criteria for treatment at a partial hospital level of care are quite specific. Often, a client no longer meets these criteria but has been certified for additional days of treatment. The right thing to do is to discharge the client to a less structured level of care, but this is not what happens in every case. When I deem that the continued care of the client for 1 or 2 days will prevent or forestall a relapse or rehospitalization, I may make this choice. In the same way, I would advocate for a client who was being discharged before receiving maximum benefit from the intervention if I believed that he or she could benefit from additional treatment.

The concept of ethics lies outside of the scope of this chapter, but I mentioned it as another aspect of the complexity involved in clinical reasoning. The decisions practitioners make about what they do need to be reasoned about in terms of whether they are the right things to do. Ethical reasoning is a part of this process.

NARRATIVE REASONING

> Whether I shall turn out to be the hero of my own life, or whether that station will be held by anybody else, these pages must show. (Dickens, 1849/2000)

People are all the heroes of their own lives, and the way in which their stories come out has a lot to do with health and illness. Mattingly and Fleming (1994), Schell (2003a), and others have stressed the importance of the client's meaning-making in clinical reasoning. Each client's story is unique and carries the seed of intervention. *Narrative* is the story one tells of illness and wellness and how the practitioner fashions a view of the client's future world. Often, a disparity exists between this vision and the reality of the ensuing course of treatment (Mattingly & Fleming, 1994; Schell, 2003a). In the story of Roxanne, I envisioned her bonding with her children and teaching them an activity. What occurred on the surface was what I had envisioned, but its meaning for Roxanne was worlds apart from my view.

Listening for the meaning in the narrative requires the skills of an experienced clinician. Narrative reasoning exists on two levels. First is the life story of the client as it unfolds during evaluation and continues in treatment. Second is the narrative constructed by the practitioner as intervention is designed and implemented.

The key task for the practitioner who wishes to reason in narrative form is to listen, listen, listen. The story emerges through the storytelling. A beginning student is juggling so many impressions and ideas in his or her mind that the art of active listening can be lost. As experience makes it easier for the student to focus attention, she or he can relax in the client's story. In my own work (Babiss, 2003), the story has become the method for making decisions about ways of improving outcomes. I let the client tell me how the next chapter of her or his story should proceed. This can be invaluable in those instances when a practitioner is troubled by some aspect of a client's treatment. It is always worth the time and effort to sit with a client and allow meaning to emerge. Often, the experience is quite intense when a client can see that you get it, and his or her world opens to you.

CASE SCENARIO 7.2: CHRIS

Chris is a handsome young man who was a brilliant student with a few good friends, a loving mother, and an obsession with flying. In his first year of aviation school, he began to hear voices, which continued until he was forced to leave school and enter a psychiatric hospital. After the inpatient stay, the story he had written for himself—college graduate, pilot, husband, and father—was dashed. "I was going along fine, and then I was plucked out of life," he said with tears in his eyes. Chris' story highlights the temporal quality of narrative. He believed that his life was traveling a path and that its trajectory was assured.

On hearing this narrative of an interrupted history, the practitioner reasoned that Chris's assertion that he had been "plucked" from life had some validity, but the practitioner believed that he had been removed only from the life he had envisioned. Together with Chris, the practitioner determined that the task ahead was to write a new story and allow the narrative to unfold in a new and different way.

In a review of a book of his short stories, the author William Trevor (as cited in Allen, 1998, p. 7) said,

> It's not as rose-tinted a world, as most people would like it to be. But the people in my stories and novels are not ragingly desperate; they have . . . come to terms, and coming to terms in itself is quite an achievement.

It seemed that Chris's main task would be to write a new story of coming to terms with what he could do now, and the practitioner's job would be to work with Chris on editing his life.

The practitioner's narrative was grandiose and spectacular but acknowledged the reality that Chris could not hope to fly again because of his psychiatric history. The practitioner's plan involved exploring with Chris

(continued)

CASE SCENARIO 7.2: CHRIS (cont.)

the support activities involved in aviation. Chris's loss of narrative rendered cooperation difficult initially, but eventually he determined that he wanted to become involved in the construction of airplanes. This goal set the path that permitted the practitioner to work with Chris on constructing a daily life built around purposeful activities that would ensure that Chris's story would not face a major disruption. Chris worked out a daily schedule, independently figuring out that setting the alarm on his aviator's watch would remind him to take his medications, compliance with which was critical to maintaining his stability and function. Chris had a very supportive mother who was instrumental in providing a home environment in which Chris could remain independent but supported.

Together, Chris and the practitioner researched schools, and he chose one far from the hospital. He applied to the school, visited it with his mother, and was accepted. It was determined that he would remain at home until the next school semester, 3 months away. During that time, Chris came to the hospital and worked on work and study skills. He wanted his story to be one of someone who could concentrate in school despite the voices, which still plagued him from time to time. He worked on the computer in the clinic and showed slight improvement with time.

In addition, Chris made friends with several other clients in treatment. His story of the roles that had been disrupted made it difficult for him to see himself as their peer. As time passed, however, he realized that he had more in common with them than he had at first thought. The practitioner's story of Chris's life in the clinic before returning to school contained chapters on his connecting with other people, so she constructed group experiences and even the placement of chairs in the computer room to encourage spontaneous conversations.

The story ended for the practitioner when Chris and his mother moved to another state so that he could attend school. Chris's last letter told of his moderate success in school and that he had a few friends. He was still sad about the change in his circumstances, but it seemed that he had come to terms with his new story.

Narrative reasoning helped this practitioner enter into her client's world to collaborate on the plot for future chapters. It is crucial to know what the client's story is so that effective interventions can be made.

Again, the most crucial element in narrative reasoning is listening. Without hearing what the client with a disability is saying, a practitioner is unable to place his or her reasoning skills into that person's world. Peloquin (1993) addressed some of the beliefs that interfere with the ability to establish a full understanding of the client in his or her narrative. When practitioners think of a client as, for example, "the right hemi," they are engaging in the reductionistic, monistic thinking that leads to applying techniques and rote exercises to a problem that may have more to do with a person's desire to pet her cat. Thus, to engage in meaningful narrative reasoning, one has to take the time to hear the story.

EXERCISE 7.3: CLINICAL REASONING AND ACTIVITY CHOICE

The following case scenario represents a unique instance of an individual with both behavioral health and physiological concerns. Read through the case and begin to think about the planning, performance, and reflection involved in working with this client.

CASE SCENARIO 7.3: GERARD

Gerard is a 55-year-old single man referred to the day program after an inpatient stay on the psychiatric floor of a major hospital. This behavioral health hospitalization was his first.

The information collected during the occupational profile revealed a man of many facets. Gerard is of slight build and medium height, slender, and graceful in his movements, all of which makes his story more remarkable. Gerard was a veteran of the Vietnam War, with the rank of captain. He watched as several of his men died in a helicopter that took off while he remained behind on orders from a superior. He commented that he has always felt guilty about this. After a 4-year tour, he returned home to find that his peers had gone to school, gotten married, and moved on. He joined the city fire department, where he worked for 20 years in some of the most dangerous neighborhoods in the city. On retirement, he sold the condominium in which he lived alone and moved into an apartment in the house of his sister and brother-in-law.

Gerard never married and attributed this to his use of alcohol throughout most of his life. At the time of his admission to the day program, he had not had a drink for several months. "Alcohol is the thing that destroyed anything good in my life." Gerard identified as an asset his desire to spend time with his family and as a weakness a fear of close relationships with people other than his family.

(continued)

CASE SCENARIO 7.3: GERARD (cont.)

In retirement, Gerard taught himself to use a computer and started to work in construction with his brother-in-law. This vocation contributed to his current difficulties. While working on his sister's house, he fell from the roof, fracturing his spine and crushing his right radius. Gerard's back healed, but he required surgery for his forearm, which has several internal stabilization devices in it. Gerard laughed ruefully as he said, "I set off the alarms at the airport now." Although Gerard went to therapy after the surgery, he remained unable to use his hand for carpentry and the computer keyboard. Besides computers, he identified golf and carpentry as avocational pursuits, all of which have been greatly hampered by the lack of range of motion. Frustrated with the difficulties with his hand, Gerard contemplated suicide, which necessitated the inpatient hospitalization.

As he began to realize that he would not regain full use of his right hand, Gerard began to experience what he described as anxiety attacks. He then remembered that in his last few years at the fire department he had become panicked and gone to speak with the fire department psychiatrist a few times. This was, however, Gerard's first inpatient and subsequent day hospital encounter.

It was clear that more information was needed about the prognosis for Gerard's hand. A phone consultation was conducted with the occupational therapist who had treated Gerard. She reported that Gerard's internal fixation status would limit his wrist extension to 40° forever, but she believed that he could adequately accommodate for this with respect to the computer. Carpentry work, however, would be limited, unless he was able to change handedness for the use of tools.

Case questions: What is the priority need for intervention with Gerard? Why did you make this choice? Suspend pragmatic and ethical concerns and make purposeful activity choices to provide intervention in the priority area. Reason about the importance of social components for Gerard in planning choice of occupations.

The pragmatic realities of Gerard's case greatly hampered the realization of interventions that the treatment team reasoned to be meaningful. Gerard was discharged after 2 weeks, secondary to constraints of both his insurance company and the decrease in his acute psychiatric symptoms of anxiety and suicidal ideation. The treatment team, working in a behavioral health environment, reasoned that the most important task for Gerard was to arrive at an acceptance of the restrictions in his hand's range of motion so that he could begin to move ahead with plans for avocational pursuits that took his limitation in hand function into account. Without acceptance, Gerard would have no motivation to act in a goal-directed manner oriented toward the future. Second, a review of Gerard's history seemed to suggest that he was not deeply concerned with the lack of intimate social relationships in his life and that the suggestion of 12-step attendance (Alcoholics Anonymous) would not be a good choice for him. Gerard seemed motivated to interact with family members and did not seem to value relationships outside of his family. Unfortunately, the treatment team did not get to enact many interventions with Gerard, beyond leaving him with the information about coming to terms with his hand injury.

New Directions in Clinical Reasoning

The directions being taken by occupational therapists who address clinical reasoning hold great promise. In the recent past, in my opinion, work in the area of clinical reasoning in occupational therapy took a step toward a more reductionistic view of the phenomenon. Schell (2003a) began to look at clinical reasoning as a cognitive activity, which it is, and to suggest the use of mental models as a means of making practice more efficient. Mental models were first suggested by the philosopher Craik (1967, p. 59), who posited that people used a small-scale model of reality to be able to predict events and explain phenomena. Although Schell (2003a) acknowledged a drawback to fitting people into scripts and schemata, she was supportive of mental models.

I acknowledge that a thinking practitioner can do almost nothing to avoid categorizing and pattern recognition, but grave danger exists in adopting this habit as a means of making work more efficient. Johnson-Laird, Girotto, and Legrenzi (1998) warned against the dangers of reasoning using mental models. People who create mental models make explicit very little as they focus on the implicit information in their models. This use of mental models creates an environment in which the possibility of considering alternatives that lie outside the mental model is diminished. Johnson-Laird et al. provided an example of a grievous error of this nature that occurred during the nuclear crisis at Three Mile Island. The rise in temperature in the plant was ascribed to a leak. The staff did not entertain other explorations, which would have revealed that a valve was stuck in an open position. Their actions were guided by a faulty mental model, and the result was a disaster. Practitioners with less experience may welcome the ease of mental models, but the difficulty of changing one's models can make them too strong to reject.

The art of practice is born of treating each client as if he or she were a completely new experience because he or she is a new experience. If I start out working on pattern recognition and mental models, I may remain within this framework and never grow into a seasoned professional who has the ability to look outside of the cubbyholes I have created. A "typical hemi" is never just that. Currently, Schell and Schell (2008, p. 405) are not speaking of mental models but have embraced the importance of the clinician's ability to search for evidence-based interventions as a major part of reasoning behavior.

KNOWING MORE THAN WE CAN SAY

Thinking about our thinking, the act of *meta-cognition,* is a laborious task. When asked to think about the way in which you decided to pursue a career in occupational therapy, you could probably discern a linear path that you followed in making the decision. Identifying the intangible factors that affected your decision is not so straightforward an activity. Time spent examining the way in which your mind handles information and experiences can result in a significant improvement in your ability to reason about activities.

A structured portal into your thinking about thinking is the examination of your style of learning new information. Learning-style models abound, and a student or practitioner who is interested in exploring how he or she learns what he or she knows is advised to choose a taxonomy that feels suited to his or her needs. Gardner (1983) and Kolb (1984) offered learning-style models based on, respectively, looking at seven types of intelligence and at experiential learning. Gardner (1983) asserted that intelligence is not one discrete measurement, but that it includes seven dimensions: (1) logical–mathematical, (2) linguistic, (3) musical, (4) spatial, (5) bodily–kinesthetic, (6) interpersonal, and (7) intrapersonal. For example, over time I have come to know that my strongest areas of intelligence are linguistic and spatial. Therefore, when learning new material or working with new clients, I read and observe as much as I can. It is the reason I am drawn to qualitative, narrative information gathering.

Kolb's (1984) work on experiential learning is similar to that of Schön (1983) in that it is based on doing and reflection. He reasoned that people learn through doing and thinking about what they have done. For further information on learning styles, readers are referred to Schell and Schell (2008).

A practitioner who wants to expand his or her ability to know without knowing and improve his or her prowess in the intuitive leaps that characterize a seasoned clinician is advised to practice some form of self-awareness technique. Meditation, yoga, and journal writing are all satisfactory means of expanding one's inner life through occupation. The more awareness you have of the ways in which you make sense of the world, the better your ability to understand how this view affects your reasoning.

FOUR-QUADRANT MODEL

Greber, Ziviani, and Rodger (2007a, 2007b) have presented a model of facilitated learning that uses teaching–learning approaches. They contended that this approach, the Four-Quadrant Model, can enhance clinical reasoning and help to organize choice of intervention with clients.

The theoretical framework of the model is Bandura's (1977) Social Learning Theory, which serves as the foundation of some acquisitional frames of reference (Mosey, 1986). The four quadrants, as a schematic (Greber et al., 2007a, p. S32), contain several continua, ranging from learning that is initiated by the facilitator to learning that is initiated by the learner, from direct teaching methods to indirect teaching methods, and from teachers moving from leading learners to fading from them. This results in a gradation of ability much like that from novice to experienced therapist, but it clearly incorporates methods of learning that are based in social learning. Greber et al. explored several learning strategies to create the four strategy clusters that make up the quadrants. Thus, they contended that the model provides a scaffolding for making clinical decisions about interventions with clients and that it enables therapists to make accurate choices in interventions. An occupational therapist can begin working with a client in direct teaching methods, demonstrating how things are done, and giving concrete instructions and move all the way to the fourth quadrant in which the client is engaging in problem solving and questioning his or her own progress. The usefulness of this organization as it is applied to the teaching of occupations remains to be determined.

CASE STUDIES: CLINICAL REASONING IN ACTION

I conclude this chapter with two examples of treatment interactions contributed by two occupational therapists. I asked each to think and reason about the choices they had made. The narratives provide a glimpse into the activity reasoning of a novice practitioner and an experienced practitioner, respectively. As you read, think about how you might have reasoned about each situation.

CASE SCENARIO 7.4: JANE

The following description of an assessment, treatment plan, and intervention was conducted by Ann Winter, an occupational therapy student who had worked many years as a certified occupational therapy assistant but was beginning to negotiate the transition to the role of occupational therapist. Much of what she wrote included her reasoning, and I also asked her to think and write about the decisions made in collaborating with this client. What follows is both a wonderful account of a creative novice practitioner

(continued)

CASE SCENARIO *7.4:* JANE *(cont.)*

and a meta-cognitive exploration of clinical reasoning. Winter's musings about her choice, made after the treatment, are presented in italics.

Jane is a 17-year-old girl adopted from Korea. She was diagnosed with left hemiplegic cerebral palsy at age 8 months and acquired Prader–Willi syndrome when she was 3 years old in addition to an inoperable tumor on her hypothalamus. She has many of the symptoms and signs of congenital Prader–Willi syndrome, including low muscle tone, short stature, cognitive disabilities, problem behaviors, and a flaw in the function of the hypothalamus, resulting in chronic feelings of hunger.

Jane's brother, also adopted by the same U.S. parents, displays no cognitive or physical disabilities. The ethnic disparity in the family is reported to have had no effect on Jane's social or school experiences. Jane's father has a drug and alcohol dependency and has emotionally abused Jane's mother for the past 15 years. Consequently, Jane's mother has assumed the majority of the responsibilities associated with Jane's care since infancy and currently has an order of protection against her husband. He has been out of the house for the past 6 months. There is no history of physical abuse to either child.

Jane's room is on the ground floor of a home that has been environmentally adapted to suit her needs in terms of bathroom requirements and front-door accessibility. She requires moderate assistance to rise from a sitting position; ambulate; and perform bed transfers, oral hygiene, dressing, showering, and toileting. She is able to navigate independently in a motorized wheelchair when outside of her home. Her bedroom is adjacent to the den, which houses a television, computer, and stereo system, all of which Jane is able to operate.

Jane attends a Board of Cooperative Education Services high school and participates in its 6-week summer session. She has been taking part in a prevocational program at her school where she assembles parts for test tubes 1 full day once a week and receives a weekly paycheck. She spends the other days working on academics. Jane reads at a third-grade level, and she can perform single-digit addition and subtraction problems. Jane is unable to speak and must use an augmentative communication device to converse. She acknowledged that she enjoys communicating over the Internet and stated that she loves "looking things up." Jane's IQ was measured on a standardized intelligence test as 77. She continues to receive physical therapy at school, but much to her mother's opposition, occupational therapy services were discontinued 3 years ago because her therapist believed that Jane had reached a plateau in terms of skill acquisition. Jane displays enthusiasm for school, and as long as her routine is not interrupted, she moves willingly through her day. Any change in routine, however, such as a different bus driver, brings on an emotional meltdown in the form of a temper tantrum, according to Jane's mother. In fact, a change in the bus driver has on a few occasions resulted in Jane's mother having to miss a day of work.

Jane has two close female friends she has known since kindergarten, and whenever possible their mothers take them to the mall. According to her mother, Jane has not demonstrated an interest in or curiosity about boys. The mother's extended family lives in New Jersey, and they visit whenever possible. Jane receives home health care 3 hr a day, 4 days a week, and 8 hr on Saturday to help alleviate the strain placed on her mother. Jane's father does not visit, nor does he contribute financially to the family.

Jane presents as a grossly overweight adolescent girl of short stature. At the onset of the evaluations, she did not appear timid or fearful in the presence of the evaluating therapist and did, in fact, seem to be excited by the attention. Although Jane is nonverbal, she demonstrated exuberance by displaying a broad smile and waving her arms up and down. Jane's left arm is significantly weaker than her left leg and only moves slightly in momentum with her body during her excitement. She is able to use her left arm as an assisting extremity for stabilization of objects in various tasks, such as eating or writing.

During the interview, Jane was cooperative for approximately 15 min, oriented to the reason for the interview, and adept in the use of her communication device. She used her right index finger to operate her communication device and computer. Jane's cooperation lasted for a brief period, and her mother had to complete various portions of the interview process with Jane's approval. Jane made frequent nonverbal sounds, which her mother understood to mean that she wanted food. According to her mother, Jane requests food all day long, and as soon as she comes home from school, she either listens to music, logs on to the Internet, or watches television, while repeatedly making requests for food. Jane's mother spoke with the therapist to point out that Jane has an ongoing obsession with the stories she had watched on the Lifetime network. She speaks incessantly to her teachers about the melodramas, claiming that specific actors are actually involved in her life.

Evaluation. Jane was observed eating a lunch of scrambled eggs, using a gross grasp of her fork. Although she continually requests food and is morbidly obese, she is reportedly an extremely finicky eater and will eat particular food items, such as eggs and pizza, without demonstrating satiety. After the evaluation, Jane was seated on the floor in front of the television set in

(continued)

CASE SCENARIO 7.4: JANE *(cont.)*

the den with moderate physical assistance from her mother. She was clad in a T-shirt and underpants, which her mother stated is her usual attire for home. Jane is unable to toilet herself independently, and this state of undress is a convenience strategy. Jane ambulates in a waddling, unsteady gait and exhibits classic Prader–Willi traits of obesity, hypotonia, and dried saliva at the corners of her mouth. She wears bilateral ankle–foot orthotics to enhance ambulation stability while at school and outside. Jane only requires contact guarding when wearing the orthotics. At home, she requires minimal to moderate assistance for all transfers and ambulation and does not wear the orthotics.

Evaluation was performed in the home because Jane had finished the school year and had not yet begun the summer program. The two assessments used in this evaluation were the Canadian Occupational Performance Measure (COPM; Law et al., 1998) and the Comprehensive Occupational Therapy Evaluation (COTE; Brayman, Kirby, Misenheimer, & Short, 1976).

I chose the COPM for this client because it is a client-centered interview, one in which the therapist elicits information that the client identifies as pertinent. This particular adolescent has not had many opportunities in her life to be heard in her own voice. She has had few opportunities to make her own choices; because of her physical, communicative, and mental limitations, she rarely gets a chance to express her desired occupations, dreams, and desires as an adolescent girl. At her age, many girls have already started to choose elective classes in school, get a driver's license, research potential colleges, and think about what to do on a Friday or Saturday night. This tool enabled Jane to call the shots in terms of desired roles and satisfaction with the roles in which she currently engages in the home, school, and community. Although her mother was available to add information on issues that Jane was not interested in answering, such as household management, Jane clearly had much to say about her desired occupations. I did not want to oblige Jane to answer structured questions that limited her thought process or imagination.

I selected the COTE scale for Jane because given the time allotment, it allowed me to observe Jane and look for specific behaviors that would be pertinent to her occupational performance in interaction with people and objects in the environment and in daily life tasks. The COTE is relatively easy to administer, and Jane's behaviors were observed throughout the entire process of interview, lunchtime, watching television, ambulating from kitchen to den, and operating her communication device. Therefore, the COTE seemed to be an appropriate complement to the COPM because it required no additional effort on Jane's behalf with regard to the overall assessment, and it still afforded me very pertinent data regarding

Jane's behaviors, such as appearance, activity level, interpersonal behaviors, and task behaviors.

The COPM includes three sections consisting of self-care, productivity, and leisure. The client or caregiver prioritizes the occupations that the client needs or wants to perform within the client's typical daily routine. The respondent then rates the importance of each activity on a scale ranging from 1 to 10. Jane was able to participate in the interview by means of her communication device, and her mother continued when Jane decided that she was finished.

As noted earlier, I chose the COPM because Jane has had limited opportunity to express her wishes for direction of treatment and self-selected priorities. Jane initially appeared to enjoy the fact that the interview was directed toward her and that she had the power to answer without judgment or censure.

The problems identified as Jane's priorities offer valuable insight. Jane would like to spend more time on prevocational skills; improve her ability to cope with changes in routines; expand her range of socialization; participate in more school activities, such as cheerleading, chorus, and acting; and increase her scope of hobbies beyond that of television and computer. Jane indicated that she would like to be an actress and that although she is in chorus and cheerleading at school, she does not get as many chances to participate in these activities as she would like. In addition, she only has prevocational training 1 day a week in which she assembles test tubes. As indicated on the scoring section of the COPM, Jane believes that she does a good job at her prevocational activity but is not satisfied with the work.

I postulated that an increase in activities that Jane finds interesting, satisfying, and meaningful would lead to enhanced socialization opportunities, coping strategies, and variation in recreational hobbies because motivation is a key element in the treatment of people with Prader–Willi syndrome. Thus, in pursuing activities that Jane finds interesting, valuable, and enjoyable and melding them into the repertoire of her desired occupations (as outlined in the COPM), I hypothesized that she would be more likely to participate actively in those occupations and with a greater degree of satisfaction.

The COTE is a behavioral rating scale used as an observation tool to identify behaviors relevant to a client's occupational performance in interaction with objects in the environment and daily life tasks. The COTE consists of a single-sided sheet of paper that incorporates 26 behaviors divided into three areas: (1) general behavior, (2) interpersonal behavior, and (3) task behavior. The occupational therapy practitioner applies a rating scale ranging from 0 to 5 to the client's level of functioning for each compo-

(continued)

CASE SCENARIO 7.4: JANE (cont.)

nent of behavior (Brayman & Kunz, 2000). I used the COTE throughout the entire process of the interview, during which time Jane ate lunch, watched television, operated her communication device, and ambulated from the kitchen to the den. This tool was extremely helpful in evaluating Jane because it documented valuable information about Jane's behaviors while imposing no further demands on her attention. Evaluating observed strengths and weaknesses makes treatment planning easier.

Jane's major identified areas of difficulty are independence, attention-getting behaviors, concentration, cooperation, decision making, coordination, and frustration tolerance. These behaviors correspond to the deficits indicated on the COPM and, in particular, the problems that Jane experiences in coping with changes. Challenges presented to Jane in the form of a new task, alteration in a task, or unfamiliar peers and personnel may elicit an extremely negative response. It is therefore easier for those around her to play it safe rather than risk evoking a tantrum reaction from Jane.

Jane might benefit from treatment using interventions based on the Model of Human Occupation (MOHO; Kielhofner, 1995). According to the MOHO, the person is perceived as an open and dynamic system in which the organization of cognitive processes, musculoskeletal integrity, and nervous system influences the person's ability to successfully explore the environment. The MOHO suggests a human system that is not only in a constant state of organized process but also encompasses three subsystems: (1) the volition subsystem, which refers to a person's ability to anticipate, choose, experience, and interpret his or her own occupational behavior; (2) the habituation subsystem, which occurs when the human system acquires automatic and familiar performances as a result of recurrent patterns of occupational behavior; and (3) the mind–brain–body performance subsystem, which incorporates the biomechanical components of the person's physical and mental features.

This is also the reason why I chose MOHO as a frame of reference for Jane's treatment. For example, interests, attraction, and preference for certain occupations and aspects of performance are vital components of MOHO. The primary method for arousing motivation in adolescents with Prader–Willi syndrome is to focus on their interests. Another component of MOHO, values, will generally follow suit after interest has been established within the adolescent's personal convictions and sense of obligation toward an occupation that he or she finds pleasant or interesting. The MOHO also incorporates occupational choice, and one of the key aspects of choosing the COPM was to allow Jane to give voice to what she finds meaningful and valuable in her life. Knowing Jane's personality traits and those of other people with Prader–Willi, I believed that motivation for occupation (Kielhofner, 1995) was the only way to elicit Jane's incentive to engage in desired occupations.

Activity reasoning and use of evidence-based support. In completing the COPM, Jane was given an opportunity to prioritize her interpretation of the volitional structure of her life's routines. Providing a rationale for motivation is a key element in the treatment of people with Prader–Willi syndrome. Weber (1993, p. 6) found that "based on past experiences, a combination of social reinforcement and token economy incentives work well to control and change behaviors" (p. 6). In exploring occupations that she might find valuable, enjoyable, and interesting, I projected that Jane's sense of self-efficacy would improve. Moreover, the adolescent with Prader–Willi syndrome is most comfortable with routine and repetitiveness in daily occupations. To meld the performances that Jane chooses into a habituation process, the collaborative team involved in her progress will "provide opportunity for increasing emotional adaptability by systematically and slowly changing structure" (p. 5). Jane has many physical issues that must be considered when planning treatment, and her performance is greatly affected by the impairments associated with her dually diagnosed conditions. "Occupation requires us to use our bodies to traverse the geography and act upon the objects of a physical world" (Kielhofner, 1995, p. 116). Jane's mind–brain–body subsystem has affected her actions in an inefficient manner as a result of low tone, neurological deficits, and decreased cardiopulmonary energy. With the introduction of activity choices that address her volitional needs, I anticipated that she would move along the continuum from the current state of parent-asserted helplessness, observed incompetence, and inefficacy toward occupational exploration. It is likely that she will gain a sense of competence and eventual mastery over chosen occupations.

Jane demonstrates a zeal for occupations that she enjoys and for independent thought processes pertaining to attractions and interests that trigger personal convictions. According to the COPM, Jane has the ability to attribute significance to certain occupations in which she would like to be engaged. The COTE scale revealed an adolescent girl who has a generally appropriate orientation to her situation and surroundings and the desire for increased socialization along with a highly animated and appealing affect.

After examination of the results of the COPM and COTE, the primary areas in which Jane exhibits deficits are socialization, play or leisure exploration, and vocational exploration. These skill areas were clearly prioritized in the initial COPM assessment, and the deficits observed in interpersonal behav-

(continued)

CASE SCENARIO *7.4:* JANE *(cont.)*

iors and task behaviors on the COTE further support the concentration of intervention on these areas. Jane exhibited a lack of independent actions and self-assertion and a plethora of attention-getting behaviors (noisemaking and waving her arms) during the meal and interview process. Her task behavior demonstrated poor concentration, poor coordination, and inadequate decision-making abilities. She lost interest in the interview and had no coping mechanisms to implement when frustration emerged. Jane could benefit from activities that provide an opportunity to develop a sense of efficacy and control in achieving desired behavior outcomes (Kielhofner, 1995).

Socialization was deemed a priority to be addressed within the treatment plan, and vocational exploration was the next concern. The most likely scenario for Jane's future is to reside in a group home and work in a sheltered workshop. Jane is presently dissatisfied with the work that has been chosen for her. Thus, the sheltered workshop activity in which she engages does not facilitate a sense of personal causation, values, and interest. A disconnection exists between the reality of her current and projected life management. Play and leisure exploration are Jane's concern and her mother's. It would benefit Jane both physically and socially to broaden her range of hobbies to include fewer sedentary interests. Adolescents with Prader–Willi syndrome can benefit from activities involving muscular strength, endurance, cardiovascular endurance, and coordination (Weber, 1993). Her current lack of incentive to actively explore her environment reflects a dysphoric attitude toward physical activity.

Treatment planning. To facilitate improved socialization skills, performance components that must be focused on include increased problem-solving skills, attention span, interests in activities that Jane enjoys and that may be shared with others, social conduct, interpersonal skills, self-expression, coping skills and self-control for improved frustration tolerance, and assumption of roles for societal demands. Jane's strength, endurance, and gross motor coordination need to be addressed to enhance participation in many social activities.

When planning treatment for vocational performance, the occupational therapist must take into account many areas of concern, including deficits in fine and gross motor coordination, endurance, strength, attention span, problem solving, initiation of activity, role assumption of worker, interest in task, social conduct, interpersonal skills, self-expression, coping skills for transitioning to new tasks, time management, and the self-control to modulate behavior in response to new demands. Jane's present play and leisure activities require very little physical exertion. She identified interests in acting and cheerleading. She will have to work on improving strength and endurance, gross motor coordination, postural control, attention span, initiation of activity, and problem solving. She also needs to assume the role of an active participant; assess her values in determining that an activity is worth her effort; share her interest in the chosen activity; and improve social conduct, interpersonal skills, self-expression, coping skills, and self-control.

First short-term goal. With moderate verbal assistance, Jane will within 2 weeks identify two alternative strategies that she may implement when presented with a group task that she either is not interested in or does not want to complete, to enhance her problem-solving skills within a social context.

Second short-term goal. With moderate assistance, Jane will within 1 week compile a list of at least five activities that she is interested in attempting and that require more than one person to perform to increase self-expression pertaining to a social setting.

Long-term goal. Jane will, within 4 months, demonstrate an improved ability to interact with peers in an appropriate contextual and cultural manner by participating in a group task consisting of at least three other group members, with close supervision for 20 min and requiring fewer than three verbal prompts to stay on task, to promote her role as social participant.

Activity: Guess What I Am Doing? This activity is a form of charades, but it takes the game a few steps further into occupational reality. A minimum of two participants is needed.

- The occupational therapist or occupational therapy assistant prints on index cards different tasks and activities that occur in everyday life. For example, a card could specify brushing one's teeth, washing dishes, or making a bed.
- Each participant gets a card when it is his or her turn, and he or she must act out the task on the card.
- The other participants write down what they think the actor is doing.
- The actor then tells the group what he or she has performed.
- The participants are encouraged to applaud the actor at this juncture.
- After the performance, with the practitioner's assistance, the group discusses whether any components of the task have been omitted in the performance. For example, if the task is brushing teeth, perhaps the actor has forgotten to replace the toothpaste cap or rinse off the toothbrush.
- It is then the next person's turn to give a performance.

I selected this activity for Jane because as indicated on the COPM, she desires to participate as an actress in plays and make more friends. This activity gives Jane an opportunity to act and exhibit self-expression while

(continued)

CASE SCENARIO *7.4:* JANE *(cont.)*

integrating socialization skills into the group process. The game also gives Jane a chance to be part of the audience; therefore, she may practice waiting her turn, attending to task, and implementing problem-solving strategies if necessary during the course of the activity.

Guess What I Am Doing has a great deal of significance relating to Jane's projected future in a group home. Although I anticipated that she would enjoy the experience of role playing within the socialization of a small group, the tasks that are to be enacted mimic activities that are a part of Jane's daily routines. In fact, many of the tasks on the index cards can be modified to correspond to the COPM's self-care and productivity sections. To become a successful member of a group home, it is in Jane's best interest to practice situations and tasks that may be expected of her. In this manner, she will help to establish a sociocultural fit that will apply to current and future relationships and environments.

Intervention. The second visit with Jane took place in the late afternoon on a day on which she did not attend the summer program. Jane's mother invited Jane's two close girlfriends over, who knew ahead of time that they would be trying out a game. The activity encouraged participation and engagement because the girls appeared motivated to act out the situations and were eager to respond with their deductions. They giggled at each other's portrayals and were able to identify the tasks. The tasks were purposely very simple, such as brushing hair or washing face, to reduce possible frustration. The game addressed the priorities and goals because Jane was observed to wait her turn, interact appropriately, express herself, and clearly maintain attention for a full 10 min before she required redirection to the activity. She began to ask for food, and her mother told her that she would have to wait.

I would have preferred to field test the activity within the setting of Jane's summer program where there would have been more adolescent participants. The benefit to testing the game in Jane's home was that there was a high comfort level. Nonetheless, the Board of Cooperative Education Services would have been a better environment in which to observe the efficacy of the game's components and how they relate to Jane's goals. The discussion component of the game (Step 6) is one that would be reserved for a group with a relatively high attention span and frustration tolerance. It was apparent that each participant wanted to take her turn as soon as the previous actor's task was identified. They did not have the tolerance or interest in discussing whether any aspects of the represented task were omitted in the performance.

CASE SCENARIO 7.5: MR. LAMB

The following vignette was provided by Donald Auriemma, MSEd, OTR/L, BCN, who is an assistant professor of occupational therapy at York College of the City University of New York. He was pleased to write this case scenario because of his belief that the skill of reasoning about activities connects directly to the elegance of practice. (Case reprinted with permission.)

Mr. Lamb, at age 78, was referred for occupational therapy services through a certified home health agency. I began this journey with a review of the documentation package. A broadly written referral requested both evaluation and treatment of challenges to activities of daily living. Frequency of treatment was set at two to three times per week for 9 weeks. Mr. Lamb had arrived home after an inpatient stay for an exacerbation of congestive heart failure (CHF). His hospital stay was just one of several in the past few years for heart failure. An exacerbation of CHF was his primary condition; severe osteoarthritis was the secondary condition. Cardiac precautions were clearly indicated. Mr. Lamb's medication list was extensive. A preliminary picture was drawn of a person facing the challenges that the later stages of his diseases posed. I made an appointment for an initial evaluation.

As I approached his front door, I made my way up his four-step stoop, and the absence of handrails stood out. In response to my knock, he called out for me to just walk in. A frail-appearing, well-spoken gentleman welcomed me. The sight of this unkempt person sitting on a stained and tattered couch struck me. A musty smell and strong body odor permeated the room. Signs of years of neglect marked the first floor of his home. Mr. Lamb immediately offered an apology for not being able to walk over to open the door. A combination of limited range of motion and multiple sclerosis in both lower extremities along with compromised cardiovascular endurance had left him unable to ambulate.

Who was this man sitting in front of me, and how did his life situation lead to this unsettling picture? Mr. Lamb, an effective historian, provided a vivid history. As a child, he emigrated to the United States from South America. Raised by his grandmother, he lived a childhood marked by extreme poverty and a strong religious tradition. As a young adult with limited education, he learned a trade and worked as a machinist, an occupation he loved. It afforded him the ability to live out the dream of purchasing a home and raising a family. His two grown children live out of state. Proudly, he explained how in his middle years he converted his oversized garage into a machine shop. There, for more than 20 years, he was able to support his family. Advancing CHF and osteoarthritis slowly robbed him of the ability

(continued)

CASE SCENARIO 7.5: MR. LAMB (cont.)

to continue his business, maintain his home, move about, and ultimately per-form much of his self-care. He had been married for more than 40 years. His wife needed to work long hours in a hair salon she was trying to sell. Som-berly, he described how he spent both day and night on his living room couch. For approximately the past 3 years, his wife had provided him with breakfast, lunch, a clean urinal, and a bed pan. He would stay alone until she returned from work. Recreation was watching television and an occasional visit from a friend or neighbor. His elderly wife usually returned home visibly exhausted. Because he was reluctant to further burden his wife with the assistance he needed, several days would go by before he had a bath or changed his clothes. A dust-covered standard walker stood in the corner of his room. It was the only piece of therapeutic equipment Mr. Lamb had.

Evaluation. During this visit, I completed the initial evaluation. The informa-tion I obtained helped me to better understand Mr. Lamb's challenges and assets. His roles as a husband, provider, friend, and neighbor were no longer satisfying. His ability to spend time in his machine shop as a leisure pursuit was gone. Participation in home maintenance, cleaning, and shopping was no longer possible. Rolling and sitting up in bed was possible, but ambulating was not. Physical assistance to transfer was required. If food was brought to him he could feed himself. He could manage to dress his upper body, but he required assistance with his pants, shoes, and socks. Bathing was limited to sponging with assistance. He would toilet himself with the use of a bedpan and urinal. Deterioration in key performance components appeared to have significantly contributed to these performance area declines. Significant limi-tations in range of motion were present in all extremities and trunk, more so in his lower extremities. General strength was fair-plus to good-minus. His endurance was significantly limited, with an estimated muscle endurance test level of 2.0 to 2.5. The high value he placed on self-reliance; his ability to cope with demanding situations, interest in learning, and strong interpersonal skills; and liberal health insurance were some of the outstanding assets.

Reasoning and treatment planning. I believed that a client-centered approach and early successes would lay down the foundation for allowing Mr. Lamb to believe change was possible. This approach could motivate optimal par-ticipation and create an effective therapeutic relationship, thus maximiz-ing his functional potential. Collaboration with Mr. Lamb revealed that functional mobility was his number one priority. My thoughts focused on adaptations, equipment, and instructed skills. Mobility options needed to match his physical capabilities and not place a dangerous demand on his compromised cardiac function. Sliding transfers and manual wheelchair use were chosen. Both could use the greater strength of and range in his upper extremities and allow for a rest period at any point when the physiological demand became too challenging.

Intervention. Mr. Lamb's couch no longer confined him. Independence was achieved by providing a hospital bed, drop-arm commode, and a manual wheelchair. He now slept on an electric hospital bed set up in his living room. Sleeping became more restful, and Mr. Lamb found it easier to breathe in a semireclined position. Using all four extremities, he could move about in a manual wheelchair, in a slow and effort-filled manner. Access to his living room, dining room, and kitchen was regained. Within 2 weeks, his world had expanded from his couch to the entire first floor of his home.

Mr. Lamb's next priority was to reduce the burden on his wife by gaining a greater capacity to perform his own self-care. A focus was placed partially on what compensatory treatments would best help meet his desires. Through training with the use of a dressing stick, sock aid, reacher, long-handled shoehorn, and buttonhook, he regained the ability to dress himself. Long-handled devices provided access to the distal parts of his body that limited joint range prevented him from reaching. Commode use replaced the need to use a urinal and bedpan. Wheelchair access to the kitchen sink afforded Mr. Lamb a consistent opportunity to sponge bathe and groom regularly. Now able to reach his refrigerator, Mr. Lamb could choose from a variety of prepared or simple-to-prepare foods. A reacher provided access to lightweight objects placed in closets.

During this same period, Mr. Lamb engaged in an exercise program designed to remediate endurance, range of motion, and muscle strength. Because of his frail health, frequent, brief, and mild bouts of exercise were thought to be the most beneficial and least risky. Therefore, the remediation program was split between being provided as a portion of the three-times-a-week visits and a home exercise program that was performed on nontreatment days. I believed that even small gains in these components of performance would positively contribute to Mr. Lamb's regaining both the quantity and the quality of his functional abilities, and they did. Gains contributed to achieving independence in more physically demanding, modified stand-pivot transfers. Manual wheelchair propulsion was performed with greater ease. Self-care activities were performed with a reduction in the number of rest periods required. Once again, Mr. Lamb was strong enough to open and close his heavy front door. Successes gained in the 6 weeks of the program continued to motivate Mr. Lamb.

Mr. Lamb was encouraged to broaden his thinking. A 3-week window for occupational therapy was left. Cognizant of the limited remaining time and

(continued)

CASE SCENARIO *7.5:* MR. LAMB *(cont.)*

projected discharge date, his interest shifted to regaining access to his community. I judged his limited endurance and the four steps to enter his home to be his greatest challenges. The acquisition of a power wheelchair and a ramp constructed by a neighbor met these challenges. Power wheelchair use afforded Mr. Lamb access to his beloved machine shop. Traveling four blocks to the local shopping area became possible. Moving through his community allowed him to engage again with friends and neighbors with whom he had lost touch. His power wheelchair served him well for neighborhood travel. A solution for traveling longer distances was desired. Returning to driving seemed impossible. Car-related costs and the physical demands of placing a wheelchair into a car were beyond his economic and physical capabilities. Cab service costs could not fit within his limited budget. A referral to a city-based transportation service was pursued. This low-cost service broadened access beyond Mr. Lamb's immediate community. For the price of public transportation, he was able to travel throughout the city.

Termination of occupational therapy services occurred, as planned, in the 9th week of sessions. Contact with Mr. Lamb was maintained informally after his discharge through an occasional visit or crossing paths while I traveled through his neighborhood providing services to others. Despite the continuation of the destructive course of the CHF and osteoarthritis and several more hospitalizations, greater participation filled his remaining years. For years, it made my day brighter seeing him talking to neighbors in front of his home or traveling about his neighborhood.

These two cases are very different. What they have in common was the therapists' desire to enter the client's world so that they could collaborate in the creation of a meaningful environment for the client. Each therapist used different forms of clinical reasoning to achieve his or her objectives.

Summary

In this chapter, I explored the many facets of reasoning about activity. My goal was to increase awareness of the nature and importance of how you reason about what you do with clients. The enormity of the responsibility for decisions made in collaboration is mitigated by a conscious attention to the task of clinical reasoning. One day, a student or client may ask why you did or said something as you go through your day as a practitioner. If you can answer the question, you will be on the way to becoming an expert practitioner who can balance self-awareness with an awareness of the client's needs within the realities of the environment. It seems a worthwhile goal to strive for the ability to reason with awareness.

Acknowledgments

I acknowledge the invaluable contribution of Ann Winter and Donald Auriemma, occupational therapists who willingly examined their practice and gave of their words and time.

References

Allen, B. (1998, September 6). Fatal attraction [Review of the book *Death in Summer*]. *New York Times Book Review,* p. 7.

Babiss, F. (2003). *An ethnographic study of mental health treatment and outcomes: Doing what works.* New York: Haworth.

Bandura, A. (1977). *Social learning theory.* Englewood Cliffs, NJ: Prentice Hall.

Brayman, S. J., Kirby, T. F., Misenheimer, A. M., & Short, M. J. (1976). Comprehensive occupational therapy evaluation scale. *American Journal of Occupational Therapy, 30,* 94–100.

Brayman, S., & Kunz, K. (2000). The Comprehensive Occupational Therapy Evaluation. In B. J. Hemphill (Ed.), *The evaluation process in psychiatric occupational therapy* (3rd ed., p. 270). Thorofare, NJ: Slack.

Craik, K. (1967). *The nature of explanation.* Cambridge, England: Cambridge University Press.

Cohn, E. S. (1991). Nationally Speaking—Clinical reasoning: Explicating complexity. *American Journal of Occupational Therapy, 45,* 969–971.

Coster, W. J. (2008). Curricular approaches to professional reasoning for evidence-based practice. In B. A. B. Schell & J. W. Schell (Eds.), *Clinical and professional reasoning in occupational therapy* (pp. 311–334). Baltimore: Lippincott Williams & Wilkins.

Csikszentmihalyi, M. (1990). *Flow: The psychology of optimal experience.* New York: HarperCollins.

Dickens, C. (2000). *David Copperfield.* New York: Modern Library Classics. (Original work published 1849)

Dreyfus, H., & Dreyfus, S. (1986). *Mind over machine: The power of human intuition and expertise in the era of the computer.* New York: Free Press.

Duncombe, L. (2008, December). *Nurturing professional and personal growth through reflective inquiry: A gift to fieldwork students and yourself.* Paper presented at a meeting of the Metropolitan Occupational Therapy Council, New York.

Gardner, H. (1983). *Frames of mind: The theory of multiple intelligences.* New York: Basic.

Greber, C., Ziviani, J., & Rodger, S. (2007a). The Four-Quadrant Model of facilitated learning (Part 1): Using teaching learning approaches in occupational therapy. *Australian Journal of Occupational Therapy, 54*(Suppl. 1), S31–S39.

Greber, C., Ziviani, J., & Rodger, S. (2007b). The Four-Quadrant Model of facilitated learning (Part 2): Strategies and applications. *Australian Journal of Occupational Therapy, 54*(Suppl. 1), S40–S48.

Joint Commission on Accreditation of Healthcare Organizations. (2008). *The Joint Commission accreditation process: Hospital leadership.* Retrieved January 19, 2009, from www.jointcommission.org/Standards/SII/

Johnson-Laird, P. N., Girotto, V., & Legrenzi, P. (1998). *Mental models: A gentle guide for outsiders.* Retrieved September 24, 2003, from www.si.umich.edu/ICOS/gentleintro.html

Kielhofner, G. (1995). *A Model of Human Occupation* (2nd ed.). Baltimore: Williams & Wilkins.

Kolb, D. A. (1984). *Experiential learning.* Englewood Cliffs, NJ: Prentice Hall.

Law, M., Baptiste, S., Carswell, A., McColl, M. A., Polatajko, H., & Pollock, N. (1998). *Canadian Occupational Performance Measure* (3rd ed.). Ottawa: Canadian Association of Occupational Therapists.

Mattingly, C., & Fleming, M. H. (1994). *Clinical reasoning: Forms of inquiry in a therapeutic practice.* Philadelphia: F. A. Davis.

Mattingly, C., & Gillette, N. (1991). Anthropology, occupational therapy, and action research. *American Journal of Occupational Therapy, 45,* 972–978.

Mosey, A. C. (1985). A monistic or a pluralistic approach to professional identity? [Eleanor Clarke Slagle Lecture]. *American Journal of Occupational Therapy, 39,* 504–509.

Mosey, A. C. (1986). *Occupational therapy: Configuration of a profession.* New York: Raven.

Peloquin, S. M. (1993). The patient–therapist relationship: Beliefs that shape care. *American Journal of Occupational Therapy, 47,* 935–942.

Polanyi, M. (1974). *Personal knowledge: Towards a post-critical inquiry.* Chicago: University of Chicago Press. (Original work published 1962)

Rogers, J. C. (1983). Clinical reasoning: The ethics, science, and art [Eleanor Clarke Slagle Lecture]. *American Journal of Occupational Therapy, 37,* 601–616.

Schell, B. A. B. (2003a, October 6). Clinical reasoning and occupation-based practice: Changing habits. *OT Practice, 8,* CE-1–CE-8.

Schell, B. A. B. (2003b). Clinical reasoning: The basis of practice. In E. B. Crepeau, E. Cohn, & B. Schell (Eds.), *Willard and Spackman's occupational therapy* (10th ed., pp. 131–139). Philadelphia: Lippincott Williams & Wilkins.

Schell, B. A. B., & Cervero, R. M. (1993). Clinical reasoning in occupational therapy: An integrative review. *American Journal of Occupational Therapy, 47,* 605–610.

Schell, B. A. B., & Schell, J. W. (Eds.). (2008). *Clinical and professional reasoning in occupational therapy.* Baltimore: Lippincott Williams & Wilkins.

Schön, D. (1983). *The reflective practitioner: How professionals think in action.* New York: Basic.

Weber, R. C. (1993). Physical education for children with Prader–Willi syndrome [Electronic version]. *Palaestra, 9*(3).

8

Application of Activities to Practice

Nancy Robert Dooley, PhD, OTR/L

Every day, occupational therapists and occupational therapy assistants must choose the best activity or occupation to meet the therapeutic goals of the client who sits in front of them. For students and beginning therapists, this choice can be a scary and overwhelming prospect. Clients in health care, education, and community settings have performance problems affecting their brains and bodies in endless combinations. They come from extremely diverse backgrounds and environments that may be very different from the practitioner's. Clients and families expect practitioners to be expert at providing therapy yet also client centered to respect their particular wishes, needs, and interests. Payers and employers expect practitioners to fill specified numbers of therapy minutes, and they must do all this with limited resources or planning time.

Occupational therapy beliefs and presumptions focus on the value of activity as an effective tool for facilitating change and growth. The profession of occupational therapy supports the use of activities to enhance people's ability to engage in the occupations that they need and choose to do. Engaging in activities requires interaction with other people; the social environment; and the physical environment, including natural or built objects and spaces (American Occupational Therapy Association [AOTA], 2008). In occupational therapy practice, activities are the tools used to acquire skills, to complete tasks, to fulfill life roles, and to resume participation in meaningful occupations. Just as music therapists use music and art therapists use various forms of artistic expression to achieve therapeutic goals with clients, occupational therapists use occupation or activities. The number of possible activities that one can use is limited only by the imagination. Occupational therapists continually meet new clients and populations with unique needs, and therapists and clients combine and modify ideas in endless variations to meet the demands of each unique situation.

CASE SCENARIO 8.1: TOM

After Tom's shoulder injury and rotator cuff repair, his occupational therapist focused on wanting him to gain another 30° of shoulder flexion and return to normal strength. Tom, however, cared about moving normally when he took off his suit jacket at work or when he wrote on a whiteboard during presentations and meetings. He was concerned about his ability to perform normal daily activities. During a therapy session, his wife stated that she wished Tom could resume his usual role of maintaining the yard. Tom agreed that he enjoyed yardwork and looked forward to assuming responsibility for it. He also really wanted to go along when one of his sailing friends needed a crew member. In this case, the occupational therapist's goals, focusing on physical limitations and providing treatment to address specific deficits, were not consistent with the client's priorities and desires. They did not address the occupations that made Tom's life meaningful. Engagement in occupations makes people human and gives their lives meaning.

Being occupied generally results in a more satisfying life. Some activities are old and familiar and have great personal meaning, privately or publicly. Other activities can be newly acquired, giving new meaning and satisfaction to people's lives as life roles shift. New occupations are explored and adopted throughout life. Occupations help people maintain their desired roles and sense of self.

Using Activities to Facilitate Engagement in Life Roles

In this chapter, I present real-life examples of activities used in occupational therapy practice. I illustrate various ways to create and adapt activities to meet clients' needs. I encourage readers to use the learning activities to stretch their thinking about activities and occupations. Practice with these ideas and questions will make you more comfortable in intervention planning so that making activity choices becomes easier.

Practitioners must collaborate with the client, caregivers, or both in choosing activities for use in practice settings. Obtaining an occupational profile is a key element of the occupational therapy evaluation process: Who is the person, and why is he or she seeking services? What circumstances have caused a change in his or her ability to engage in daily occupations? What are the person's priorities, and what is his or her occupational history? All of these factors give the occupational therapist a baseline for establishing context for each client. The challenge for occupational therapists is to continually develop activities that are meaningful to the client and relevant to his or her life, experiences, hopes, and dreams, which results in therapy that is tailored to the person via activity choices.

CASE SCENARIO 8.2: ROBERT

Robert, a 64-year-old, otherwise healthy right-handed man, had joint reconstruction surgery of the right carpometacarpal joint to ease pain and regain mobility lost as a result of osteoarthritis. The therapist's goal, based on a biomechanical frame of reference, was for Robert to achieve full thumb opposition to all finger tips. He had most trouble opposing to the fifth digit. Robert's occupational therapist asked him to complete simulated activities, such as using a peg board or nuts-and-bolts board, at the outpatient clinic. Robert was bored and did not see the point of occupational therapy. At home, he wanted to resume activities that he valued such as cooking, gardening, caring for his dog, helping with household chores, and playing cribbage in a weekly league. He also had to go back to work soon, where he would need to handle money, complete paperwork, and use a computer smoothly and efficiently.

EXERCISE 8.1: ADAPTATION—EVERYDAY ACTIVITIES

Create some purposeful activities for Robert to replace enabling or simulated tasks. Because you are seeing Robert in an outpatient clinic for 30 minutes at a time, most of Robert's hand use will happen in the course of his daily activities at home rather than in the brief intervention with you. Recommend some activities that Robert can complete as he goes about his day so that he can continue to gain pain-free opposition. You may need to suggest adaptations to his usual movements so that the desired motions are included.

Activities are therapeutic when they are used as directed by a frame of reference or other theoretical guidelines for intervention. A therapist skillfully uses activities as directed by the frame of reference to ensure that the client's therapeutic goals are achieved. The activities, although selected to relate to a person's occupations, must be expertly applied so that the client accomplishes his or her goals. At times, the goal is the ability to perform an occupation. At other times, the goal is to participate with adaptation or modification. Unfortunately, at still other times, the therapeutic goal is to replace the occupation with one the client is able to perform. In all cases, therapy is directed by sound theoretical principles.

In this learning activity, you created purposeful activities for Robert. Purposeful activities are one type of intervention used in occupational therapy. These activities have both meaning and purpose in the client's eyes and a therapeutic purpose for the therapist. By recommending ways for Robert to incorporate therapeutic hand movements into his everyday routines, you suggested occupation-based interventions that will help stretch the benefits of occupational therapy well beyond Robert's 30-minute visits. More important, using real occupations in the intervention plan will help him to see occupational therapy's importance and role in helping him return to his valued life roles.

The choice of activity is crucial to a successful outcome for the occupational therapy process, namely that the client be able to engage or reengage in desired roles. Therapists' activity choices also affect the relationships that they are trying to build with clients. Asking a child to do things that he or she does not like or does not find fun will often result in refusal, tears, or limited attention. Adults are more likely to initially go along with activities they do not value or understand, but they may later complain that their occupational therapy session was stupid, childish, or boring. Adolescents, however, will often express the same complaints loudly and immediately. When this occurs, therapists have to work extra hard to provide meaningful activities to rebuild any therapeutic rapport that they may have established up to that point.

Listening to clients and their caregivers helps therapists create solutions that enable them to engage in their own recovery process. Consider these case scenarios:

CASE SCENARIO 8.3: JACK

Jack is a 28-year-old man diagnosed with autism who attends an adult day program where most of the other clients have mental illness or acquired brain injuries. Jack's occupational therapy program was based on a developmental frame of reference with a focus on skill development. Level II occupational therapy assistant students at the center noticed that Jack had a hard time concentrating in many group activities such as crafts and games. When he was overstimulated or having trouble engaging in an activity, Jack sought almost constant reassurance from group leaders and began to make odd noises that got louder and louder. He had a history of occasionally being physically aggressive when he was very frustrated. The occupational therapy assistant student noticed that Jack was always eager to push people in wheelchairs and do other tasks that involved movement or resistance. He asked the staff for jobs to complete and said that he liked to help. Remembering the principles of sensory integration, the students, Jack, and the occupational therapist tried to find activities for Jack to do that included heavy work: carrying groceries, moving boxes of holiday decorations, pushing the lunch cart, and carrying plates. Jack's success at these activities has led to part-time employment in a janitorial position at the adult day program.

CASE SCENARIO 8.4: GERRY

Karen met Gerry when she was a young therapist working at a long-term-care facility where he resided. Gerry was 22 when a diving accident left him with a spinal cord injury and quadriplegia. His parents' home was not physically accessible, and he had many assistance needs. He had been living at the facility for about 6 months when Karen began her long campaign to reengage Gerry in life. At first, she only stopped by his room to talk because Gerry would not come out of his room or attend any activities. Eventually, Gerry agreed to go to the break room with Karen while she had some coffee. They talked about common interests and began to establish rapport. Gerry would not have a beverage because he was embarrassed about needing an adapted cup as a result of his limited hand grasp.

Eventually, Karen got Gerry to try playing table tennis. With the paddle strapped to Gerry's hand, they played brief games on half of the table. His strength and endurance improved as they played for many weeks. When Gerry began beating Karen at every table tennis game, he had to find more worthy opponents. Gerry began to see himself as a capable person again when he participated in the popular and age-appropriate game. This participation was the start of Gerry's engagement in a series of new activities that helped him to live a more satisfying life. He eventually got a job working as the facility's telephone operator.

Our society expects young adults to be productive. Besides lacking the proprioceptive input that Jack needed, the existing groups at the day program did not provide him with a feeling of satisfaction, productivity, or self-worth. When he began to work for the center, got paid, and had people depend on him, however, Jack could see himself as a whole person. For Jack, purposeful activities suggested by the occupational therapy staff led to the creation of a new occupational role. The case of Gerry is another example in which an occupational therapist used activities to help a young adult reestablish a productive place in society.

Real purposeful activities require a complex interplay of physical, cognitive, perceptual, and psychosocial skills and have the potential to produce change in a person. By choosing tasks in the areas of social participation and leisure, Karen used real occupation to help Gerry gain the physical and emotional skills needed to engage in some of the roles he had lost.

The intervention modalities that practitioners use reflect back on the occupational therapy profession as a whole. If practitioners choose interventions that look a lot like what the physical therapist does, then why should insurance companies pay for both services? Yes, strengthening upper extremities can contribute to someone's ability to dress and bathe themselves. Many clients, however, do not find lifting weights in rote exercise a meaningful activity. Moreover, a substantial body of evidence is accumulating that shows that participation in real activities in context is most effective in building motor skills and cognitive skills (Ma & Trombly, 2002). It is critical that occupational therapists demonstrate their unique and valuable contribution to the rehabilitation process.

The best way to effect change and restore meaning in life is to listen carefully to clients and to tailor interventions to each person's life and contexts. That being said, it is not possible to incorporate purposeful activity or intervention in all therapeutic interventions. Preparatory methods are appropriate and effective occupational therapy interventions (AOTA, 2008). For example, scapular mobilization may be needed before a client with hemiplegia can use her affected arm while dressing or putting dishes in an overhead cabinet. A child with attention or learning differences may participate more efficiently in class after receiving joint compressions or other sensory stimulation as part of a sensory diet. Ultrasound and splinting are effective techniques for people recovering from hand injuries or surgeries. The caveat with preparatory methods is that they generally do not stand alone as occupational therapy for billing purposes or for the integrity of the profession. Whenever a therapist is providing a preparatory modality or activity, it is critical that the client and his or her caregivers understand the relationship between participation in the activity and the long-term therapeutic goals.

Occupational therapists often use simulated or enabling activities as part of the intervention process (Early, 2006). Simulated or enabling activities provide opportunities for the client to practice motor, cognitive, or psychosocial skills. The value of this practice is supported by various theorists who have reported that clients need repetition to incorporate new skills or performance patterns into their daily lives (Ma & Trombly, 2002; Mosey, 1986). Simulated activities were popular in the 1980s when occupational therapists were trying to make the profession more objective and measurable so that it would fit more easily into the dominant medical model. At that time, it became popular to use cones, blocks, puzzles, and other therapeutic activities to try to develop subcomponent skills. Recently, occupational therapists have embraced the use of real-life and community-based activities, which is considered by many therapists to be consistent with the fundamental assumptions of occupational therapy. Moreover, such activities support the use of contextually relevant activities that facilitate a client's use of physical, cognitive, perceptual, and psychosocial skills to interact with his or her environment. In the next example, the therapist has devised an activity that promotes social and cognitive skills in a teenager who has autism.

CASE SCENARIO 8.5: JULIAN

Cyndi is a registered occupational therapist who specializes in working with children with severe developmental disorders. Cyndi wanted to find an activity that would allow Julian, a 16-year-old with autism, to practice communication skills, organization, following directions, and completing multi-step tasks. She has selected a cognitive frame of reference that focuses on problem solving and organizational skills. The teachers and therapy staff of Julian's school order a take-out lunch every Friday. Julian's job is to knock on each classroom door, make eye contact with the teacher, and ask "Are you ordering lunch today?" Cyndi has created an order sheet that Julian follows. He crosses off the staff member's name if he or she is not ordering. Otherwise, the staff member writes in the order and gives Julian the money. Julian repeats this process for each classroom. Before Julian could carry out his assignment in the context of the real school hallways and classrooms, Cyndi coached him through various parts of the task in the occupational therapy room. Then she accompanied him on the job and gradually withdrew her support.

In other years, students who lacked reading skills would keep track of orders using a form with each staff member's picture. Next year, when Julian moves on to another job within the school, the lunch-ordering activity will be adapted again to meet the needs of another student.

People perform better under normal, contextually relevant circumstances. As this example illustrates, school-based (and home-based) occupational therapy provides opportunities to help clients participate in real-life roles. Everything takes place in the client's actual environment, and visits can often be scheduled so that they coincide with daily routines. An early morning visit can address bathing and dressing routines. In the afternoon or early evening, cooking a meal makes sense. Observing a student at school recess gives the occupational therapist real information about the child's physical and social adaptation in the playground. An outpatient clinic, however, has clients scheduled throughout the day, often around their usual daily occupations. The setting is often relatively plain and sterile, and there may be postsurgical protocols to follow. Some occupational therapy settings place constraints on the performance of real occupations. Thus, time, space, and resources may be limited by the intervention setting. Here is an exercise to explore the influence of the environment on intervention.

EXERCISE 8.2: RESTRICTIVE ENVIRONMENT

An occupational therapy assistant is working in a rehabilitation hospital with Damon, who has cognitive and physical impairments after a traumatic brain injury caused by a motorcycle accident. In collaboration with his occupational therapist, they have developed an intervention plan based on a cognitive frame of reference. Damon has progressed through several purposeful activities related to shopping and money management. The occupational therapy assistant would like to challenge her patient with the unpredictable distractions and physically close quarters of a real urban convenience store. She knows that Damon will be returning to that environment in about a week. Facility policies related to payment and liability say that patients cannot leave the hospital grounds. Describe at least five ways for the occupational therapy staff to further challenge Damon without violating this policy. Compare your thoughts with your classmates' answers.

You are likely to find that this learning activity prompts a wide variety of ideas and possibilities. Indeed, your professional colleagues are great resources for imaginative activity ideas. Everyone's brain works a little differently, and everyone has different life experiences to call on. In Damon's case, the setting that seemed restrictive may still provide opportunities for occupation-based interventions. For instance, does the hospital have a cafeteria or a gift shop?

Practitioners' use of activities in the real world involves creating the "just-right" match among the client, the frame of reference that guides intervention, the context, the activity, and the service delivery model. The ultimate goal of an occupational therapy intervention is for the client to engage in occupations, and as stated throughout this book, one specific and valuable tool is purposeful activity.

A therapist selects purposeful activities consistent with the theoretical base of the frame of reference. When an activity is selected to be therapeutic, it has two distinct sets of goals. First are the client's goals. These client-centered goals are influenced by the client's desires, abilities, needs, desires, motivations, and limitations. Second are the therapeutic goals set by the therapist, which are influenced by the service delivery model and where it is applied, the resources that are available to support the intervention, and the practitioner's knowledge and skills (Schell & Schell, 2007).

At times, occupational therapists will say that they are too busy or stressed to create new treatment activities for every client, so they fall back on a small repertoire of exercises and enabling or simulated activities. The idea that "one size fits all" does not tend to work well in occupational therapy. One-size-fits-all activities lack the elements that Dunton identified when the profession was just beginning in 1918 (Peloquin, 1991). Attention to individual and group needs and goals is a key element distinguishing occupational therapy services from the unskilled provision of activities. Florence Clark and her colleagues at the University of Southern California quantified this difference in their 1997 Well Elderly Study in which community-dwelling older adults benefited significantly more from occupational therapy than from activities supervised by nonprofessional staff.

Recognizing Occupation-Based Intervention Cues

Occupational therapists and occupational therapy assistants do not always have to generate novel activities for clients. Often, the client and his or her family have an existing set of activities that will work well to facilitate desired changes. Familiar and routine tasks are often easier to engage in than new ones. Moreover, recipients of occupational therapy services often have difficulty following through with home exercise programs; one way to overcome this problem is to use familiar everyday tasks instead.

When practitioners work in skilled nursing facilities, a common complaint takes the form of "I can't get Mrs. Smith to do anything." Karen, an occupational therapy assistant with 33 years of experience, sees it as a personal challenge to take on these clients. She does not have any magic tricks but instead uses some simple ideas to get residents moving again. The first is talking and listening. What does this person value? Who are the important people in his or her life? What can be learned by observing the person and his or her room, personal items, or photographs? If someone just wants to talk, Karen will use the conversation as an opening to begin to create rapport and wait for a natural activity to present itself. The resident may discuss a valued occupation or role; for example, Mrs. Smith might say that she misses her grandchildren. Karen will then use that information to synthesize an activity that supports the desired role and incorporates a therapeutic goal. In the case of Mrs. Smith, her limited standing balance and upper-extremity strength could be addressed while baking cookies for her grandchildren's visit.

EXERCISE 8.3: HOME ACTIVITY PROGRAM

Consider a working adult who also has responsibilities in child rearing and other instrumental activities of daily living. Think about all the possible everyday activities that could be used or adapted so that he or she works on shoulder strength. Name at least 15 ways for the client to incorporate your suggestions into his or her daily routine so that a home exercise program just happens and is not an added chore in already busy days. How would you upgrade or downgrade these activities?

EXERCISE 8.4: RESPONDING TO A CLIENT'S ACTIVITY CUES

Think about an older adult who has been admitted to a skilled nursing facility for short-term rehabilitation. She is debilitated after a hip replacement and pneumonia. What occupations are suggested by these client statements?

"I'm thirsty."
"I'm cold."
"It's too hot in here."
"I look terrible."

What performance skills could be observed by enabling the client to participate in the occupations you described for each statement?

As a means of engagement, it is often easier to convince people to help others than it is to convince them to do something for themselves alone. For example, Karen might say "I know you don't feel like exercising today, but I need help with all these plants." Mrs. Smith could work on her standing balance and upper-extremity strength by watering the plants in the occupational therapy clinic. As Mrs. Smith's tolerance for standing activities improves, the activity could be expanded to include trimming dead leaves, transplanting plants, or weeding outdoors at a raised flower bed.

Karen often tells students that she does not mind when a skilled nursing facility resident says "I have to go to the bathroom." Students tend to wonder why she wants to facilitate an activity that may be difficult, smelly, or dirty. What Karen knows is that she has the chance to help the resident engage in a purposeful activity of his or her choice while Karen observes the resident's abilities and difficulties with various underlying skills. Because the resident requests the activity and it takes place in his or her current home environment, it not just an activity but a true occupation.

Marsha is a registered occupational therapist working in an urban school system. She has a large caseload of elementary school children and relatively few resources. The school system requires therapists to intervene with children in the classroom whenever possible. One of Marsha's favorite places to work with her clients is the art classroom. In collaboration with the art teacher, Marsha can ensure that children with special needs participate in the same projects and activities as the other children by suggesting activity adaptations. The art teacher can also use these activity adaptations to enhance participation for children who do not qualify for occupational therapy services.

EXERCISE 8.5: SCHOOL-BASED ACTIVITIES

Divide into small groups. Compete with classmates to see which group can identify the greatest number of activities that would help facilitate handwriting in an elementary school student. In your groups, consider the various reasons why a child might have a problem with handwriting. Now, create a list of activities for addressing difficulties with handwriting when it is not caused by difficulty with fine motor coordination. Compare the activity list.

As discussed in Chapter 1, activities need not be glamorous or fancy to be useful in occupational therapy. Consider Case 8.6 of Erika.

Another case manager at the shelter might have gotten the bus pass for Erika more quickly, but she would not have helped her client accumulate new skills and self-confidence. It is often easy to pick out practitioners working in nontraditional roles by their propensity to do things *with* clients instead of *for* clients, as Erika's case illustrates.

CASE SCENARIO 8.6: ERIKA

Erika was a 33-year-old mother of three children living in a family shelter. She was able to live there for up to 8 weeks while looking for permanent housing. The shelter director told her that she would qualify for a public transportation pass to save money when she rode the bus. A few days later, the director could not understand why Erika had not gotten the bus pass. Cecilia, an occupational therapy assistant and case manager at the shelter, met with Erika to help her break up the activity of getting a bus pass into manageable tasks. Cecilia learned that a major barrier was Erika's anxiety about taking the bus into the city to get the pass. Erika came from a rural area and had forced herself over the past several months to take local buses after she lost her car. Cecilia seized the opportunity to help Erika expand her skills and confidence in using public transportation. They planned and timed their route, made transfers, and rode together to obtain the bus pass. Cecilia gradually withdrew her support until Erika could go anywhere by bus. Afterward, Erika said it was not as bad as she thought it would be but admitted she did not know whether she would ever have done it without Cecilia's help.

CASE SCENARIO 8.7: ALEX

Alex, who has depression and anxiety, had been a member of a psychosocial clubhouse for 18 months, yet he had become involved with very few activities. When art students from a local design college began working with
club members on a Halloween haunted house, someone mentioned that
they should have spooky music. Alex sheepishly said that he had an electric
keyboard that might work. After discussing music one-to-one, the occupational therapist learned that Alex had taught music lessons for many years
and still played now and then at home. He saw that this might be a perfect
way to get Alex more involved in the clubhouse activities and arranged for
the van driver to bring the keyboard to the center. Alex played for 3 hours
during the haunted house event. He got so much positive feedback that
he decided to leave the keyboard at the clubhouse, and he now leads sing-
along groups every week and takes pride in being a teacher again.

Even when clients cannot communicate verbally, they can usually express their activity preferences. Clients will select participation in specific activities they enjoy when they are given choices or opportunities.
Many years ago, when working in a long-term-care setting for adults
with developmental disabilities, Karen, an occupational therapy assistant, had a client named Sara who was unable to find her way to any
of the places she routinely visited, such as the cafeteria or recreation
room. On the basis of the Model of Human Occupation (Kielhofner,
2008), Sara had an occupational therapy goal related to topographical orientation. Sara could not even walk from place to place with a
group because she would stop anywhere along the route or just wander
off. Whenever Karen brought Sara to the recreation room, which had
a piano in it, Sara always gravitated toward it and she would "play"
the piano by pounding on the keys and laughing with delight. They
did this for months while addressing a variety of other issues. One day
Karen decided to watch from behind as Sara began walking through the
building in a goal-directed manner. She went up a stairway, down a cor-
ridor, made two turns, descended a few more steps, and arrived at the
recreation room. She went straight to the piano to play it. Eventually,
Sara was able to meet her goal of finding her way around the hospital
grounds.

Modifying Existing Activities to Meet Therapeutic Goals

When working with clients of any age, adapting activities to address their
therapeutic goals may be necessary. For example, clients with orthopedic

conditions, traumatic conditions, or burns may commonly have to execute specific actions in therapy. Rather than asking the client to participate in rote exercises that focus on the problem areas, the practitioner can creatively adapt one of the client's own purposeful activities or occupations to see that it includes the required actions. Listening to the client, caregiver, or both is still very important when adapting or modifying activities. Moreover, if activities become too contrived, they may become meaningless and thus not therapeutic. The choice of activities and the client's ability to participate in an activity program will depend on the client's interest, ability, and needs. The activities could be part of any area of occupation as defined by AOTA (2008): activities of daily living, instrumental activities of daily living, rest and sleep, education, work, play, leisure, and social participation.

Cases 8.8 and 8.9 illustrate the use and adaptation of people's existing activities to work toward therapeutic goals and allow them to engage in their desired occupations and roles (Figure 8.1). These scenarios also illustrate how the occupational therapy intervention for the co-occupation of caregiving may benefit clients and family members.

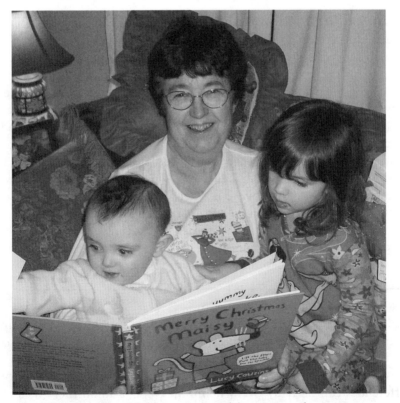

Figure 8.1. Grandchildren are powerful motivators for activity.

CASE SCENARIO 8.8: PATRICIA

Patricia is a 65-year-old, newly retired financial planner who has osteoarthritis and is troubled by pain and stiffness in her hands and knees. Patricia's most cherished role is being a caregiver for her only granddaughter. It is difficult for her to manipulate the sticky tape on disposable diapers, and a squirming and crying baby made the situation more taxing. A lot of the baby clothes her son and daughter-in-law sent over had multiple snaps in the inseams of pants and pajamas. Working with her occupational therapist, who decided to use an ecological theoretical perspective, Patricia found that diapers with Velcro tabs were easier to handle and more adjustable. The therapist also suggested finding baby clothes with fewer snaps. Patricia was thrilled to follow that recommendation because it reinforced her valued and longstanding leisure occupation of thrift store shopping. Patricia loves to buy the baby gently used clothes that she knows she will be able to use.

CASE SCENARIO 8.9: IAN

Ian was born at 28 weeks' gestational age and was being seen by an occupational therapist in a neonatal intensive care unit (NICU). Although this situation is always stressful, Ian's mother was having additional difficulty with her son's premature birth because she had previously had another son who died in the NICU after living only 1 day. She also reported that she felt guilty and wondered what she had done to precipitate another premature birth. When the medical team agreed that Ian should try bottle feeding, the occupational therapist sat with the mother and baby to evaluate and facilitate the process. The occupational therapist showed her how to hold Ian to maximize his breathing and swallowing. When his suck was weak, the therapist showed her how to use her fingers to support Ian's oral musculature and control his chin. In a few days, the therapist encouraged Ian's mother to show another relative the special techniques for feeding him. These positive experiences helped Ian maximize his nutrition and increased his mother's sense of self-efficacy in caring for her son.

In early intervention programs, therapists use everyday tasks in their natural settings to help children from birth to age 3 engage in their appropriate occupations of play, self-care, and social participation. Parenting can itself be stressful, but meeting the needs of a child with medical or developmental differences can be truly overwhelming. Occupational therapists in early intervention use a family-centered approach to help parents and caregivers maximize their children's abilities and minimize disruptions in daily routines. Parents and caregivers may need to learn how to hold a child, position a child, and engage a child in play.

CASE SCENARIO 8.10: KARA

At 30 months, Kara was receiving early intervention occupational therapy services to help bring her fine motor, visual–perceptual, and self-care skills to an age-appropriate level (Figure 8.2). Kara had a new baby brother and was having trouble coping with the new demands on her parents' attention. The occupational therapist saw that Kara liked playing with a baby doll, emulating what her mother and father did. The therapist suggested they provide real diapers, clothes, and a doll stroller so Kara could take care of her doll. They were able to address all of Kara's problem areas with creative play that the toddler loved. Kara's engagement with caring for the doll helped to give her mother a break so that she could feed the baby or put him down for a nap. As Kara's fine motor and perceptual skills improved, the therapist talked to her mother about the next steps, for example, introducing doll clothes with snaps or buttons.

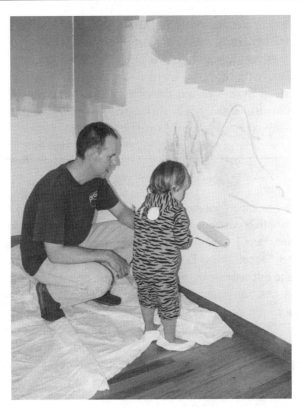

Figure 8.2. A child paints.

CASE SCENARIO 8.11: MR. SWEENEY

Mr. Sweeney, who had mild to moderate Alzheimer's disease, lived with his wife in their own home. He was retired from his job as a journalist and editor. His wife has already cared for his mother, who had Alzheimer's and had died several years earlier. She was cheerful and patient with her husband but also recognized his decline and dreaded going down the road that she had traveled with her mother-in-law. Paying the bills had always been one of Mr. Sweeney's jobs, and he got upset when he saw his wife doing it. Mrs. Sweeney was frustrated because she knew he would make mistakes in bill-paying tasks or get angry when he could not recall the next step in the activity. The consulting therapist used cognitive and contextual evaluation and activity analysis to suggest ways to structure the activity and break down the tasks so that Mr. Sweeney could still participate. Mrs. Sweeney maintained control of the finances to prevent errors, and Mr. Sweeney signed the checks and applied stamps and return address stickers to the envelopes. They felt satisfied that they could do a purposeful activity together, and the stress level around this household chore decreased significantly.

At the other end of the lifespan, adults with dementia or other degenerative diseases also require care from others. Case 8.11 is an example from a home-based occupational therapy consultation in a memory disorders clinic.

Anyone who has had a new baby or a frail elder in his or her home knows that sleep is an easily disrupted part of daily life that is extremely important. Lack of restful sleep makes other activities more difficult and contributes to a lower quality of life. Case 8.12 illustrates how an occupational therapist helped restore sleep to the life of a family caregiver.

CASE SCENARIO 8.12: MRS. D'AMBRA

Mrs. D'Ambra was caring for her husband, who had moderate dementia. She felt relatively satisfied with their daily routine, in which Mr. D'Ambra went to an adult day program 3 days a week so that she could run errands and have a few hours to herself. Mrs. D'Ambra thought her husband was relatively content, but she felt worn out. He would take a short nap most afternoons, but she felt that she could never nap herself and leave him unsupervised. They lived in an apartment on the first floor off a long hallway. The problem came at night when Mr. D'Ambra tended to get out of bed and wander into the hallway. Once in the hallway he could not recognize his own door because they all looked the same. Also, all the apartment doors would be locked, and the only door that would open was the fire door at the end of the hall-

(continued)

CASE SCENARIO 8.12: MRS. D'AMBRA (cont.)

way, leading him out to the cold night, close to the road, in his pajamas. Mr. D'Ambra had been discovered by chance outside one night, and his wife was terrified that he could die or be seriously injured if it happened again.

She told the occupational therapist who made a home visit that she did not sleep well because she knew from experience that she might not wake up if her husband got up at night. Mrs. D'Ambra had begun to push the kitchen table against the apartment door and pile the chairs on and around it. If he tried to get out the door, she would hear him moving the furniture and get up. The occupational therapist discussed her concern that blocking the door, although it seemed to help keep Mr. D'Ambra inside the apartment, was dangerous in other ways. The neurologist had previously suggested a door alarm, but Mrs. D'Ambra felt it was too expensive. The occupational therapist suggested attaching a string of large bells to the door so that Mrs. D'Ambra would hear the door opening. Mrs. D'Ambra was not sure that this would work, but then she remembered that her daughter had used a baby monitor for her children. Mrs. D'Ambra liked her own solution best because she could keep the monitor right on her bedside table and control the volume herself. A follow-up call a month later revealed that the monitor was working well, Mrs. D'Ambra was sleeping better, and she felt more effective as a caregiver.

Power of Activities

As illustrated in this chapter, activities at an appropriate level of challenge that fit the needs and desires of the client and his or her family and work well within their life roles and contexts can be very powerful in building a sense of competence. When therapists, clients, and families can harness that power, the full range of motor, cognitive, emotional, and social benefits of activity engagement are easy to see. It is hoped that a heightened level of participation and sense of competence carry far beyond the walls of an occupational therapy clinic or intervention setting, as seen in the cases in this section.

CASE SCENARIO 8.13: SEAN

Sean was born at 28 weeks' gestational age weighing 2 pounds, 10 ounces. He required a ventilator for several days and supplemental oxygen for about 8 weeks. He was later diagnosed with bronchopulmonary dysplasia and plagiocephaly for which he wore a cranial remolding orthosis (helmet). Sean did very

(continued)

CASE SCENARIO 8.13: SEAN (cont.)

well at home and needed occupational therapy only from the early inter-vention team. With early intervention his upper-extremity muscle tone gradually normalized, and he was more capable of transitioning to devel-opmentally appropriate positions using typical movement patterns. Sean was always attracted to a wooden rocking horse that belonged to his older sister. When he was about 15 months old, he would creep over to the rocking horse and pull himself to stand. He relied on his parents to put him on the horse and safely support him while he rode on it. He did not like to wait for help; he was intrinsically motivated to get on that horse and stay on it. He built his strength, balance, coordination, and other skills while his mother and father gradually downgraded the level of support they provided. When he mastered the activity of riding the rocking horse, Sean had to show his skill to everyone who came to the house (Figure 8.3).

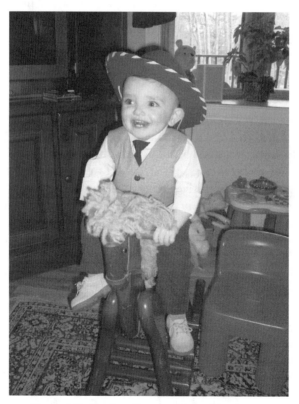

Figure 8.3. Cowboy Sean on his rocking horse.

CASE SCENARIO 8.14: MATT

Matt is an 8-year-old boy who has cerebral palsy with left hemiparesis. He began receiving occupational and physical therapy as an infant and has since been diagnosed with attention deficit hyperactivity disorder and sensory-processing disorder. Matt's parents tried to get him involved with various activities and sports with little success until they found martial arts. Matt has been participating in karate classes three times a week since age 4. His differences were never seen as a barrier to his participation in all the class activities, just as challenges to overcome. A few activities were initially adapted for Matt's participation, but now he engages in classes, tournaments, and social events at the martial arts academy independently. Matt has been discharged from all therapies. He has earned his adult brown belt and is adept at cartwheels, flips, and other acrobatics. Not bad for a boy whose doctors thought might never walk!

EXERCISE 8.6: DEVELOPING FINE MOTOR COORDINATION

Think about all the possible everyday activities that could be used or adapted to help a 3-year-old boy develop fine motor coordination. They could be part of self-care, play, or any other area of occupation. Name at least 20. How would you upgrade or downgrade these activities? What suggestions could you make to his caregivers to help incorporate your suggestions into the family's daily routine?

Arts and crafts activities were a primary focus at one time in occupational therapy history. Over time and with an increasing emphasis on working within the medical model, many practitioners abandoned or deemphasized the use of arts and crafts. Engagement in arts and crafts activities reinforces hand skill development, builds the ability to concentrate and follow written directions, and fosters values for creativity and effective use of leisure time. Arts and crafts projects can build self-esteem at any age through the completion of a project, either to keep or to give as a gift.

CASE SCENARIO 8.15: ALICE

Alice attends an adult day program and receives help with several daily activities. She has a history of strokes and many other medical problems. She uses a wheelchair but transfers independently and lives in her own home with support from aides. Alice was one of the first people at the adult day

(continued)

CASE SCENARIO 8.15: ALICE *(cont.)*

program to get involved in making blankets for recent immigrants who lacked warm clothes and household goods. The occupational therapy assistant students and I taught Alice and several others to make "no-sew" fleece blankets and adapted the tasks as needed so people with many different functional abilities and impairments could participate. Alice became an advocate for the project, recruiting her many friends at the center to help. It was very important to her to feel useful, and she often discusses her gratitude for the help she has received from others.

The blanket donation project was completed, but Alice was just beginning. She asked for help getting to the fabric store so she could make blankets for her home health aides. She altered the shape and size so that she could make herself a cape that she wears in cold weather when she rides in the van in her wheelchair. She explained how coats were never very practical considering her size and physical limitations. The cape keeps her hands and whole body warm. After being away from the center for several weeks, I returned one morning to hear Alice calling me and wheeling right over. It was a rainy day, and she had to show me her latest creation—a new cape with water-repellent fabric on one side and fleece on the other.

In other situations, occupational therapists and occupational therapy assistants do not have to provide new activities for their clients. They may facilitate someone's engagement in client-identified activities through adaptations or contextual changes, as shown in Case 8.16.

CASE SCENARIO 8.16: JOSH

Josh was a 6-year-old boy who had received chemotherapy for his leukemia and experienced hair loss and peripheral neuropathy. He worked with an occupational therapist to find a new personality for himself in the classroom. He found a cool hat. The splints that supported his wrists during classroom activities were the newest shade of neon. He covered his splints with stickers of space heros. Josh invented a spaceship captain personality for himself. He got to write using a special multicolor pen grip. He had a laptop computer that allowed him to interface with the "mothership" main frame about whatever the class was learning each day. Using play and re-establishment of a special role in a familiar situation, the occupational therapist helped Josh build self-esteem and peer acceptance of his differences.

CASE SCENARIO 8.17: MARCUS

At an adult day program for people with acquired brain injuries, Marcus was the comedian of the group and said he wanted to be on stage. He tried appearing at an open mic night at a local comedy club and got some laughs. Now his goal was to win the cash prize offered once a month. He worked with some occupational therapy students to use a computer to write down and fine tune his jokes. While practicing his act, they found that he would remember the beginning, but his attention skills were not perfect and he would begin to ramble toward the end. Marcus's stand-up comedy was actually sit-down comedy because he used a power wheelchair. He and the students collaboratively determined that he could tape a cue card to his pants and refer to it to keep on track while on stage. Marcus invited everyone to the next open mic night, and he has won several cash prizes since then.

Staff at the day program knew that Marcus made some female day program members uncomfortable when he told sexually inappropriate jokes during leisure or cooking groups. With prompting, Marcus recognized that he needed to learn the proper time and place for his jokes. The occupational therapist developed a cuing system that was agreed on by Marcus and the staff so that he could receive the limit setting he sometimes needed, without embarrassment.

CASE SCENARIO 8.18: WALTER

Walter, a 53-year-old man with bipolar disorder, was an active participant in a psychosocial clubhouse. He was very sociable and funny, but his participation in social activities was limited by his need to leave three mornings a week to go to renal dialysis. Having gained some insight into his tendency to ramble in conversation, he admitted that he did not always know when he needed to "reel it in." He wanted to make the most of his time at the center and did not like it when other members interrupted him so that someone else could talk. As a consulting occupational therapist, I suggested that when we were in group activities together I would do a hand motion to simulate reeling in a fish. Walter thought that was a great idea because it appealed to his sense of humor and pride. After trying the agreed-on cue, we decided that the first cue would simply be the reeling-in gesture. If Walter did not notice that, the group leader would speak his name, then make the hand signal. It worked like a charm.

Case Scenario 8.19: Preventing Repetitive Strain Injuries in the Workplace

In a workplace in which people use computers all day, an occupational therapist may recommend changing the height of monitors, the ergonomic demands or position of the keyboards, or the amount of time spent at computer terminals. Desks and chairs can be changed or adjusted to provide adequate ergonomic seating support. Occupational therapists can teach workers to regularly schedule rest and stretch breaks. One way to do this would be to use timers that go off at certain intervals. The timer would cue workers in that area to stand up and do some stretches derived from yoga poses. These or other fun activities encourage changes in posture and gross mobility rather than concentrated use of the hands. Evidence-based practice has shown yoga to be an effective, nonmedical intervention for carpal tunnel syndrome (Garfinkel & Singhal, 1998; Michlovitz, 2004). Additionally, an occupational therapist could recommend that the management team bring in a yoga instructor to conduct classes on a weekly basis or reimburse employees for the cost of yoga classes.

Use of Activities at the Organization Level

Thus far, the examples in this chapter have dealt with occupational therapy for individuals or groups. Occupational therapy services may also be provided to organizations such as employers (AOTA, 2008). A common application of occupational therapy expertise in this arena is in suggesting activity or workstation adaptations when carpal tunnel syndrome or other repetitive strain injuries are prevalent. Consider the example in Case 8.18.

Similar routines could be incorporated into the work days of hair stylists, dentists, and dental hygienists, who spend long hours in repetitive hand use, often with awkward wrist positions or stooped shoulder postures. Also, in those professions a real break is provided between appointments or tasks. These breaks, although short, could be used to perform neck, shoulder, and arm circles that help counteract the static postures that contribute to repetitive strain injuries. If these exercises are to be successfully incorporated into the day's routine, all members of a work unit need to follow them. Signs around the workplace, computer screen savers, and other cues could be used to make hand-saving techniques just as normal as hand-washing behaviors in health care, childcare, and food preparation settings.

Use of Activities at the Population Level

Occupational therapy interventions for populations are meant to help an entire group of people rather than individuals (AOTA, 2008). For example, occupational therapy faculty and students at the New England Institute of Technology have developed a summer day camp program for children living in a nearby family shelter. The camp provides safe and developmentally appropriate play and social participation opportunities for homeless children living at the shelter. Innumerable unserved or underserved populations could benefit from occupational therapy services in some form. A few examples are in Case 8.20.

To say that adolescents or young adults have a lot to adjust to after a spinal cord injury is an understatement. One very important change is the limited access they have to social and recreational activities. Community organizations exist around the country that help people with spinal cord injuries adjust to their new lives. Organizations like Shake-A-Leg in Newport, Rhode Island,

---

CASE SCENARIO *8.20:* THERAPY MISSIONS

In 2007, Carol Doehler, Dahlia Castillo, and other occupational therapists offered their services to the Fundacion de Integra in Juarez, Mexico. Integra is a community-based agency established by the families of people with disabilities. In Mexico, children with disabilities other than blindness are not allowed to go to school. Many children would thus not leave their homes. Rehabilitation for adults with physical disabilities is very limited. Some may be given a wheelchair, but few buildings or public services are wheelchair accessible.

Parents and other family members bring people to Integra, where they learn and carry out therapeutic exercises and participate in horseback riding or water activities. Integra has intermittent services from a physiatrist, but it has no professional rehabilitation therapists.

The U.S. occupational therapists quickly noticed that many of the children who visited Integra had no outlets for play. One of the first interventions for this population was to teach parents and other caregivers how to help the children access toys and play in developmentally sound and therapeutic ways. Various toys and positioning devices were purchased or created so that the children could try to play. By helping the parents think about play as a normal and beneficial occupation for their children, the therapists empowered parents to expand therapeutic activities into their home lives and to strengthen their community by sharing ideas with each other. Although Integra has functioned as a home base for the visiting therapists, the entire population of people with disabilities in Juarez, Mexico, is being served by the education of families and other caregivers. Several of the therapists who have visited Juarez have formed Therapy Missions, a nonprofit organization that aims to provide occupational and physical therapy to underserved populations around the world.

and Crested Butte Adapted Sports in Colorado provide much-needed services to teens and adults with paraplegia and quadriplegia. Some of the possibilities for wheelchair sports were shown to the general public in the documentary film *Murderball* (Shapiro, Mandel, & Rubin, 2005), which showcased athletes playing wheelchair rugby at an international level. Although no occupational therapists are depicted in the movie, many opportunities for professional or volunteer involvement with these and other sports exist.

Summary

All activities have the potential to be important and meaningful therapeutic modalities when used by occupational therapists. Guided by theoretically based frames of reference, occupational therapists and occupational therapy assistants promote change through the use of purposeful activities, in the context of real life. Purpose in doing the activity must be inherent for activity participation. Practitioners skillfully use activities to facilitate a client's participation in his or her daily life. The variety of activities and intervention settings is limited only by one's imagination.

References

American Occupational Therapy Association. (2008). Occupational therapy practice framework: Domain and process (2nd ed.). *American Journal of Occupational Therapy, 62,* 625–683.

Clark, F., Azen, S. P., Zemke, R., Jackson, J., Carlson, M., Mandel, D., et al. (1997). Occupational therapy for independent-living older adults: A randomized controlled trial. *JAMA, 278,* 1321–1326.

Early, M. B. (2006). *Physical dysfunction practice skills for the occupational therapy assistant* (2nd ed.). St. Louis, MO: Mosby.

Garfinkel, M. S., & Singhal, A. (1998). Yoga-based intervention for carpal tunnel syndrome. *JAMA, 280,* 1601–1603.

Kielhofner, G. (2008). *Model of Human Occupation: Theory and application* (4th ed.). Philadelphia: Lippincott Williams & Wilkins.

Ma, H., & Trombly, C. A. (2002). A synthesis of the effects of occupational therapy for persons with stroke, Part II: Remediation of impairments. *American Journal of Occupational Therapy, 56,* 260–274.

Michlovitz, S. L. (2004). Conservative interventions for carpal tunnel syndrome. *Journal of Orthopaedic and Sports Physical Therapy, 34*(10), 589–600.

Mosey, A. C. (1986). *Psychological components of occupational therapy.* New York: Raven.

Peloquin, S. M. (1991). Occupational therapy service: Individual and collective understandings of the founders, Part 2 [Historical Article]. *American Journal of Occupational Therapy, 45,* 733–744.

Schell, B. A. B., & Schell, J. W. (2007). *Clinical and professional reasoning in occupational therapy.* Philadelphia: Lippincott Williams & Wilkins.

Shapiro, D. A. (Director & Producer), Mandel, J. (Producer), & Rubin, H. A. (Director). (2005). *Murderball* [Motion picture]. Los Angeles: THINKFilm.

9

◈

Occupation and Activities in Groups

Jeff Tomlinson, MSW, OTR, FAOTA
Deborah Moore, MA, OTR/L

Activities are the building blocks of occupation. Because humans are social animals, many of the activities involved in the various areas of occupation are naturally performed in groups. For example, children gather to play in playgrounds or parks equipped with climbing frames and swing sets and in open play spaces or a tenants' or homeowners' association holds meetings to provide a forum for discussion, decision making, and action on issues affecting its members. Such group activities may fall under social participation, leisure, or any other area of occupation, depending on the design, purpose, and context of the group. Common to all groups are the necessary communication and social skills and emotional regulation skills (American Occupational Therapy Association [AOTA], 2008).

The environment, performance context, and cultural considerations are critical to both naturally occurring groups and therapy groups. A naturally occurring group such as a tenants' or homeowners' association is formed to deal with the issues of a particular neighborhood; a parent–teacher organization at a local school is operated for the benefit of the children who attend that particular school; or ice skating lessons are given at an indoor skating rink or outdoors in a local park during the winter. These groups are all formed for a particular purpose unique to their environmental context, and they function accordingly (Figure 9.1).

Several useful definitions of *group* are found in the occupational therapy literature. A group is "a gathering of three or more people joined together for a joint face-to-face purpose for a continuous period of time" (Donohue & Greer, 2004, p. 226). According to Barbara Posthuma (2002), "a group is a sum of its parts: a collective of individual persons participating together" (p. 17). Gail Fidler (1969) declared that a group is a therapeutic agent. The purpose of any group is for people to engage in activities together.

Naturally occurring groups can be formal or informal. *Informal groups* often occur spontaneously in playgrounds, in school and work settings, in religious centers, in health clubs and Internet cafes, and within families.

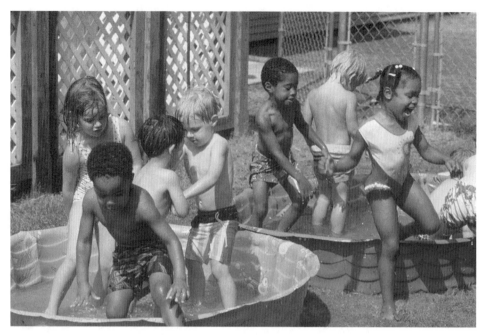

Figure 9.1. Naturally occuring groups form around children's play.
Note. Photograph courtesy of the Public Health Image Library, Centers for Disease Control and Prevention. Photo by Jim Gathany.

Wherever people gather, groups form. Examples of more structured or formal naturally occurring groups are families, classrooms, school sports teams, special interest clubs (e.g., chess, gardening), scouting organizations, volunteer community task forces, political action groups, and teams and committees in the workplace. Many social venues, such as parties, concerts, plays, tours, movies, and sporting events, are examples of large, structured, *formal groups* created for particular purposes (Figure 9.2). Groups such as these are often planned by large organizations, well in advance, for the purpose of fundraising or as profit-making business ventures. An increasing number of groups are Web-based, such as online learning sites, blogs and forums, shopping sites, e-mail groups, and social and personal sites, some formal and some informal. Available through the Internet, these virtual groups do not require the "face-to-face" aspect crucial to earlier definitions of groups.

An occupational therapist functions as a member of many groups in the workplace. Therapists are often part of a large organization—a school system, a hospital, a home care agency, or a university. They are also part of the smaller group of their occupational therapy department, and often they are one member of a rehabilitation team composed of people from several professional disciplines. Membership on a committee or task force may be an additional type of group participation in which therapists engage at work. Occupational therapists also lead or colead therapy groups for their clients. Thus, the awareness of the nature and structure of groups, of group process,

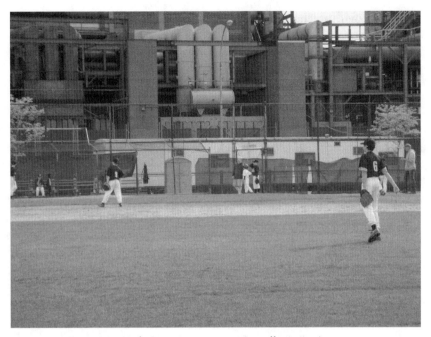

Figure 9.2. Little League game—a naturally occurring group.

and of the stages of group development and group roles is critical knowledge for all occupational therapists.

Therapy groups are planned, structured groups that are held in a particular setting or treatment environment context, designed for a therapeutic purpose with a specific, selected population of participants. Groups may be designed around members' interests, common needs and problem areas, or similar treatment goals. Occupational therapy groups are usually named after the primary activity that will be used therapeutically or the performance skills that will be enhanced during the group treatment sessions. Some common examples of occupational therapy groups are exercise, cooking, and dressing groups in rehabilitation centers. Schools often have gross motor skills and sensory–motor skills groups. Community day treatment programs frequently use budgeting and stress management groups. Some settings include assessment or evaluation groups and treatment groups. Participation in a therapy group is most often voluntary but may sometimes be required as part of a treatment plan or treatment program.

The participants in a group are usually called *members*. Occupational therapy groups are run by one or two therapists, who are the designated group leaders, and usually consist of between 5 and 10 group members. In the occupational therapy literature, 8 is mentioned as the optimal number for therapy groups (Fidler, 1969), but smaller and larger groups may be designed for specific purposes in many treatment settings. One challenge facing occupational therapists and occupational therapy assistants is that they must design therapy groups that meet the needs, concerns, and treatment goals of both the individual members and of the entire group. In addition, they must consider the following:

When providing therapeutic activities, occupational therapy practitioners attend to five major components: (1) the activity, (2) the occupational therapy practitioner's use of self as a leader, (3) the group members as participants, (4) the group's process or interactions, and (5) the group's culture and physical context. (Donohue & Greer, 2004, pp. 226–227)

In occupational therapy groups, the focus is often primarily on the activity (as opposed to the self, which is the primary focus in psychotherapy or social support groups). This focus on activity stimulates interest and often leads to continued, sustained group participation. Engagement in an activity allows clients to focus on the tasks and to work toward the achievement of successful end results. Group activities are designed by occupational therapists to incorporate individual treatment goals, such as working on cognitive, fine motor, and visual–motor integration performance skills during grooming, woodworking, cooking, or beading activity groups. Group activities also provide a forum for the observation of a person's behavior in the here-and-now of the group (Mosey, 1970). Group process, although often seeming to be focused primarily on the tasks of the group and participation within the group, also provides the occupational therapist and other group members with critical opportunities to provide behavioral feedback to individual group members. Feedback to individual members and to the group as a whole is usually concrete, task focused, and behavior based, but it may also be about the process observed within the group (Figure 9.3). We discuss group process feedback in greater detail later in this chapter.

EXERCISE 9.1: NATURALLY OCCURRING GROUP HISTORY

In a group of three or four students, briefly describe some of the naturally occurring groups in which you participated during early childhood, childhood, adolescence, and young adulthood. Note similarities and differences, including the environmental or cultural context of the groups. Alternatively, interview another student, a neighbor, a friend, or a relative about their participation in groups while growing up.

EXERCISE 9.2: RELATIONSHIP OF ACTIVITY GROUPS TO AREAS OF OCCUPATION AND PERFORMANCE SKILLS

For the groups you recalled in Exercise 9.1, delineate the group activities in which you participated, and classify them by the areas of occupation under which they fall. Where possible, also state the performance skills involved in the activities performed in these groups. Prepare to share this information in a group discussion.

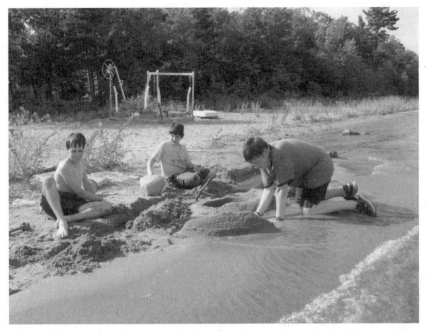

Figure 9.3. Boys give each other feedback then return to task-focused behaviors.

CASE SCENARIO 9.1: YOHANAN

Yohanan is an occupational therapist in a mental health day program treating adults with chronic mental illness. The clients in the day program have myriad deficits, including social skills and activities of daily living performance. Yohanan leads two to three groups each day that address these deficits, including social skills, cooking skills, problem-solving skills, instrumental activities of daily living skills, exercise, cognitive skills, and a men's mutual support group. Each group takes advantage of group interaction around purposeful activities.

Group Development

Many social scientists have studied groups and identified stages in the development of group interaction. This information has been well summarized elsewhere in occupational therapy texts (Cole, 1998; Howe & Schwartzberg, 2001; Posthuma, 2002). Three pioneers in analyzing and articulating phases of group development are Bruce Tuckman, Roy Lacoursiere, and William Schutz.

Tuckman (1965) named the stages of group development as *forming, storming, norming,* and finally *performing.* Lacoursiere (1980) labeled these stages *orientation, dissatisfaction, resolution, production,* and *termination.* The stages described by Tuckman (1965) and Lacoursiere (1980) have been given convenient, self-explanatory descriptive names. Each theorist identified an initial formative phase. Note that during the second stage of group development, each of these authors articulated a period of turbulence and disagreement, followed by more smooth periods during which most of the group's work is accomplished.

Schutz (1958) described the stages as *inclusion, control,* and *affection.* During the inclusion stage, group members are concerned with acceptance and belonging in the group as the group forms. During the control stage, they are focused on issues regarding leadership and authority. During the final affection stage, group members are primarily concerned with the emotional attachments between members.

Schutz's (1958) theory of group development is innovative in that he identified these stages as a cycle that reoccurs during the life of the group (Posthuma, 2002; Schutz, 1958). At times of stress or crisis in the group, a reversion to one of the earlier group phases (often that of turbulence or control) frequently occurs. Because of this movement, the group stages can be viewed as swinging like a pendulum or as moving through stages in recurrent cycles. In therapy groups that have many members with impaired social skills, it is possible that the turbulent second stage and the camaraderie of the production or affection stages cannot fully develop. Most authors who study group development have now also incorporated Lacoursiere's (1980) idea of a final termination or adjourning stage, in which the group moves toward a sense of closure. The termination phase occurs as the group completes its work (e.g., planning a special project), when the allotted number of sessions for the group ends (e.g., the end of a semester or the school year), or whenever group leaders or group members change.

The relationship between group leader and group members evolves with each developmental stage of the group. Early in the group's development, members often demonstrate some level of dependence on the leader. At later stages, group members may be quite independent. The leadership role will usually be challenged by group members at some point, most frequently during the phase of discord in the group's development. We discuss group leadership challenges later in this chapter along with the therapist's role in groups, group roles, and common group problems.

EXERCISE 9.3: IDENTIFYING GROUP STAGES

Reflect on and briefly describe one team experience or group project in which you have participated. How did the initial forming phase feel? Was there a phase of discord? Did the group achieve a sense of unity and affection as tasks were worked on? Was there a clear termination phase? Compare your notes with a partner, in class discussion, or with a supervisor.

Group Norms

In any group involving occupation, implicit and explicit rules guide behavior and actions within, and at times outside, the group. These rules of behavior are called *norms*. The norms of the groups may, in part, be handed down by the institution that the group works within. Other norms may be dictated by the group's leaders, and then additional norms may be generated by the group members. Group norms of the greatest importance usually relate to the safety and dignity of the group members and to the maintenance of the group's existence and functioning.

Implicit norms are often regular attendance and punctuality. Important *explicit norms* usually include confidentiality within the group and that the members all speak to one another and to the leader. Group norms operate in a manner similar to the laws of grammar in that most group members are generally not consciously aware of these norms, particularly the implicit ones. At the same time, group norms have a strong influence on shaping group members' behavior (Figure 9.4). The need for individual members to be accepted by the group and maintain their membership in the group strengthens the force of norms on shaping behavior and conformity within the group. When membership in the group is very attractive, the group's norms will hold greater influence over the members.

In occupational therapy groups, certain values are implicit norms. These values include engaging in purposeful and productive occupa-

---

CASE SCENARIO 9.2: CHRISTOPHER

Christopher is a 14-year-old high school freshman who has a diagnosis of conduct disorder. Christopher is struggling with destructive and attention-seeking impulses that have made it very difficult for him to attend to and participate in the activities in a classroom. Christopher has been invited to join an after-school group that is coordinated by an occupational therapy assistant. The group uses skateboarding; interactive party video games; and popular music such as house, hip-hop, and reggae to facilitate social interaction between the members. Christopher is immediately very attracted to both the activities and the other members, and he finds himself looking forward to getting together with the other members of the group. Initially, he starts to act up in the group, trying to dominate materials and attention. Other group members, through both verbal feedback and modeling, give Christopher a clear message about the group's implicit norms of sharing and taking turns. Although Christopher struggles to control his impulses, he finds the group very important to him and works harder to follow the group's norms around these behaviors.

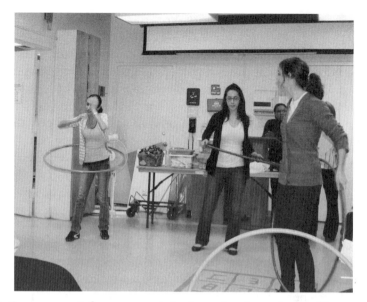

Figure 9.4. Group norms influence group behavior and each member's willingness to engage in the activity.

tions, interdependence, and a client-centered approach to therapeutic relations. The group setting provides an invaluable opportunity for refining members' perceptions of independence. Through collaborative relations with others in groups, the members have the opportunity to realize the existential reality of interdependence—that is, the reality that in human society people are never completely independent but rather rely on each other for the satisfaction of many of their needs. Therefore, one of the core values of occupational therapy groups is not independence but, more accurately, successful and balanced interdependence. For group members who may be adjusting to diminished abilities or radically changed life circumstances, this reframing of values is critical.

Therapist's Role in Groups

The therapist is most often a leader, coleader, or organizer of occupational therapy groups. Gail Fidler (1969) advocated that the group leader's overall role is not that of a treatment giver but rather that of an agent in maximizing the group's therapeutic learning potential. The group leader's responsibilities may include the selection of group members, the provision of adequate meeting space and materials, the initial establishment of the rules and nonexplicit norms for the group, and the responsibility to function as a technical expert and a role model for appropriate participation in the group.

Some effective techniques that may be used by the leader to model appropriate group behaviors are self-disclosure ("I wonder if anyone else felt. . . . "), self-reflection ("I felt . . . when. . . ," "I thought. . . ," or "What do you think of Joe's idea?"), and empathy (Cole, 1998; Posthuma, 2002). The therapist's role is to be an effective helper in the group, which Davis (1989) has described as facilitating and assisting rather than controlling, using active listening, and using empathy. *Active listening* involves restatement of the problem, a statement of reflection on it, and a statement clarifying it. *Empathy* is described as listening to others with the "third ear," which is attuned to the feelings of others and the meaning of the feelings for others, so that the leader can describe what it is like to be in the situation of another group member.

The relationship between group leaders and group members has also been studied, and stages in the development of this relationship have been identified. The relationship of members to the group leader is known as the *authority cycle* (Posthuma, 2002) . This cycle has been found to evolve in similar ways to those described in the earlier section on the stages of group development. The stages of the authority cycle are *dependence, counterindependence, counterdependence, independence,* and ultimately *interdependence. Dependence* is the stage in which the group obtains its information from the leader and imitates the leader's behaviors. *Counterindependence* is marked by a moving away from the leader; it may be accompanied by emotions of fear and anger because the leader may be seen as not doing his or her job and the group may feel like a rudderless ship (Posthuma, 2002). *Counterdependence* is the stage in which the leader is rejected, and members' feelings of hostility and tension may predominate as a struggle for authority and leadership ensues. The next stage, *independence,* is characterized by cohesion and socializing among members while the leader is left out and the group's work tasks are often ignored. A great deal of positive interpersonal learning may occur during this stage. *Interdependence* is the highly functional stage in which unity and confidence exist among members, and the leader is no longer excluded from the group. It is notable that in the second and third stages of the authority cycle, turmoil exists as the leadership role is challenged, which is also reflected in the second stage of group development (dissatisfaction, control, or storming), as described earlier. As with the stages of group development, the group may move back and forth among the stages of the authority cycle, swinging particularly during times of stress within the group.

All group members and leaders can facilitate development of maturity in groups by attending to and modeling appropriate member behaviors during group sessions. Some particularly important behaviors, in addition to paying attention to feelings, are further role-modeling behaviors (Figure 9.5). This modeling of behavior often involves being an active participant rather than a silent observer, giving objective and constructive positive or negative feedback to others, and being receptive to feedback oneself (Cole, 1998). In groups that use activities, interactions develop around the tasks. (We discuss levels of group interaction further later in this chapter.) These interactions occur in behaviors, feelings, and group roles. Three distinct

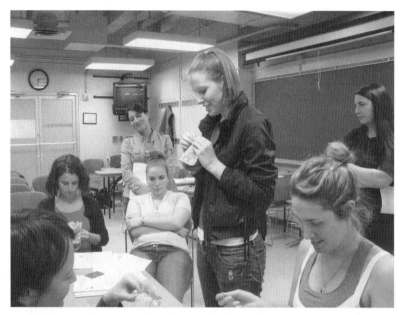

Figure 9.5. As the group leader models behavior, others in the group copy it while one member does not participate.

types of group roles exist—*group task roles, group building and mainte-nance roles,* and *individual roles*—each of which may be modeled by the group leader and is discussed in detail later in this chapter (Cole, 1998; Posthuma, 2002).

Group Membership and Roles

One of the immediate considerations in planning a group is its membership. In a naturally occurring group, the members select each other. This formation is either through an attraction between the members (a social desire

---

EXERCISE 9.4: GROUP LEADERSHIP

Select two or three groups you have been part of and reflect on the relationship between the group leader(s) and group members. Did this relationship follow the pattern outlined in the stages of the authority cycle? If not, reflect on the differences in your group(s). If you have been a leader in a group, reflect on the relevance of the authority cycle to your role as leader. Which stages stand out most in your recollection of the group and why? Share your thoughts in classroom discussion or with your supervisor.

to spend time together), a perception that the group will help them in some manner, or an attraction to the group's activity. In the latter scenario, the members come together out of a shared interest in the activity itself, and most often group members have been drawn together without knowing each other before their participation in the group (Figure 9.6).

Groups may have either formal or informal membership. Many therapy groups are formal in membership; the clients are selected by the therapist or by other staff, they are clearly identified, and their participation in the group is formally recognized. In groups with formal membership, norms and expectations about attendance are usually formalized as well. In groups that have informal membership, such as a cancer survivors' support group, the therapist allows members to attend or not attend group sessions as they desire.

In groups that have formal membership, the group may be either closed or open to new members. Open groups will allow new members to join throughout the group's lifespan. Closed groups, however, will begin with a set membership and will not allow any new members to join. A group that is designed so that members acquire new information or skills in a sequential or developmental manner, such as an introductory pottery class, may choose a closed format because new members would be entering in the middle of a process and might not benefit fully from the group.

In planned groups, the therapist must consider many factors in the selection of the group members:

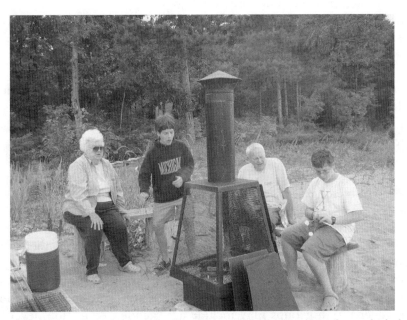

Figure 9.6. Families enjoy spending time together engaged in an activity from which they receive pleasure.

CASE SCENARIO 9.3: FLO

Flo leads both a social skills training group and a psychoeducational group in which she is currently teaching budgeting skills at a mental health day program. The social skills training group encourages members to bring to each group examples of difficult interpersonal situations that they have encountered since the group last met. The group then selects a different social situation, and each member works at mastering communications that are more effective. The format of the group is consistent from week to week; however, the specific content of the group varies and often has little relationship to last week's group session. In the psychoeducational group, Flo is teaching budgeting skills that build developmentally on the content learned from the previous session. In the first group session, the members learned how to keep records of money they spent. In the second session, the members learned how to separate these expenditures into different categories, and in the third session the members learned how to collect the different expenditure categories into fixed monthly expenses and variable expenses. Any client who asked to enter the budgeting skills group at the third session would be at a significant disadvantage because he or she would not have learned the content of the previous group sessions. The psychoeducational social skills group, however, could function as an open group, admitting new members at any time.

- Clients' therapy needs and individual goals,
- Whether the clients' needs are better served in a group or in individual sessions, and
- The clients' ability to participate in groups.

In some settings, the therapist may begin the treatment planning process by collecting data on the service needs of the population in the setting. The therapist then matches the service needs of the clients with the existing therapy programming and ultimately identifies unmet areas of treatment need, which should lead to the planning of new treatment programming, including groups. During this process of identifying unmet treatment needs, a potential group of members will most likely have already been identified.

One aspect of group membership that should be considered is homogeneous vs. heterogeneous group composition. *Homogeneous group composition* means that certain relevant qualities of the group members are the same or very similar (e.g., a particular diagnosis). *Heterogeneous group composition* means that certain identified qualities in the group members are significantly different. The relevant qualities or client factors to consider for homogeneity in groups may include age, gender, education, level of experience in an occupation, common treatment problems and goals, medical diagnosis, or level of functioning. Both types of group composition have advantages and disadvantages. A more homogeneous group may be better able to identify with each other and develop group cohesion quickly, so that group tasks are more readily accomplished. Heterogeneous groups, however, provide a variety of experiences, knowledge, and unique contributions that can be used to stimulate the group and may provide a richer problem-solving base when difficulties in task performance or other conflicts arise.

The size of the group should be carefully considered, as discussed previously. For many occupational therapy groups, six to eight members is considered optimal. In psychoeducational groups, in which more of a class process exists, the group may be much larger and still work successfully. The therapist should take into consideration how much assistance the members may need during tasks and the nature of the activity to engage an adequate number of members in relation to the number of group leaders.

Member Roles

In groups, members will assume different *behavioral roles,* or patterns of behavior, as a result of their character and individual needs or through the group's dynamic pressures and demands. This process of assuming a certain role or roles in a group usually occurs without the member's awareness. Benne and Sheats (1948) set forth a long list of the roles that frequently occur in groups. More recently, three main types of roles have been identified (*task roles, group building and maintenance roles,* and *individual roles;* Cole, 1998; Posthuma, 2002), which we briefly summarize here.

Task roles are those that relate to facilitating completion of the group's tasks:

- *Initiator–contributor*—helps provide initiative in the group, suggests new ideas, and contributes frequently
- *Information seeker*—often asks for information from others in the group
- *Information giver*—frequently provides information to the group
- *Opinion seeker*—often solicits opinions from other group members
- *Opinion giver*—frequently expresses his or her own opinions and beliefs
- *Elaborator*—often further explains a point made by another member of the group
- *Coordinator*—organizes information, plans, and events for the group
- *Orienter*—summarizes to help keep the group organized and points out when the group strays from its original focus
- *Evaluator–critic*—provides judgmental feedback to the group or its members
- *Energizer*—provides encouragement or a boost to help the group move forward with tasks
- *Procedural technician*—provides detailed information about how to get tasks done and may give out task supplies

- *Recorder*—keeps notes or records of events in the group, either in writing or by memory.

Group building and maintenance roles are those focused on the functioning of the group process:

- *Encourager*—provides verbal encouragement and support to group members
- *Harmonizer*—tries to smooth over conflicts in groups and maintain peace
- *Compromiser*—gives up a position or power to help resolve group conflict
- *Gatekeeper–expediter*—facilitates communication between members
- *Standard setter*—communicates standards for performance in the group
- *Observer–commentator*—makes comments on observations of events in the group
- *Follower*—more passive than the other members, goes along with group decisions.

Individual roles are those focused on the individual members and their own issues and needs. These individual roles frequently disrupt or impede progress in group process:

- *Aggressor*—forceful and outspoken in the group, often to the detriment of others or to the group
- *Blocker*—frequently raises negative objections, opposition, or obstacles to group movement or group efforts
- *Recognition seeker*—frequently acts in ways that draw attention to him- or herself
- *Self-confessor*—uses the group to get personal issues off his or her chest
- *Playboy or playgirl*—stays on the periphery of the group; offers little to the group, as if above or different from the rest of the group; often jokes off topic
- *Dominator*—often tries to control the events or members in the group
- *Arguer*—frequently takes an opposing viewpoint for the purpose of disagreement to continue group discussion; may plead special interests or causes.

Roles are not mutually exclusive. Members may take on multiple roles within the group, either simultaneously or on an alternating basis. One group member may be both an information giver and an information seeker (task roles), a harmonizer (group building and maintenance role), and occasionally a self-confessor (individual role). Communication within the group may be enhanced or disrupted by the roles individual group members take on during the group's activity performance. We discuss group interaction and communication further in the following sections of this chapter, including levels of group interaction, task groups, group process, group decision making, and common group problems.

Levels of Group Interaction

Communication is a process of information exchange among people using a mutual system of signs, symbols, or behavior in the interaction. Thus, by definition, communication in groups is an interactive process, using behavior in addition to the symbol system of language for verbal communication. For optimal communication, it is crucial that the communication be consistently and appropriately interactive during activity groups.

Five levels of communication have been analyzed and envisioned as a pyramid, known as Powell's pyramid, with its tip labeled *peak communication* and its base labeled *cliché conversation* (Davis, 1989). The levels of communication in this hierarchy above the base of cliché conversation are *reporting facts*, then *personal ideas and judgments* and then *feelings and emotions*, and the pyramid is capped by *peak communication*. Thus, the highest level of the pyramid of human communication is peak communication, which is used in intimate relationships and is the least frequently occurring type of human communication. The lowest form of communication is cliché conversation, which is the most frequently occurring type of human communication.

As with the stages of group development and of the authority cycle, movement between levels of communication often occurs in a nonhierarchical manner. Levels of communication can rapidly and frequently shift between levels, and simultaneous communication at more than one level may also occur. Usually, verbal communication between therapists and group members would be at several levels, with some cliché conversation but with most verbal interactions residing in the middle three pyramid levels; that is, communication regarding facts, ideas, and feelings. It would be inappropriate for therapists to engage in peak communication or only in cliché conversation in work situations. The communication pyramid is a good foundation for beginning to analyze verbal interactions in any activity group.

Interaction skills have also been considered in relation to activity groups in occupational therapy. Anne Mosey (1970) described five categories of developmental groups that are distinguished to assist in the development of group interaction skills in a sequential manner. These group levels can also be used as a framework by which the relative maturity of a group's interaction may be gauged. Thus, Mosey's developmental groups can serve as a structure for creating, organizing, and understanding the social interaction skills in other types of activity groups as well.

Mosey (1970, 1986) identified the types of developmental groups as *parallel, project, egocentric–cooperative, cooperative,* and *mature,* listed in order from the simplest level to the highest level of interaction among group

---

EXERCISE 9.5: DEVELOPMENTAL GROUPS AND LEVELS OF COMMUNICATION

From your own experience of participation in groups, find examples of each of Mosey's (1970, 1986) developmental group types. Identify the levels of communication most often used in each group type. Compare your findings in a group discussion.

---

members. The role of the leader and interactions with the leader are considered in this framework. In *parallel groups,* minimal conversation and minimal sharing of activities occurs, so the therapist encourages and reinforces appropriate behaviors and social interactions. *Project* groups have limited shared interaction and cooperation among members; therefore, the therapist sets up, encourages, and reinforces social interaction and sharing of tasks. In *egocentric–cooperative* groups, members are beginning to engage in joint decision making and interact with others with more social awareness, and so the therapist encourages group problem solving. *Cooperative* group members share ideas and feelings and are able to fulfill one another's interaction needs; however, the activity becomes secondary to these group members, and so the therapist is an advisor and coparticipant in the group. In *mature* groups, members take on a variety of roles, and a balance exists between the activity and member need satisfaction. Therefore, the therapist functions simply as a group member and provides mutual reinforcement of appropriate behavior within the group. Using this framework in occupational therapy groups, group members' interaction abilities and limitations are matched with the activity group leaders' interactions. We discuss Mosey's (1970) taxonomy of activity group types further in the section on task groups.

Group Process

The structure, the task behaviors, and the process of the group are three intertwining aspects of an activity group (Posthuma, 2002). In any group that interacts around a task, many phenomena exist of which to be aware (Figure 9.7). The first and most obvious element of this interaction is the content of the communication—the objective record of what is stated between members of the group. The second set of phenomena that requires attention is the process of group communications—how events unfold in the group and what unspoken meaning these events may have. Process considerations would include questions such as "Who made the statement?" "To whom was the statement made?" "What was the timing of the communication?" "What was the tone of the communication?" and "What could be a manifest reason for the communication?"

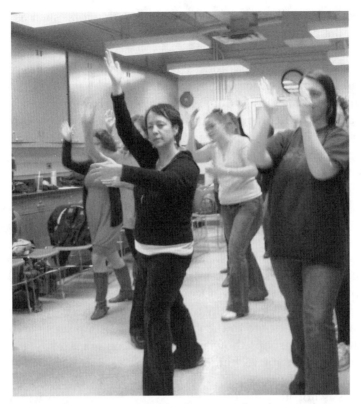

Figure 9.7. Yoga provides a group activity that is structured so that members respond to each other while focusing on their own actions.

> Therapists who are process-oriented are concerned not primarily with the verbal content of a patient's utterance, but with the "how" and the "why" of that utterance, especially insofar as the how and the why illuminate aspects of the patient's relationship to other people. Thus, therapists focus on the meta-communication aspects of the message and wonder why, from the relationship aspect, a patient makes a statement at a certain time in a certain manner to a certain person. (Yalom, 1995, p. 131)

The occupational therapist has additional interests in group process. Beyond the communication process between group members, the occupational therapist is also concerned with the effect of the activity demands on the process of the group. In other words, how do the activity demands of the group's occupation affect communication? Does the activity facilitate or require communication? How much communication? What style of communication? How frequent? Does the task require collaboration? Do the group's activity demands require communication and collaboration at the beginning of the activity only, or during several steps of the activity? In addition to imposing communication demands on the members, the inherent qualities of some activities will elicit different member behaviors, such as quiet individual parallel performance, serious outcome-driven team collaboration, or loose and boisterous play.

The literature on group process is focused mostly on psychotherapy groups and groups in which verbal interaction is the primary or sole group activity. In psychotherapy groups, a technique called *process commentary* becomes a central therapeutic intervention. *Process commentary* involves the giving of immediate feedback to the group on its current group process. Process commentary is used for developing insights and changes among group members. Initially, the therapist leading the group will introduce the technique of process commentary to the group by stopping the current group activity and making comments about what seems to be occurring. Eventually, clients may contribute to this effort to gain insight by offering their own comments on what seems to be happening in the group. Process commentary is not a natural social behavior in most groups. In ordinary social groups, members do not normally make comments on the group's process and underlying events. Occupational therapists involved in facilitating natural activity groups in more natural contexts may find process commentary inappropriate to the group type or group setting. In many occupational therapy groups, however, process commentary is a critical and fundamental therapeutic technique.

> Process is not just one of many possible procedural orientations; on the contrary, it is indispensable and a common denominator to all effective interactional groups. . . . A process focus is the one truly unique feature of the experiential group . . . where else is it permissible, in fact encouraged, to comment, in depth, on the here-and-now behavior, on the nature of the immediately current relationship between people? (Yalom, 1995, p. 137)

When does the occupational therapist use process commentary? In many types of groups engaged in occupations, the occupational therapist may rarely or never use process commentary as an intervention strategy, as noted earlier. The therapist may determine that the activity demands, the communications, and the relationships that evolve around the activity are therapeutic in themselves. In some group scenarios, the members of the group may not have the capacity to use or benefit from an insight-oriented meta-cognitive task such as process commentary. Process illumination may raise group members' anxiety levels, may initially cause some confusion, or may be met with some resistance from group members. With some populations who respond to stress poorly or in a nonadaptive manner, this type of intervention may not be indicated. In addition, during the early stages of group formation and development, members may not be ready for the task of receiving and considering process comments. As the group members become comfortable with process commentary and experiences, they may eventually welcome this exercise and benefit from this intervention, and the members may even occasionally initiate their own process.

In other instances, however, the therapist may conclude that the group members can certainly benefit from process commentary. When group members have the cognitive ability to reflect on the comments regarding current events within the group, to gain some new understanding or insights, they will learn from such reflection on events. This reflective learning most often occurs when the group members' abilities and goals are consistent with this therapeutic technique. Renee Taylor (2008), in discussing the therapeutic intentional relationship in occupational therapy, recommended that the therapist balance the group's "activity focus" with an "interpersonal focus." Occupational therapists may use process comments at any point during the group. When process comments are introduced during the activity, the activity is usually stopped. The comment may be made during the activity when a problem has arisen or when a significant event has occurred in the group relations and communications. At other times, the therapist may find that the activity is proceeding smoothly and that stopping the group to make comments would be disruptive. In this case, the therapist may decide to wait until the end of the session to comment. The therapist must then leave adequate time at the end for group members to respond to and discuss the therapist's comments.

Group Decision Making

Any group that is involved in occupations will have to make decisions, including what occupation to select. Other decisions regarding occupation may include time, place, materials, procedures, division of labor, roles, and the projected outcome. Early formative group decisions may have to be made by group leaders. The pre–group session decisions about a therapy group's purpose and membership criteria will be made by group leaders, sometimes before group members are identified.

The process by which the group makes decisions can itself be an important therapeutic modality. Who will assume leadership roles in the occupation? How will group members be involved in decisions? Providing group members with an opportunity to resolve these decisions, whether individually or as a group, can offer an excellent opportunity for personal growth. Johnson and Johnson (2009) listed seven methods for group decision making:

1. Decision by authority without discussion
2. Decision by authority after discussion
3. Identification of an expert member who leads the group decision
4. Identification of an average of the members' opinions
5. Decision by a minority of the group

6. Democratic decision—a majority of the group by vote
7. Consensus.

Another form of decision making, similar to the democratic decision, is the supermajority (two-thirds) vote. This approach helps to empower the subgroups that tend to be in the minority in many of the group's decisions and requires the group to discuss a matter and negotiate long enough to build a larger subgroup of support for a position.

It is well understood that member involvement in group decisions improves interest and motivation. Involvement in group decisions helps members to feel that they are part of the group, enhancing their sense of affiliation and thereby improving group cohesion. In addition, involving group members in the decision-making process improves the amount and quality of information included in the decision. Each member brings a unique combination of knowledge and experience to the group. Groups that are more heterogeneous in background and experience have the advantage of a broader knowledge base for group decision making. The collective knowledge of the group, and the diversity of that knowledge, should be identified as one of the group's main assets and should be used when making group decisions.

Throughout the course of a group, the group leader must make careful decisions concerning when it is appropriate for group problems and decisions to be delegated to the group. Although the democratic process of voting to make group decisions may seem to make the most logical sense, scholars of democratic government have talked at length about the tyranny of the majority, the concern that members of a group who find themselves in the minority on repeated votes or on key issues may feel estranged or disenfranchised from the group. Whenever votes are being used to reach group decisions, the group leader should be actively concerned about the impact of voting on group cohesion and membership. In fact, the group leader may find that even when the group uses voting for some decisions, other decisions central to individual rights and membership must be made by consensus.

Group decision making by consensus is often considered the gold standard because all members have, by definition, reached agreement on a decision, and the estrangement of group members is therefore avoided. Consensus decision making is often a very lengthy deliberative process that requires extensive collaboration and compromise, or even conflict resolution between members or subgroups. When decisions have to be reached in a timely manner, a consensus process may not be feasible. Many decisions may not practically be reached by consensus, particularly in larger groups. On more serious or controversial issues, true consensus decision making in which all members in a group agree may be rare.

A group's effectiveness in decision making is, of course, dependent on the quality of the group's overall functioning. Groups that are very large might find that consistent involvement of all members in all decisions is too cum-

---

CASE SCENARIO 9.4: CARLA

Carla, an occupational therapist leading a group in a day program for elderly people, found that the members often disagreed on many matters on which the group had to decide. Many of these decisions seemed rather simple and could easily have been made by herself—for example, what activities the group would engage in at the next session. Presenting each decision to the group, however, provided the members with an opportunity to discuss the matter and develop stronger relationships within the group and feel more ownership for the group's activities. At one point, however, a subgroup of women in the group expressed the idea that the group was involved more in female gender–related activities and felt that the minority subgroup of male members might be more comfortable with forming a separate group to pursue activities that were more related to their gender. One more vocal female member suggested that this issue be put to a vote. Carla suggested that this was a very important issue and should be discussed further and decided by full consensus because any of the individual male members might feel a strong affiliation with the group and choose not to leave. In addition, Carla recognized that there might be some underlying gender relationship issues that should be explored and discussed further.

---

bersome and difficult. In these instances, delegating certain decisions and re-sponsibilities to a committee or subgroup may be a more appropriate use of time and resources. Groups that are experiencing repeated or extreme conflict around an issue at hand, or around other issues, will usually have difficulty with the decision-making process. At such a time, the therapist must make a thorough assessment of the nature of the conflict and the group's process and development. Any thoughts about changing the group's method for making decisions at this time must be given careful consideration. Another important aspect of group decision making is the client factors supplied by the members. For example, the capacity for clients to cognitively participate in decisions varies. Groups that have members with cognitive impairments may depend on many decisions made at an authority level by the group leader.

Creativity and Problems in Decision Making

For a group to solve a problem or work productively in a creative manner, the initial steps described for problem solving must be followed within a very cooperative group context. The group should be supportive and not overly pressured. If group members feel threatened or not supported, they will be less likely to take risks with creative suggestions. Diverse viewpoints and suggestions must be encouraged. Controversy and debate must be allowed, supported, and tolerated. Finally, the group must also be allotted appropriate time to reflect on the diverse ideas developed in the group.

Johnson and Johnson (2009) described seven symptoms of defective decision making. Therapists can use these indicators to assess difficulties with the group's approach to problem solving:

1. Incomplete survey of alternatives
2. Incomplete survey of objectives
3. Failure to examine risks of preferred choice
4. Poor information search
5. Selective bias in processing information at hand
6. Failure to reappraise alternatives
7. Failure to work out contingency plans.

Group engagement in decision making is an excellent opportunity for teaching and modeling effective problem solving because it parallels individual problem solving. The therapist can lead the group through the steps of problem solving: clear identification of the problem and its implications; brainstorming potential actions or solutions; assessment of the different possible solutions; selection of that solution; and, ultimately, implementation and reassessment.

Therapeutic Factors

A variety of processes inherent to working in a group foster learning, growth, and development for individual group members. Yalom (1995) described 11 of these therapeutic factors that make group membership and group treatment so potentially powerful, efficient, and dynamic:

1. Instillation of hope
2. Universality
3. Imparting information
4. Altruism
5. Corrective recapitulation of the primary family group
6. Development of socializing techniques
7. Imitative behavior
8. Interpersonal learning
9. Group cohesiveness
10. Catharsis
11. Existential factors.

A brief discussion of each therapeutic factor follows. In addition to Yalom's list we have added two more therapeutic factors specific to groups that use occupation:

1. Effectance (Schwartzberg, Howe, & Barnes, 2008; White, 1959, 1971) and
2. Experiential learning (Schwartzberg et al., 2008).

INSTILLATION OF HOPE

Groups provide mutual support and assistance that inspires hope in their members. Often members will find hope in observing other group members with similar problems who have made progress. Yalom (1995) recommended that group leaders capitalize on this dynamic by pointing out members' progress or achievements.

UNIVERSALITY

Many people come to groups feeling isolated and quite different from others, whether this feeling is related to their illness, their disability, or their unique set of life problems. Even though an individual may have some knowledge of stories and demographics of others in similar situations, the group experience delivers this information in a more intimate and personal format. Members have the opportunity to hear directly from each other and may realize that they are not completely alone in their experience. Members may begin to see that others are struggling, and perhaps also progressing, with similar problems. *Universality* is this consensual validation, which can be very comforting to group members and may foster feelings of connection.

IMPARTING INFORMATION

The group is a natural context for the sharing of information by both group leaders and group members. Group leaders are a great source of information. They may have added experience or educational resources to which the members have not yet had access. At the same time, one potential pitfall arises when the group leader is identified as an expert. In groups in which people are struggling with disability and dependency on others, the group expert may encourage or prolong that dependency role, which may in turn stunt the group's development. In addition, the establishment of the leader as an expert risks creating an informational orthodoxy that prevents the introduction of alternative views or suggestions.

Group members should thus be recognized as invaluable sources of information. In the early stages of group development, when the members first assume that the leader(s) will simply deliver the information and resources necessary for the group, group members may not recognize that they themselves may hold most of the information and resources needed to accomplish the group's tasks. The group may slowly begin to realize its own potential, a process that may need to be facilitated by the group leaders. This process begins with the group leader's genuinely recognizing each group member's unique value and imparting this information to the group. A Socratic approach to the collective knowledge of group members is one method used by group leaders to facilitate information sharing. A group therapist using the Socratic method recognizes that as a collective, the group has extensive knowledge, and through carefully formed questions, the group can reveal its knowledge. This approach goes against an assumption often manifest in group members that the therapist or group leader is the expert and that they are in attendance to learn from the leader. The group members indeed begin to realize that they can learn from each other. This realization of group efficacy helps to both promote group development toward more advanced levels of functioning and to promote group therapeutic factors. The realization that group members can learn from each other may also dispel assumptions that both therapists and members have about disability and knowledge.

Altruism

Group endeavors in occupation provide great opportunities for members to assist each other. During this process, members may experience giving and receiving firsthand. The act of helping others can be very cathartic in itself and often spurs the giver on toward further development of interpersonal relationship skills.

Corrective Recapitulation of the Primary Family Group

The family is the very first social group to which a person belongs. The person's experiences in the family group, both positive and negative, shape cognitive schema and thus influence his or her perceptions, understanding, and responses in all subsequent social groups. A carefully led therapeutic group provides opportunities for members to reexperience patterns of behavior and interpersonal interaction in previous relations and opportunities to reflect on those patterns, to develop insight into the meanings within these patterns, and to eventually work to correct social responses that have been unsuccessful for the person in previous groups.

Development of Socializing Techniques

The group, especially when engaged in occupation, provides a rich social laboratory for members to learn social skills. For members who are extremely anxious in social situations, occupation offers an opportunity to divert the focus from eye contact and verbal response to a task. This task focus then provides a context and natural reason for required interpersonal interaction.

Imitative Behavior

The group provides a natural context for the development of social skills. It also provides members with opportunities to observe others and to imitate the actions of others, and it then offers repeated opportunities to practice and develop social perceptions and shape each person's repertoire of behaviors.

INTERPERSONAL LEARNING

Groups provide opportunities for members to learn about themselves through interactions with others. In their most intensive format, groups may even provide for a corrective emotional experience through which individual members develop insight and make transformative changes in their relations with others.

GROUP COHESION

Although we discuss group cohesion as a therapeutic factor, it is also a critical aspect of group development and function. *Group cohesion* is the extent to which members feel connected to each other and feel a bond with the group as a whole. Cohesion reflects the quality of the individual member's relationship with the group. Group cohesiveness is a critical underpinning for sustaining membership when problems or conflicts arise and a critical foundation for the effective operation of many other therapeutic factors.

CATHARSIS

The group can provide stimuli for catharsis for its members. Such stimuli may include the recapitulation of previous relationships, which leads to the expression of deeply held feelings about previous life events and current events within the group.

EXISTENTIAL FACTORS

Yalom (1995) added this 11th therapeutic factor. He suggested that the group provides opportunities for its members to identify core life issues that have more meaning and relevance than day-to-day trivialities. Thus, members learn that they are ultimately responsible for how they live out their lives.

EFFECTANCE

Effectance is the idea that people are naturally drawn toward activity. Therefore, the availability of the opportunity to participate in activity is in itself strongly self-motivating (Schwartzberg et al., 2008; White, 1959, 1971).

EXPERIENTIAL LEARNING

In groups in which members participate in occupation, the group provides not only opportunities for learning social skills but also a forum for learning about occupation through interaction with the activity. These activities provide members with safe, supported opportunities to explore occupation, to interact with the materials and particular qualities of activities, and to realize their own interests and the other individual client factors that affect performance (Schwartzberg et al., 2008).

Groups engaged in occupation may include any of these therapeutic factors, although those involving more intensive psychodynamic processes, such as recapitulation of the family or catharsis, are less likely to be operative in occupation-focused groups. The immense potential power of group treatment is largely the result of therapeutic factors, whether in a psychodynamic group or a task group.

Task Groups

The history of the task group focus in occupational therapy can be traced back to its roots in the moral treatment movement of the 1830s, when groups of people worked together on particular activities that were important to maintaining their community. By the mid-20th century, occupational therapists recognized the importance of socialization and group process in task groups. Group cohesiveness is now believed to be needed for effective treatment using activities in groups (Howe & Schwartzberg, 2001).

Gail Fidler (1969) posited that task groups consist of active involvement in doing. Her seminal article described the relationship among feelings, thoughts, actions, and group task performance as creating excellent learning opportunities. For example, task groups can be structured to allow sharing of responsibilities and accomplishments, behavioral trial and error, problem solving, and feedback on actions within the group. Task groups can also be structured for gradation of engagement in concrete social interactions; new learning; engagement with nonhuman objects and the environment; and sheltered opportunities for reality testing of behaviors, actions, feelings, and perceptions of both self and others. Task group members become aware of their limitations and abilities and develop their functional capacities through concrete, reality-based task achievement.

Anne Mosey (1986) developed a taxonomy of treatment group types used in occupational therapy and also articulated the differences between task groups and verbal groups. Task groups have a centrality of activity, an immediacy of events (the here and now), and a circumscribed focus of the group on the task group itself—a characteristic that distinguishes task groups from verbal groups. The six types of occupational therapy groups identified by Mosey are (1) evaluative groups, (2) task-oriented groups, (3) developmental groups, (4) thematic groups, (5) topical groups, and (6) instrumental groups. *Evaluative groups* identify client assets and limitations and help set treatment goals. *Task-oriented groups,* similar to Fidler's (1969) task groups, develop awareness of the relationship among thoughts, feelings, and actions. Mosey (1986) emphasized that importance be placed on the way in which the tasks are carried out, not on the particular tasks involved in the task-oriented groups. *Developmental groups* emphasize social interaction, as discussed in the previous section of this chapter on levels of group interaction. *Thematic groups* are concerned with gaining skills and knowledge to master performance skills and occupations; thus, they have less focus on group process dynamics. *Topical groups* are primarily discussion groups concerned with the learning of new skills, which may be anticipatory or concurrent, and are useful for the developmental levels of egocentric–cooperative and higher. *Instrumental groups* are concerned with maintaining function and meeting health needs but are not focused on change, and their purpose is simply to have fun socializing and to enjoy performing tasks (Mosey, 1986). Focus on tasks is central to all of Mosey's group types, just as activity is central to occupation and forms the core of the practice of occupational therapy.

Common Group Problems

Groups provide many therapeutic intervention opportunities for the group leader. Leading groups, however, also presents the therapist with a unique set of problems.

CASE SCENARIO **9.5**: RUTH

Ruth is newly retired and lives alone; she keeps very busy with a variety of activities. Her clowning class is her favorite activity. This group meets every other week and shares ideas on costumes, tricks, and antics that are involved in clowning. Although the group is focused on the task of learning how to be a clown and these thematic aspects, it also has instrumental process aspects that are even more important to Ruth. She finds that participating in these activities with others is very beneficial for her. The clowning class allows Ruth a liberating permission to be playful and spontaneous and have fun. In addition, the group provides her with an opportunity to socialize and form new friendships in her postwork retiree life.

EXERCISE **9.6**: FORMULATING A GROUP PROTOCOL

For one of the group types delineated by Anne Mosey (1986), create an occupational therapy group. Succinctly state the type of group and its name; describe the population for which the group is designed; describe group membership; state the group's purpose; list group goals (two short-term goals matched with two long-term goals); briefly list the group activity procedures (for an activity to be performed in *one* group session); specify requirements for space, supplies, equipment, and cost; and list any references or sources needed for the creation of the group.

Problems With Group Formation

Many issues affect group functioning and successful participation in occupations. Some of these issues arise early in the formation of the group, particularly in occupational therapy settings in which group membership is involuntary. This issue arises most commonly in penal and mental health settings. Involuntary membership is in itself antithetical to the inherent values of the profession and compromises the therapeutic factors of activity groups, including effectance. In this setting, the occupational therapist, while enforcing the rules of the institution or agency, must eventually present therapeutic activity groups as an opportunity to make the best of things and use activity as a diversion from the constraints of such a setting and as an opportunity to prepare for leaving the setting.

A second common group formation issue is member recruitment. The enrollment of inappropriate members can severely affect early group development and functioning and may contribute to serious conflict within the group. Clearly articulating the criteria for group membership, both inclusionary and exclusionary, is critical to prevent such situations. In addition, when enrolling a person in a group, it is essential that the group's purpose and general goals be clearly shared with the potential member. Clients often enter groups because of an interest in being with the group leader or a particular group member. Members may also be strongly attracted to the group's activity without understanding its therapeutic purpose.

Closely related to the issue of member recruitment is the frequent challenge of activity selection in a heterogeneous group. When a group is formed of members who have a wide variety of individual interests and skills, the selection of commonly shared occupations may be very difficult. After careful discussion and exploration of different occupations, some groups may conclude that membership must be re-formed around the occupations in which the members can better share participation.

Finally, early in group formation, norms and rules regarding attendance and punctuality must be articulated clearly. Inconsistent attendance sends an unspoken message that the group is not valued and erodes group formation and the development of cohesion. Late arrivals and frequent departures from the group can be very distracting to group members. Although group leaders may negotiate attendance and punctuality rules in some groups, once the rules are set, they should be consistently enforced.

Problems in Group Process

Conflict in groups is often inevitable. As previously discussed, group theorists suggest that conflict is one of the normal stages of group development. Conflict in a group is a natural interpersonal event that provides a therapeutic opportunity for the individual members involved, and for the group as a whole, to learn from the immediate moment to develop further via successful conflict resolution. Appropriate management of conflict begins before the conflict arises, with successful development of roles, relationships, norms, and cohesion in the group. These elements help prepare the group to weather conflict and maintain a commitment to participation in the group. Rules regarding mutual respect among the members and limits on destructive language and behavior are essential in successful conflict resolution.

Once conflict has occurred, the group leader may have to actively reinforce these limits, especially when conflicts resurface. The group leader should respond positively by suggesting that conflict is natural and offering a constructive opportunity for group development. The group leader should then assist the group in a structured negotiation of the conflict, using the same steps set forth for group decision making. This problem-solving approach includes clear identification of the conflict, recognition of opposing viewpoints, brainstorming for possible solutions, and the group selection of a resolution to the conflict.

Dependency can also be a difficulty and is a dynamic common to all groups. Dependency can be seen as a developmental phase of the group. As discussed earlier with regard to the therapist's role in the group, the first stage of the group members' development in relation to the group leader is dependence (Posthuma, 2002). The group members feel and enact a dependence on the group leader. Members interact little with the other group members and look only to the leader for direction and answers. In groups made up of people with disabilities, this stage of group development may be prolonged. The group leader should recognize that this stage is natural yet at the same time, the leader should foster growth toward more functional interdependence. Group members' strengths and abilities should always be considered in the selection of group activities. These assets should be repeatedly recognized and celebrated by the group. The leader should at times redirect questions and requests back to the group members. These techniques will foster experiences within the group in which the members begin to recognize the individual and collective skills that they bring to the group (Posthuma, 2002).

Some groups may experience apathy or amotivation. When apathy or amotivation arises, the leader or facilitator should evaluate whether it is caused by the illness that group members are struggling with, such as depression, negative symptoms of schizophrenia, or residual deficits of brain injury. Apathy or amotivation may also arise from issues such as frustration with an activity in the group, selection of an activity that is not attractive to the group, or anticipation of failing by the group members. Apathy may also arise out of interpersonal conflicts within the group followed by failures at attempts to resolve those conflicts. Groups in which the members experience repeated futility in problem solving have a high potential for apathy. Apathy in the group requires careful assessment by the group leader or facilitator, along with the selection of strategies that are unique to that situation. Changes in the group's activity and the infusion of greater energy through the activity, its leaders, or new group members may be helpful in reducing group apathy.

Parallel process is another common problem in groups in which the leaders or the members also interact in another setting in addition to the activity group. The events and process in one setting can spill over to the other setting. Group leaders can be affected both positively and negatively by the organizations for which they work. When group leaders experience certain strong dynamics within an organization, it is not unusual for them to carry that experience into their work, even into the activity group. For example, in an organization in which the group leader experiences a hostile work environment and lack of support by a supervisor or coworkers, it would not be unusual for the group leader to come to the group feeling that he or she is not safe or in reasonable control of events. That feeling may be unconsciously transmitted to the group members in a variety of ways. Parallel process can also occur among group members. Issues that have arisen elsewhere in the treatment milieu or in previous groups may easily spill over into the activity group. Careful evaluation and recognition of these problems is essential. When the group leader is bringing organizational problems into the group, the leader must recognize that he or she is doing so and work to prevent it from occurring again (Figure 9.8). When the leader recognizes that members are bringing issues into the group from other settings, this issue should be confronted. Whenever possible, group members should be encouraged to maintain the boundaries of the group and prevent outside matters from infringing on its tasks. In occupational therapy

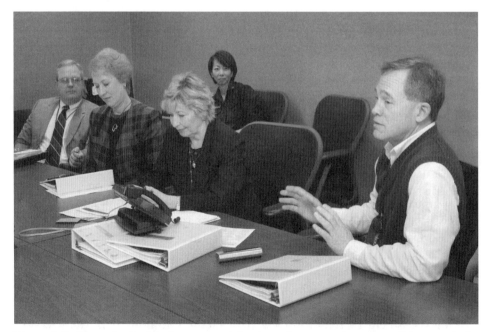

Figure 9.8. Group leadership is an essential role and ensures the accomplishment of the group's goals.

Note. Photograph courtesy of the Public Health Image Library, Centers for Disease Control and Prevention. Photo by Jim Gathany.

groups, this encouragement can be especially important for clients who need to develop the ability to focus on an activity and complete it despite the existence of current problems or stressors.

Summary

Therapeutic activity groups present multidimensional opportunities for individual member interpersonal development and growth during engagement in occupation. Many levels of interpersonal communication, a variety of roles, multiple therapeutic factors, and opportunities for group leadership and decision making are some of the critical areas of learning that are experienced during the complex process of treatment in a therapeutic activity group. Group treatment using occupation can be one of the most efficient and dynamic means of achieving individual goals in many treatment settings.

References

American Occupational Therapy Association. (2008). Occupational therapy practice framework: Domain and process (2nd ed.). *American Journal of Occupational Therapy, 62,* 625–683.

Benne, K. D., & Sheats, P. (1948). Functional roles of group members. *Journal of Social Issues, 4,* 41–49.

Cole, M. B. (1998). *Group dynamics in occupational therapy* (2nd ed.). Thorofare, NJ: Slack.

Davis, C. M. (1989). *Patient–practitioner interaction.* Thorofare, NJ: Slack.

Donohue, M., & Greer, E. (2004). Designing group activities to meet individual and group goals. In J. Hinojosa & M. Blount (Eds.), *The texture of life* (2nd ed., pp. 226–261). Bethesda, MD: AOTA Press.

Fidler, G. S. (1969). The task-oriented group as a context for treatment. *American Journal of Occupational Therapy, 23,* 43–48.

Howe, M. C., & Schwartzberg, S. L. (2001). *A functional approach to group work in occupational therapy* (3rd ed.). Philadelphia: Lippincott.

Johnson, D. W., & Johnson, F. P. (2009). *Joining together: Group theory and group skills* (10th ed.). Upper Saddle River, NJ: Pearson Education.

Lacoursiere, R. (1980). *The life cycle of groups.* New York: Human Sciences Press.

Mosey, A. C. (1970). The concept and use of developmental groups. *American Journal of Occupational Therapy, 24,* 272–275.

Mosey, A. C. (1986). *Psychosocial components of occupational therapy.* New York: Raven.

Posthuma, B. H. (2002). *Small groups in counseling and therapy* (4th ed.). Boston: Allyn & Bacon.

Schutz, W. (1958). The interpersonal underworld. *Harvard Business Review, 36,* 123–135.

Schwartzberg, S. L., Howe, M. C., & Barnes, M. A. (2008). *Groups: Applying the functional group model.* Philadelphia: F. A. Davis.

Taylor, R. R. (2008). *The intentional relationship: Occupational therapy and the use of self.* Philadelphia: F. A. Davis.

Tuckman, B. W. (1965). Developmental sequence in small groups. *Psychological Bulletin,* 63(6), 384–399.

White, R. W. (1959). Motivation reconsidered: The concept of competence. *Psychological Review,* 66, 297–333.

White, R. W. (1971). The urge toward competence. *American Journal of Occupational Therapy,* 25, 271–274.

Yalom, I. D. (1995). *Theory and practice of group psychotherapy* (4th ed.). New York: Basic Books.

10

The Ability–Disability Continuum and Activity Match

Lisa E. Cyzner, PhD, OTR

> The totality of the impact of serious physical impairment on conscious thought, as well as its firm implantation in the unconscious mind, gives disability a far stronger purchase on one's sense of who and what he is than do any social roles—even key ones such as age, occupation, and ethnicity. These can be manipulated, neutralized, and suspended, and in this way can become adjusted somewhat to each other. (Murphy, 1990, p. 105)

In his book *The Body Silent*, Robert Murphy (1990), a retired professor from the Department of Anthropology at Columbia University in New York City, described his experiences living with a chronic illness as the most challenging journey of his life. Invoking this metaphor of a journey, he took his readers with him as he related how every aspect of his life was affected after learning that he had a spinal cord tumor that eventually caused him to develop quadriplegia. If life is the journey, the body is the vessel through which we experience life. The body is our physical, psychological, philosophical, and sociological connection to the world through which we strive to create meaningful lives.

As occupational therapists or occupational therapy assistants working with people who have disabilities, we must also incorporate this multifaceted approach in incorporating the physical, psychological, sociological, and philosophical perspectives into our evaluation and intervention using purposeful activities. By helping people engage in purposeful activities, we operate within the domain of our profession by "supporting health and participation in life through engagement in occupation" (Americal Occupational Therapy Association [AOTA], 2008, p. 626). In a sense, we can embrace Murphy's (1990) anthropological perspective as a way to individualize our approach. The journey is different for each person: For some, it begins at birth; for others, it begins after a traumatic event. The families, friends, and significant others of people with disabilities are part of this journey as well, often engaging in co-occupations, such as caregiving, with the individual. For many, the journey is a lifelong process of living with a chronic illness. Regardless of the timing or process of this journey, we must recognize how essential occupations, and the activities that compose them, are to a person's identity and sense of competence and meaning in his or her daily life (AOTA, 2008).

This chapter is divided into two major sections. In the first section, I discuss each of the four life perspectives that occupational therapists and occupational therapy assistants should explore during the evaluation, intervention, and outcome processes for people with disabilities. In the latter half of this section, I present a graphic representation of the four continua integrating these perspectives. The second section includes a framework with explanations about how practitioners can help people construct or reconstruct their lifestyle using purposeful activities, guided by the belief that for many, the process of reconstructing a lifestyle is an evolving, ever-changing process affecting engagement in occupations. The appendix includes a worksheet developed from this framework that can be used in daily practice.

Four Perspectives: Physical, Psychological, Philosophical, and Sociological

Drawing from these four perspectives, an exercise that allows each to be addressed in turn, makes it possible to dissect, at least in part, the constructs and the thinkers who have developed them. Nonetheless, for the people involved in working with people with disabilities, all of these perspectives must inevitably be merged into one because they are inextricably linked for the whole person. Although practitioners deal with many models and ways of looking at the problems of disability and recovery, for the person experiencing them, they represent his or her life and only some of its problems.

WORLD HEALTH ORGANIZATION MODEL

In an effort to provide a framework for health professionals providing services for those with disabilities, the World Health Organization (WHO) first published the *International Classification of Impairments, Disabilities and Handicaps* (*ICIDH*) in 1980. Complete with definitions and information regarding the consequences of disease, WHO presented a continuum—an illness trajectory—through which health professionals could communicate by using more uniform terminology than had been used in the past (Knussen & Cunningham, 1988; Rogers & Holm, 1994; Wood, 1980). As Wood (1980) described, one can view this continuum as it is depicted in Figure 10.1.

Impairment, disability, and handicap are all considered to be consequences of disease. Related to the *ICIDH* definitions, Rogers and Holm (1994) cautioned that WHO defined these concepts only in terms of dysfunction. Its

Disease ⇒ Impairment ⇒ Disability ⇒ Handicap

Figure 10.1. World Health Organization's *International Classification of Impairments, Disabilities and Handicaps* continuum.

definitions present aspects of neither remediation nor compensation; however, they are useful in laying the groundwork for exploring the physical, psychological, and sociological perspectives affected by disability. Moreover, Coster and Haley (1992) noted that although WHO's continuum is hierarchical in that each of the four components represents "increasingly complex, integrated activities" (p. 13), health professionals should not necessarily view it as linear. Coster and Haley (1992) explained that even though a person presents with problems indicative of a certain component or level of the WHO model, one cannot presume that person also has problems indicative of another component along the continuum. They provided the example of a child with a below-elbow amputation resulting from trauma (an impairment) who can perform all activities of daily living (ADLs) independently with his prosthesis. Thus, according to the WHO system, although this child has an impairment, he would not also be considered disabled because he is able to perform all of his ADLs independently. Therefore, occupational therapists and occupational therapy assistants have to think and question themselves about what a person is and is not able to do. They also need to take into account what a person chooses to do and what level of assistance may or may not be needed.

Coster and Haley (1992) continued to explain that other models of disablement have been both suggested and noted to be conceptually clearer than the WHO model, such as that proposed by Nagi (1965, 1991). They described that, unlike the WHO model, Nagi's (1965, 1991) model essentially appeared to link impairment with disability through *functional limitations,* which encompass a person's ability to perform tasks and to carry out those obligations that are part of his or her roles or daily activities.

When WHO published the *ICIDH* in 1980, it was done for trial purposes. After multiple revisions based on field testing and international consultation, WHO approved the latest version—the *International Classification of Functioning, Disability and Health* (ICF; WHO, 2001)—for use on May 22, 2001. The one continuum including the concepts of impairment, disability, and handicap was replaced with a two-level or two-part system: Part I, Functioning and Disability, and Part II, Contextual Factors. Each part has several components. Within this classification and further breakdown of the components, the concepts of impairment and disability are still used; however, they are paired and grouped with other concepts related to functioning so that the presentation and relationship of all of these concepts are no longer linear as the original continuum suggested (see Figure 10.2). Most important, the *ICF* is intended to apply to all people, not just those with disabilities (WHO, 2001). Essentially, the *ICF* embodies what Coster and Haley (1992) discussed relative to models of disablement more so than did the original *ICIDH*.

The 10th revision of the *ICF*, the *International Classification of Diseases, Tenth Revision*, or *ICD–10* (WHO, 1990), which was also developed by WHO, is used to classify health conditions such as diseases, disorders, and injuries. The *ICD–10* and the *ICF* are therefore complementary because the *ICF* can provide information on a person's ability to function with his or her health conditions. Because of this, the *ICF* is now viewed more as a component of health classification rather than of consequences of disease. According to WHO, it is considered to be a multipurpose classification and conceptual framework that can be used in a variety of contexts related to health care, including management of health care systems, prevention and health promotion programs, and research related to such entities as health care evaluations, health care policy, and applied research to meet the changing needs of society (WHO, 2001).

Figure 10.3 provides an overview of the *ICF* (WHO, 2001, p. 14), outlining its overall organization and structure. One can see that the *ICF* provides information related to human functioning and to restrictions of human functioning that can be used by a variety of disciplines. Part I of the *ICF*, Functioning and Disability, has two components: (1) body functions and structures and

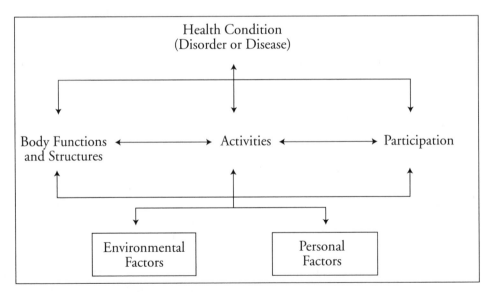

Figure 10.2. Interactions among the components of *ICF.*

Note. From *ICF: International Classification of Functioning, Disability and Health (short version)*, by the World Health Organization, 2001, p. 25. Copyright © 2001, by the World Health Organization. Reprinted with permission.

	Part 1: Functioning and Disability		Part 2: Contextual Factors	
Components	Body Functions and Structures	Activities and Participation	Environmental Factors	Personal Factors
Domains	Body Functions Body Structures	Life Areas (Tasks, Actions)	External Influences on Functioning and Disability	Internal Influences on Functioning and Disability
Constructs	Change in Body Functions (Physiological) Change in Body Structures (Anatomical)	Capacity Executing Tasks in a Standard Environment Performance Executing Tasks in the Current Environment	Facilitating or Hindering Impact of Features of the Physical, Social, and Attitudinal World	Impact of Attributes of the Person
Positive Aspect	Functional and Structural Integrity	Activities Participation	Facilitators	Not Applicable
	Functioning			
Negative Aspect	Impairment	Activity Limitation Participation Restriction	Barriers/ Hindrances	Not Applicable
	Disability			

Figure 10.3. Overview of *ICF.*

Note. From *ICF: International Classification of Functioning, Disability and Health (short version),* by the World Health Organization, 2001, p. 14. Copyright © 2001, by the World Health Organization. Reprinted with permission.

(2) activities and participation. What directly applies to occupational therapy is the information related to activities and participation, which encompasses a range of domains covering many aspects of functioning, including looking at functioning from both the individual's and society's perspective. Therefore, the components of Part I can be used to indicate a problem, impairment, activity limitation, or participation restriction, which can all be summarized under the umbrella concept of disability. These components can also be used to indicate aspects of health that are not related to a problem or impairment, which can be summarized under the concept of functioning (WHO, 2001). Therefore, as mentioned earlier, it is very important that practitioners continue to ask themselves what an individual both can and cannot do. It is also vital to

include evaluation and related questions regarding contextual factors, which I explain in the next section, and how these, too, affect a person's performance of ADLs. The information gained from this questioning is integral to evaluation, treatment planning, and treatment provision itself.

Part II of the *ICF*, Contextual Factors, includes environmental factors and personal factors. A person's level of functioning and disability is looked on as an interaction between health conditions, such as disease, illness, or injury, and contextual factors, such as how the environment affects functioning and disability. Placing value and emphasis on context is also the main focus of the Ecology of Human Performance Framework developed by Dunn, Brown, and McGuigan (1994; Dunn, Brown, & Youngstrom, 2003). According to this framework and similar to what WHO (2001) described, as outlined earlier, equal value is given to four constructs that are essential for treatment: (1) person, (2) context, (3) task, and (4) performance. This framework emphasizes the role of context because, according to its developers, context is often neglected by occupational therapists and by other programs and professions (Dunn et al., 1994, 2003). Tham and Kielhofner (2003) agreed and noted that, specifically regarding research related to disability, occupational therapy as a profession lacks empirical documentation of how social context influences occupational performance for those with disabilities.

According to WHO (2001), environmental factors are those factors from a person's immediate and surrounding environments that affect all of the components of functioning and disability. Although personal factors are included and would be considered here, they are not classified in the *ICF* because, as WHO explained, they contain too much variance related to social and cultural differences to include them in *ICF*. Yet, information related to both social and cultural factors is vital to practitioners because these factors can greatly affect how they work with people and their families and what practitioners' and families' expectations are relative to treatment. Social and cultural factors can also affect a person and his or her family's view of functioning and disability, which again has a direct influence on treatment choices, activities integrated into the treatment itself, modifications to the person's environment, or all of these.

As described earlier, those *ICF* sections and components particularly related to activities and participation and contextual factors have direct application to occupational therapy practice. It is recommended that readers consult the short version of *ICF* (WHO, 2001) for further detail on all of the *ICF*'s components, multiple usages of the classification, and other applications to practice.

To expand on this relationship of the *ICF* to occupational therapy practice, as Donald J. Lollar (2003) described in his foreword to the text *Perspectives in Human Occupation: Participation in Life,*

> Two major tenets of the new system are that the environment and contextual factors play a crucial role in human function generally

and in disability specifically. Second, the outcomes for all people are framed as societal participation. These two components of the new *ICF* have been the essence of occupation and occupational therapy since their inception: (a) participation and (b) society. This framework allows occupation and occupational therapy to take a leadership role as the field of health and disability moves beyond body function to embrace the assessment of classification of health status. The coding system will allow both positive and negative elements of the environment to be included for research, policy development, and program implementation. Evaluation of activity limitations can now be balanced between domains of individuals and their environment. New assessment tools and procedures will grow from this model, and occupational therapists will be at the forefront. (pp. vii–viii)

As noted, many of the *ICF*'s components appear similar to those areas of human experience in which occupational therapists and occupational therapy assistants have expertise. They reflect elements of the domain of concern (Mosey, 1996) and the *Occupational Therapy Practice Framework: Domain and Process*, which replaced *Uniform Terminology–III* in 2002 when it was officially adopted by the AOTA Representative Assembly. AOTA published the second edition of the *Framework* in 2008. The *Framework–II* includes language to aid practitioners in explaining occupation to their community, particularly how occupation relates to the provision of occupational therapy intervention. Furthermore, it was designed to help the profession to profess its role in "promoting the health and participation of people, organizations, and populations through engagement in occupation" (AOTA, 2008, p. 625). The *Framework–II* was also designed to be more universal, in that it incorporated terminology from the *ICF* so that other health professionals could understand it and in turn understand more about the profession of occupational therapy, its domain of concern, the client populations with whom practitioners work, and the various settings in which practitioners work on a daily basis. The *Framework–II* includes revisions necessary to update language and concepts that are part of both current and emerging practice of occupational therapists (AOTA, 1994, 2002, 2008; Hinojosa, Kramer, Royeen, & Luebben, 2003; Luebben, 2003; Youngstrom, 2002). Thus, considering all of these terms, as occupational therapy as a profession has witnessed the reemphasis and, essentially, a continued return to its roots of occupation, practitioners must also consider the larger activity performance areas, the occupations as they are affected by a disability and not just their underlying performance components (Baptiste, 2003; Clark et al., 1997; Coster, 1998; Jackson, Carlson, Mandel, Zemke, & Clark, 1998; Padilla, 2003; Wood, 1998).

Whether the performance of an activity is related to occupations such as work, play, leisure, social participation, or ADLs, some members of the occupational therapy profession have advocated that practitioners should look at these areas first—along with considering context—rather than initially evaluating, and subsequently basing treatment on, problems related to the underlying components affecting the performance. This approach is known as a "top-down" approach to evaluation rather than a "bottom-up approach," which focuses on the underlying components (Coster, 1998; Ideishi, 2003; Trombly, 1993, 1995).

When using a top-down approach with a client, the occupational therapist or occupational therapy assistant initially tries to determine a person's ability to perform certain roles and the meaning attached to those roles. The practitioner ascertains this information to determine what activities the person may want to address in occupational therapy sessions. Those roles and related activities in which a person engaged before becoming disabled or before coming to occupational therapy (as a result of a recent event or more chronic disability) become the focus of evaluation. If the occupational therapist determines that a difference exists among past, present, and future role performances, then treatment should be implemented. The occupational therapist explores with the client those role performances and activities he or she wants to do and investigates why he or she is unable to do them. This exploration aids in helping the client understand the need for treatment and what the focus of treatment will be (Trombly, 1993, 1995).

Ideishi (2003) explained that an occupational therapist can organize his or her practice in essentially three ways: through implementation of (1) a top-down, (2) a bottom-up, or (3) a contextual approach. Regardless of the approach chosen, he noted that they have in common occupation and the goal of helping people engage in meaningful occupations. He stressed that

> the challenge for the occupational therapist is to transform and articulate our theoretical concepts into daily practice. If we can articulate what we do and why we do it, our clients, our communities, our colleagues in other disciplines, and the institutions that pay for our services will understand the unique contribution that occupational therapy provides society. (p. 294)

Finally, because *ICF* is a global taxonomy, it challenges the profession of occupational therapy to clarify definitions related to activities and to occupation. Occupation is considered to be the core of our profession because it is made up of the daily tasks and purposeful activities, whether mundane or of great importance, that are meaningful to people and are a part of who they are (Hinojosa et al., 2003). Throughout the history of the profession, occupation has been used as both a means during intervention processes and an end, which is essentially the goal of interventions—so that clients can return to old occupations or choose new directions regarding their choices and participation in daily life tasks. Several people at the forefront of this debate have contributed valuable discussion to this need to clarify definitions. Many have suggested that the concept of occupation be defined as a process and activity as its outcome (Hinojosa & Blount, 2009; Hinojosa et al., 2003; Ideishi, 2003; Trombly, 1995).

Whatever a practitioner's view may be, the highest goal of occupational therapy intervention is to help a person participate in meaningful occupations, resulting in participation in life (Ideishi, 2003). Yet, little documentation of efficacy regarding occupation, the practice of occupation, and the relationship of occupation to disability exists (Padilla, 2003). Furthermore, WHO (2001) professed through the *ICF* that the medical model of disability be integrated with the social model of disability. WHO defined the *medical model of disability* as follows:

> a problem of the person, directly caused by disease, trauma or other health condition, which requires medical care provided in the form of individual treatment by professionals. Management of the disability is aimed at cure or the individual's adjustment and behaviour change. Medical care is viewed as the main issue, and at the political level the principal response is that of modifying or reforming health policy. (p. 18)

It defined the *social model of disability* as follows:

> a socially created problem, and basically as a matter of the full integration of individuals into society. Disability is not an attribute of an individual, but rather a complex collection of conditions, many of which are created by the social environment. Hence the management of the problem requires social action, and it is the collective responsibility of society at large to make the environmental modifications necessary for the full participation of people with disabilities in all areas of social life. (p. 18)

If occupational therapy as a profession embraces this integration of models, which also appears to be at the core of its philosophical underpinnings, and wants to align itself with the leaders who affect health policy, management, and outcomes, then it must be clear in its definitions and able to explain its models of intervention to society at large. Practitioners need to be able to demonstrate how occupational therapy's emphasis on occupation and social justice (the support of social policies, actions, and laws that permit people to participate in occupations that are personally meaningful and purposeful) reflect larger, universally accepted models such as WHO's. The occupational therapy profession's view of health reflects that of the WHO model. WHO stated that a person's health can be affected by the inability to carry out activities and participate in life situations related to environmental barriers and by problems that occur with body structures and body functions (AOTA, 2008; WHO 2001).

PSYCHOLOGICAL CONTINUUM: THE DISABILITY PROCESS

Much of the psychological literature describing people's reactions to disability and the processes they undergo can be found in the area of bereavement and loss and stress and coping (Carroll, 1961; Clegg, 1988; Knussen & Cunningham, 1988; Lazarus & Folkman, 1991; Parkes, 1998; Parkes & Weiss, 1983). Clegg (1988) defined *bereavement* as a state that follows an actual or perceived loss. She described bereavement as including changes in all dimensions of a person's life—physical, psychological, and behavioral—as a result of this loss. People may display their reactions to this actual or perceived loss through their own social, cognitive, physical, and emotional behaviors. Thus, again, one is reminded of the integration of the models of disability both from the individual and the societal perspectives.

One particular continuum found in the literature (Parkes & Weiss, 1983) was specifically developed from research related to bereavement. Some of Parkes and Weiss's research related to the bereavement process focused on participants who had acquired disabilities. The continuum is presented in Figure 10.4.

Clegg (1988) has said that in life people tend to live each day on a set of assumptions; these assumptions can be disrupted when one faces a loss (also see the next section on philosophical underpinnings). She explained that Parkes and Weiss (1983) viewed the grieving process as part of a person's letting go of one set of assumptions and adopting another set when coming to terms with such losses as a disability. This view is reflected in the tasks of grieving continuum.

Parkes and Weiss (1983) believed that a person must go through this grieving process before truly accepting the loss. They stated that a person facing a recent loss must try to make sense of what has happened to begin to answer the omnipresent question "Why?"

People then move along the continuum toward emotional acceptance when they begin to feel less of a need to avoid reminders of the loss, which may evoke other painful feelings and emotional responses, including denial. Some people who receive occupational therapy will never fully come to this level of emotional acceptance. This may also be true for parents of a child

Intellectual recognition and explanation of loss	⇒	Emotional acceptance	⇒	Adoption of a new identity

Figure 10.4. Tasks of grieving.

Note. Adapted from *Recovery From Bereavement,* by C. M. Parkes and R. S. Weiss, 1983. Copyright © 1983, by Basic Books.

born with a disability, one who acquires a disability, or one with a disability that develops over time, such as a learning disability or autism spectrum disorder. For many of these people, the process may be slow. Each person's experience and ways of dealing with loss will be unique, and practitioners must be vigilant about and sensitive to their place along this continuum. Last, Parkes and Weiss (1983) described the adoption of a new identity as dichotomous: "maintaining one identity while acting in another" (p. 159).

In other words, if people believe that their identity reflects the set of assumptions or ideas that they have about themselves, then these are the very same ideas that affect their choices and their activity selections. This emphasis on choice, on engaging in meaningful activity, is central to the profession of occupational therapy. Whether one is using activities in evaluation or in treatment to remediate or compensate for a particular disability, the activities chosen must be meaningful to the person. Once again, practitioners are reminded that as they help people with disabilities reenter society and rebuild their lives, occupation is the process and activities are the outcome. The choice of activities for treatment as part of helping a person reconstruct a lifestyle after a disability is specific to the person (AOTA, 1993). There must be an activity match.

PHILOSOPHICAL UNDERPINNINGS: SELF, SKILLS, AND IDEAS

The concept of *figure–ground*, originating in philosophy, appears to have direct application to looking at how a disability affects a person's physical and psychological well-being and, essentially, how a person learns to cope with the loss (Bateson, 1972, 1979; Idhe, 1991; Popper, 1985, 1992). Similar to the ideas presented by Parkes and Weiss (1983), the assumptions on which people operate and carry out their daily activities are part of their *ground*, part of what they do not necessarily consciously think about throughout the course of the day. The ground is people's background knowledge; it is what they often take for granted. Even habits can become part of a person's background knowledge. It is not until a person experiences an event that brings about change—"rupture"—that he or she sees the figure (Idhe, 1991; G. Moglia, personal communication, April 22, 1998). In other words, the figure must be brought out of the background for a person to realize all that he or she does automatically. Thus, when a person becomes disabled—when he or she can no longer perform activities as before—the disability becomes part of the figure. A person may realize what he or she had taken for granted in the past. Trying to go back to the ground is often a difficult journey.

Related both to the concept of figure–ground and to the idea that people tend to live by a certain set of assumptions is that people also tend to adhere to the belief that their ideas and skills—and essentially many of their daily activities—define who they are (see Figure 10.5). Essentially, people embody ideas. If a person relinquishes an idea or a skill—especially if he or she loses a skill and can no longer perform an activity in the way in which he or she was accustomed—then a piece of who he or she is dies (Idhe, 1991; G. Moglia, personal communication, April 22, 1998; Popper, 1985, 1992).

Although it is very hard to do, people really cannot begin to critique the ideas and skills needed to engage in activities until they are able to view those same ideas and skills outside of themselves. Accepting that some of one's ideas and skills are fallible and that one often has to make mistakes to learn more about oneself is what makes the process so difficult. However, it is only then that one can improve on one's ideas and skills (Popper, 1985, 1992). This process appears analogous to a person's accepting that he or she may not be able to perform an activity the way he or she used to or learning that he or she can still perform the same activity but that modifications may have to be made for it to be carried out independently. A person may need assistance to continue to participate in an activity that was part of his or her daily occupation before becoming disabled. Furthermore, if the symptoms of those living with chronic illness progress, the level to which they may be able to perform certain activities will change. As the conditions change, so may the need for modifications or assistance.

In the occupational therapy literature, this theme of embodiment of ideas and skills is apparent. I have selected only a few works as examples for this chapter, but others exist. To illustrate, in her 1993 Eleanor Clark Slagle Lecture "Occupation Embedded in a Real Life: Interweaving Occupational Science and Occupational Therapy," Florence Clark (1993) presented the story of Professor Penny Richardson of the University of Southern California. She poignantly told of the process that Professor Richardson went through to rediscover herself, to realize how she had defined herself before surviving the traumatic event of an aneurysm and what she would have to do to discover a new self. Clark described how, by using narrative (telling stories), she was able to help Richardson through the process of recovery and "how rehabilitation can be experienced by the survivor as a rite of passage in which a person is moved to disability status and then abandoned" (p. 1067). Professor Richardson made Clark aware "that occupations were important because they marked the new you versus the old you" (p. 1072). These statements echo not only the information presented in the tasks of grieving as described by Parkes and

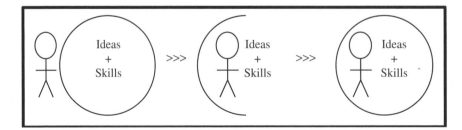

Figure 10.5. As human beings we tend to live by a certain set of assumptions and attach our ideas and skills.

Weiss (1983) but also the notion that people's ideas and skills—their occupations and the activities that constitute them—define who they are.

Similarly to Clark (1993), Price-Lackey and Cashman (1996) presented information gained from life history interviews to describe how Jenny Cashman (the second author of the work and a graduate student in library science and archeology) experienced and adapted to becoming disabled after a traumatic brain injury. They present Jenny's use of daily activities that had meaning to her and a narrative construction to help her in her recovery process to regain a sense of identity. As Robert Murphy (1990) described, Jenny also viewed her recovery process as a challenging journey. The following is an excerpt from Jenny's postscript regarding her head injury experience, which was included in the article:

> The process of healing and redefinition has also been a profound experience, providing new depth and richness to my life. The fact that my life has changed is no longer a source of grief to me, but something I embrace. I am writing again—not in the way I wrote before, but in a new way, and that feels like a gift. . . . I am—at this point, working on a book about my experience and my journey. It is somehow fitting that I celebrated my 5-year anniversary of my accident on an archeological dig in Egypt. The joy this gave me makes it clear that I have found my new path, so I have committed to working on the excavation for at least the next five campaigns. Then I'll see what happens next. Life is, after all, an eternal process of being and becoming. (p. 312)

Both Price-Lackey and Cashman (1996) suggested the following to practitioners:

- It is important for practitioners to understand what daily activities their clients engaged in before becoming ill or disabled. This information is important because descriptions of patterns of activities (occupations) may inform practitioners about their client's self-identities, and this information is integral to the recovery process.
- Goal setting should be a collaborative effort between the practitioner and the client.
- In treatment, occupational therapists and occupational therapy assistants should take into account both the doing aspects of occupations and the narrative meaning the client expresses regarding his or her daily occupations. By doing so, practitioners can truly begin to value the personal meaning that daily, purposeful activities bring to their client's lives.

In actuality, one does not have to look just to the literature to find examples of the embodiment of ideas and how people attach their ideas to themselves as a way of forming and re-forming their own identities. Occupational therapists can see this in their everyday practice and in themselves. However, until one can understand it in oneself, it is very hard to recognize the impact of attaching one's ideas to oneself in helping others.

Related to this idea, it is important that occupational therapists determine what type of learner their client may be or what type of learning style may affect his or her intervention and process of recovery. It is important to remember that a person's learning style may evolve as intervention progresses. Thus, it is key to create an environment in which people feel comfortable learning and in which people can learn through trial and error, creating their own knowledge as they begin to construct or reconstruct their lifestyle in living with a disability. Perkinson (1984, 1993) described what he called an *educative environment,* which may be helpful to practitioners as they help others learn new skills or relearn old ones in different ways. Although Perkinson mainly seemed to be describing the environment created by a teacher for his or her students, his ideas seem applicable to occupational therapists or occupational therapy assistants determining what type of treatment environment to set up for their clients, whether children or adults. Perkinson (1993) suggested that when making decisions about the environment needed to help people learn, practitioners create

- An environment in which people will feel free to "disclose their present knowledge" (p. 34);
- An environment that provides critical feedback regarding people's present knowledge (which can come from a variety of sources); and
- A supportive environment, so that people can accept criticism about their present knowledge and begin to eliminate errors.

Thus, simultaneously, practitioners must also question whether the people they work with truly understand what they have asked them to do. Again, practitioners must ask themselves "Because my client can perform a certain action while engaging in activity, does he or she really understand why I have asked him or her to perform this activity in a certain way?" (based on the understanding that the client chose the activity). In other words, can practitioners assume that if they set up behavioral Objective A, then they will get Outcome B? (Perkinson, 1993). Practitioners must be sure that the client understands why he or she is performing a certain activity and for what purpose. The person can then begin generalizing the knowledge learned from the experience of performing this activity during treatment to other activities he or she wants to do in daily life. Again, an activity match must exist among the activity itself, the underlying reasons for performing it, and the person.

Sociological Perspective and Personal Transformation

Disability can, in many ways, be described as a culture (Campbell & Oliver, 1996). In a sense, everyone can probably think of at least one activity they do that has been defined by their culture—and perhaps by society as well—or even an activity in which they may actually resist engaging because their particular culture has deemed it unacceptable. Reflecting on the disability movement in Britain and disability movements in general, Campbell and Oliver described these movements as redefining "the problem of disability as the product of a disabling society rather than individual limitations or loss, despite the fact that the rest of society continues to see disabled people as chance victims of a tragic fate" (p. 105).

For a person who has become disabled, Campbell and Oliver (1996) explained, part of this redefining is really a sociological process that includes redefining oneself and realizing that part of one's personal issues surrounding disability may also, in fact, be political. These are the issues that give rise to social movements. Therefore, the change process that affects people with disabilities is really twofold in that one looks at the changes in oneself and how these changes affect society. Campbell and Oliver (1996) described this duality as transforming both a personal and a social consciousness, "promoting self-understanding as a platform for change" (p. 145). Certainly, this very idea seems to have influenced U.S. society in such acts as the passage of the Americans With Disabilities Act in 1990 and the reauthorization of the Individuals With Disabilities Education Act in 1997 (Bailey & Schwartzberg, 1995; Johnson, 1996; Metzler, 1997, 1998). Much of the lobbying for passage of these laws came from advocacy groups, often consisting of people with disabilities and their families. Active participation in advocacy groups and other organizations often becomes a highly valued activity for people with disabilities.

Moreover, in deciding how to describe this change process to others in their book, Campbell and Oliver (1996) mentioned that they resisted separating information and issues surrounding disability, including social theory, political history, action research, individual biography, and personal experience. Each of these areas related to disability influences the other, and this is reflected in what appears to be yet another continuum regarding disability, looking at changes occurring on both a personal and a social level. Thus, there appear to be two smaller continua that are representative of the sociological perspective regarding disability and the change process associated with it. For the purposes of this chapter, I concentrate on what seems to be a personal transformation continuum that eventually affects the social transformation process as well (see Figure 10.6).

For personal transformation to occur, Campbell and Oliver (1996) suggested that first, people may deny that the existence of a problem. Their initial response may be to assimilate with the rest of society and view being disabled as part of their identity. Campbell and Oliver suggested that people must then be grateful and reasonable. By this, they mean that people with disabilities must somehow learn to balance accepting and being grateful to people who want to help them and simultaneously being reasonable and more conscious of what they should actually have to accept and even tolerate from society, including, for example, knowing when to report discriminatory

Denial ⇒ Be Grateful and Reasonable ⇒ Bearing Witness ⇒

Understanding Ourselves ⇒ Fighting Back

Figure 10.6. Personal transformation continuum adapted from ideas presented by Campbell and Oliver (1996).

acts. The next stage of the personal transformation process is that of bearing witness. This stage begins to bridge from the personal transformation to the societal transformation, which is the act of sharing experiences with others, especially those who have encountered similar problems, including those related to societal issues. Practitioners can see how activities such as these may become quite vital for those with whom they work, helping them to establish resources and reestablish connections with their world. Frequently, people learn the most from others with similar disabilities, such as information about what type of wheelchair lift to install in a van or what grocery store is the most easily accessible and accommodating to people with disabilities.

Next along this continuum is that people with disabilities must learn to understand themselves and to differentiate what Campbell and Oliver (1996) believed to be the difference between one's own personal problems and problems caused by a disabling society. Finally, these authors suggested that people can arrive at the level of fighting back, especially against societal stereotypes, by rejecting what they feel is the dominant disabling culture, getting involved in "cultural production" (e.g., the arts) as a way to express what has happened to them in their lives, and engaging in political practice by getting involved in political organizations and increasing empowerment. Speaking from their personal experience, Campbell and Oliver described, like many others, a difficult journey.

When reflecting on the four life perspectives that affect the activity performance of people with disabilities, one can begin to see the parallels among them. They seem to overlap both in the information presented regarding the change processes that take place in the person and in the fact that these processes seem to happen simultaneously. Changes occur within oneself and within one's environment. Disability can then be viewed sociologically as a "gap between a person's capabilities and the demands of the environment" (Committee on a National Agenda for the Prevention of Disabilities, 1991, p. 1). Thus, to begin looking at how to help people construct or reconstruct their lifestyle and ultimately their occupations using activities, practitioners must take into account information from all four of these perspectives. This information can be gained in many ways, most often through clinical interviews with the person, his or her family, significant others, and other caregivers. The overriding theme for the activity reasoning process goes back to the question presented in the beginning of this chapter: What is the person able and not able to do with respect to his or her ac-

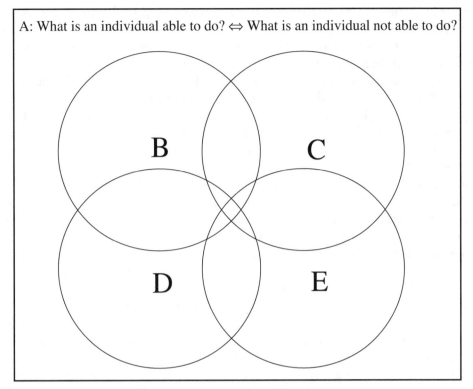

A: What is an individual able to do? ⇔ What is an individual not able to do?

B

C

D

E

Figure 10.7. Integration of the continua from the four life perspectives.

Note. A = activity reasoning process that requires occupational therapists to continually ask the question, What is the individual able to do and what is an individual not able to do regarding his or her activity performance? B = physical perspective, C = psychological perspective, D = philosophical perspective, and E = sociological perspective.

tivity performance? This continua from the four life perspectives is represented in Figure 10.7A (Figures 10.7B, 10.7C, 10.7D, and 10.7E, respectively, represent the physical, psychological, philosophical, and sociological perspectives). What practitioners may also consider includes but is certainly not limited to a person's resources; background knowledge; the client factors of values, beliefs, and spirituality; level of assistance needed; the person's own understanding of what he or she feels able to do, and the person's level of motivation. As always, each person's experiences, feelings, and life situation will be unique.

A Framework: Helping People Construct and Reconstruct Their Lifestyles Using Activities

According to the philosopher Karl Popper, to learn, human beings have to criticize their ideas and look for errors. Essentially, people often learn best through the process of trial and error. It is very difficult, however, for people to criticize their own ideas or to make other guesses about ways in which to solve problems when they are used to addressing problems in a certain way. Popper (1985, 1992) thus described one way in which people can learn more (and gain knowledge) about how to address their problems, accepting the idea that there may never be a true solution. Popper explained that once one has identified a problem, one should make guesses about how to address it and criticize each of these guesses. By discovering solutions to problems, people advance knowledge. G. Moglia (personal communication, June 1, 1998) used the metaphor of a staircase to explain Popper's ideas. People go through a process of presentation or description of the problem, make a guess, criticize the guess, and make a better guess. This process continues and evolves at each step of the knowledge staircase. Thus, as people ascend this staircase and are able to see their mistakes, they come to deeper problems and better guesses. The staircase has no finite end; it is only a process by which to reach better guesses (G. Moglia, personal communication, September 10, 1997; Popper, 1985, 1992).

The occupational therapy reflective staircase illustrates this process (see Figure 10.8). When a practitioner is near the top level of the staircase, he or she may reach the point at which the problem has to be reframed because the original problem was resolved or changed or perhaps because deeper problems underlay the original problem (Schön, 1983). An example would be when after initiating treatment, the therapist begins to realize that a person's depression is affecting physical activity performance more than the therapist had detected on initial evaluation. Thus, the person may need to address the depression before continuing treatment or concurrently with treatment, or he or she may need to seek the help of other professionals who may also be able to assist the person in addressing this problem.

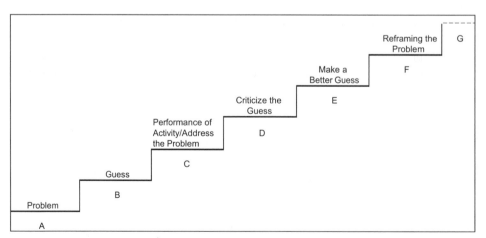

Figure 10.8. Occupational therapy reflective staircase.

Note. Adapted from the ideas for practice of Moglia (1997, 1998), Popper (1985, 1992), and Schön (1983).

Using the Staircase in Clinical Practice: The Process

Because occupational therapists and occupational therapy assistants work with people with disabilities, this process appears similar to their clinical reasoning process. When thinking about how to use activities to help people with disabilities construct or reconstruct their lifestyles, it appears applicable and useful to incorporate the use of this staircase and, essentially, the process of analysis (of the problem) and synthesis (making guesses to arrive at possible ways to address the problem).

PROBLEM

As part of the evaluation process, practitioners can ask several questions regarding the person's current and past level of activity performance. Essentially, occupational therapists seek to determine through both interview and observation of activity performance what the person is able and not able to do. More specifically, they seek to determine what the person identifies as a problem related to activity performance that is interfering with his or her ability to function as independently as possible (based on the activity he or she has chosen), and what the caregiver identifies as a problem related to activity performance. Another, related question is what purpose the activity serves. For example, is it part of the person's daily routine, is it a leisure activity, or is it an activity that aids the caregiver in assisting the person? So practitioners essentially consider the impact on both performance components, or the underlying problems, and performance skills and patterns, while always also considering contextual factors. The focus will be different for each person, and the occupation that the activity relates to may be different as well. For example, for one person, reading a book may be a pleasure; for another, it may be considered part of his or her work or education. It is important to have a clear description and understanding of the problem before proceeding with the rest of the process.

Consider the following two brief case scenarios. Embedded within them are problems the practitioner may choose to address as part of helping clients construct and or reconstruct their lifestyles using activities. More than likely, the practitioner would need more information to develop a complete intervention plan. As mentioned earlier, to provide a truly client-centered process, the therapist should include how these activities relate to a person's engagement in occupations that are purposeful and meaningful. These scenarios may, however, help stimulate your thinking in using the framework presented and in beginning to see the importance of the integration of the person with the context and environment and with his or her occupations (AOTA, 2008; Christiansen & Baum, 1997; Christiansen, Baum, & Bass-Haugen, 2005; Law, Baum, & Dunn, 2005).

After reading the case scenarios, ask yourself, What is one potential problem related to activity performance that could be addressed in occupational therapy? What occupation(s) may be affected? What other information might you need? Then describe the problem in your own words (see the worksheet in Appendix 10.A for more guidance).

CASE SCENARIO 10.1: MR. JOHNSON

Mr. Johnson is a 28-year-old man who recently developed paraplegia after a motor vehicle accident. Before his accident, he was a manager of a local business supply store. He has been referred by his physiatrist for inpatient occupational therapy now that he has stabilized; thus, it has been determined that it is safe for him to participate in a rehabilitation program. During an interview, Mr. Johnson tells you that he lives alone and plans on returning to his apartment on discharge. His nearest relatives are 400 miles away. On weekends, close friends and family have been visiting him in the hospital. His initial requests during your occupational therapy evaluation are that he wants to be able to dress and bathe himself. At this time, he is completely reliant on others to carry out these daily living tasks for him. Moreover, later in the interview, Mr. Johnson mentions having been a member of a men's sports league before his accident and that he has enjoyed competitive sports since childhood.

CASE SCENARIO 10.2: KAREN

Karen is a 5-year-old girl who attends public school in a regular education classroom. On initial evaluation, you determine that she is sensory defensive. (Sensory defensiveness is a defensive reaction to sensations that most people would not consider noxious; Wilbarger & Wilbarger, 1991, 1997). She was initially referred to you, the school occupational therapist, by her prekindergarten teacher. Her teacher reports that Karen refuses to participate in most of the daily activities in which the children engage, such as arts and crafts and snack preparation, and she becomes upset (e.g., crying, running around the room attempting to find a place to hide) when she sees that she might have to touch any type of messy materials such as glue or cookie dough. Also, she is quite fearful of playing on any moving playground equipment, resulting in her playing alone during recess. She has difficulty making friends. Her mother also tells you that Karen is unable to do many self-care activities independently, such as buttoning her shirt. You also notice that she uses a very weak grasp when drawing with crayons. Karen tells you that when she grows up, she wants to be an artist.

Guess

To begin to make a guess about how to address the problem, the initial question one should ask at this point in the process is "What is constraining activity performance?" Similar to using the top-down approach described earlier, after determining the meaning attached to a person's activities and roles, the practitioner must explore with the person (or the caregiver, or both) the possible reasons why he or she is unable to carry out certain activities described as problems. This exploration helps form the focus of treatment (Trombly, 1993, 1995). Several guesses or strategies may be used concerning how to address the problem related to activity performance. For example, the practitioner may choose to modify the activity itself, provide adaptive equipment, modify the environment, or provide physical assistance to help a person perform an activity that she or he has identified as part of his or her lifestyle. Client factors, including but not limited to values and beliefs and body functions, must be continuously taken into account as part of this client-centered process (AOTA, 2008).

Performance of the Activity–Address the Problem

Practitioners must observe people perform the activity to determine whether their guess regarding the problem was appropriate. Thus, one can reflect on the performance to move to the next step of criticizing the guess.

Exercise 10.1: Guessing

Considering the two case studies presented, think about what some of your possible guesses may be to address the problems that you have described. Again, remember that one guess is not necessarily the only correct guess; several ways to address the problem may exist. Also, when comparing the two scenarios, other issues may affect your thinking, for example, that Mr. Johnson appears concerned with reconstructing certain activities that were part of his lifestyle before his accident. This issue will have a direct impact on his occupational performance. Karen, however, may possibly never have constructed certain lifestyle activities or engaged in certain occupations because of her sensory defensiveness. For example, because she has avoided touching many objects, the musculature in her hands may not have fully developed, which would affect her fine motor performance and choice of fine motor activities and thus directly affect her play or education. You must also consider the necessity of co-occupation and these clients' interrelationship with their caregivers.

EXERCISE 10.2: PROVIDING FEEDBACK

Think about how you would provide feedback regarding errors or mistakes to both Mr. Johnson and Karen during their performance of activities. For example, if Mr. Johnson attempted to use adaptive equipment during a dressing activity, using it in such a way that he seemed to expend too much energy, how would you make him aware of this? How could you use the activity as an element of change, helping him to learn energy conservation techniques to incorporate into his lifestyle? If Karen continues to use a weak or incorrect grasp of her pencil or crayons, how will you make her aware of this? Because she is sensitive to touch, will you physically cue her to place her fingers differently on the shaft of the pencil or will you need to devise other cuing systems, such as modeling the grasp needed so that she can visually monitor the change needed for more successful activity performance? What feedback might you be able to give to Mr. Johnson's and Karen's caregivers that may help them facilitate the process in the more natural context outside of the clinic, which may ultimately affect Mr. Johnson's and Karen's choices of occupations, confidence in their performance, and level of independence?

CRITICIZE THE GUESS

This step in the process is crucial in helping a person construct or reconstruct his or her lifestyle using activities because this is the point on the staircase at which the person may see the "figure" (as described earlier in this chapter) of what he or she is still not able to do as a result of the disability.

Furthermore, if errors were made during the performance of the activity, it is important to allow the person to see the error (Popper, 1992) and to help him or her gain knowledge from the performance. Occupational therapists can also gain valuable knowledge by looking at their guesses, attempting to figure out why they were or were not appropriate or why they did or did not work in addressing the problem identified.

MAKE A BETTER GUESS

Several issues can be explored and reflected on here. Perhaps the activity in which a problem was identified was appropriate for an initial treatment activity (within the person's capabilities with or without modifications), but the conditions (e.g., the amount of time needed for performance of the activity in its entirety) or the context in which it is performed may have to be changed or modified. Maybe a different, related activity would better match the person's or caregiver's current needs. Only by making these better guesses can practitioners move people along the staircase so that they can continue to construct or reconstruct their lifestyles—and ultimately their occupations—and help them in their personal search for meaning and sense of purpose.

Reframe the Problem

This process is continuous and evolves over time. However, when guesses still do not seem to be effective, the practitioner may have to reflect on all he or she has done and reframe the problem (Schön, 1983). The original problem addressed may in fact not be the one that needs to be addressed first to effect change. As professionals, practitioners must ask themselves questions or reflect on ideas such as these:

- Did you take into account all of the possible activity demands? Is the person only physically unable to perform the activity (or elements of a larger activity), or are there other life perspectives that may be affecting performance?
- Considering the preceding question, the practitioner could then ask him- or herself whether underlying reasons explain why the person cannot perform the activity, for example, levels of motivation and meaning, difficulty reaching an emotional level of acceptance of the disability, difficulty separating ideas from self to learn, or all of these.
- What other performance patterns may need to be taken into account, for example, habits, routines, roles, and rituals? Have these changed or evolved over time as a result of the disability; living with the disability; or engaging in the occupational therapy evaluation, intervention, and outcome process (AOTA, 2008)?
- Perhaps the underlying problem is in the environment or the objects used in the activity, not the person's physical or psychological capabilities.
- Perhaps the person can perform one element of the activity, and the problem is now the next element, making the activity more complex.

Summary

Together, we have learned first how we must consider the four life perspectives and then how these perspectives can affect people with disabilities and the activity choices they make in their lives. The occupational therapy reflective staircase—incorporating the process from problem, guess, performance of activity, criticizing the guess, making a better guess, through reframing the problem—can help guide us as we learn to help people with disabilities construct or reconstruct their lifestyles using activities.

> We can bestow a meaning upon our lives through our work, through our active conduct, through our whole way of life, and

through the attitude we adopt towards our friends and our fellow men and towards the world. . . . In this way the quest for the meaning of life turns into an ethical question—the question "What tasks can I set myself in order to make my life meaningful?" (Popper, 1992, pp. 138–139)

References

American Occupational Therapy Association. (1993). Position Paper—Purposeful activity. *American Journal of Occupational Therapy, 51,* 864–866.

American Occupational Therapy Association. (1994). Uniform terminology for occupational therapy—Third edition. *American Journal of Occupational Therapy, 48,* 1047–1054.

American Occupational Therapy Association. (2002). Occupational therapy practice framework: Domain and process. *American Journal of Occupational Therapy, 56,* 609–639.

American Occupational Therapy Association. (2008). Occupational therapy practice framework: Domain and process (2nd ed.). *American Journal of Occupational Therapy, 62,* 625–683.

Americans With Disabilities Act of 1990, Pub. L. 101–336, 42 U.S.C. § 12101.

Bailey, D. M., & Schwartzberg, S. L. (1995). Section 504 and Americans With Disabilities Act. In *Ethical and legal dilemmas in occupational therapy* (pp. 31–54). Philadelphia: F. A. Davis.

Baptiste, S. E. (2003). Client-centered practice: Implications for our professional approach, behaviors, and lexicon. In P. Kramer, J. Hinojosa, & C. B. Royeen (Eds.), *Perspectives in human occupation: Participation in life* (pp. 264–277). Philadelphia: Lippincott Williams & Wilkins.

Bateson, G. (1972). *Steps to an ecology of mind.* San Francisco: Chandler.

Bateson, G. (1979). *Mind and nature: A necessary unity.* New York: Dutton.

Campbell, J., & Oliver, M. (1996). *Disability politics: Understanding our past, changing our future.* London: Routledge.

Carroll, T. J. (1961). *Blindness: What it is, what it does, and how to live with it.* Boston: Little, Brown.

Christiansen, C. H., & Baum, M. C. (Eds.). (1997). *Occupational therapy: Enabling function and well-being.* Thorofare, NJ: Slack.

Christiansen, C., Baum, M. C., & Bass-Haugen, J. (Eds.). (2005). *Occupational therapy: Performance, participation, and well-being* (3rd ed.). Thorofare, NJ: Slack.

Clark, F. (1993). Occupation embedded in a real life: Interweaving occupational science and occupational therapy [Eleanor Clarke Slagle Lecture]. *American Journal of Occupational Therapy, 47,* 1067–1078.

Clark, F., Azen, S. P., Zemke, R., Jackson, J., Carlson, M., Mandel, D., et al. (1997). Occupational therapy for independent-living older adults: A randomized controlled study. *JAMA, 278,* 1321–1326.

Clegg, F. (1988). Bereavement. In S. Fisher & J. Reason (Eds.), *Handbook of life stress, cognition, and health* (pp. 61–78). Chichester, UK: John Wiley.

Committee on a National Agenda for the Prevention of Disabilities. (1991). Executive summary. In A. M. Pope & A. R. Tarlov (Eds.), *Disability in America* (pp. 1–31). Washington, DC: National Academies Press.

Coster, W. (1998). Occupation-centered assessment of children. *American Journal of Occupational Therapy, 52,* 337–344.

Coster, W. J., & Haley, S. M. (1992). Conceptualization and measurement of disablement in infants and young children. *Infants and Young Children, 4,* 11–22.

Dunn, W., Brown, C., & McGuigan, A. (1994). The ecology of human performance: A framework for considering the effect of context. *American Journal of Occupational Therapy, 48,* 595–607.

Dunn, W., Brown, C., & Youngstrom, M. J. (2003). Ecological model of occupation. In P. Kramer, J. Hinojosa, & C. B. Royeen (Eds.), *Perspectives in human occupation: Participation in life* (pp. 222–263). Philadelphia: Lippincott Willams & Wilkins.

Hinojosa, J., & Blount, M. L. (2009). Occupation, purposeful activities, and occupational therapy. In J. Hinojosa & M. L. Blount (Eds.), *The texture of life: Purposeful activities in occupational therapy* (3rd ed., pp. 1–28). Bethesda, MD: AOTA Press.

Hinojosa, J., Kramer, P., Royeen, C. B., & Luebben, A. J. (2003). Core concept of occupation. In P. Kramer, J. Hinojosa, & C. B. Royeen (Eds.), *Perspectives in human occupation: Participation in life* (pp. 1–17). Philadelphia: Lippincott Willams & Wilkins.

Ideishi, R. I. (2003). Influence of occupation on assessment and treatment. In P. Kramer, J. Hinojosa, & C. B. Royeen (Eds.), *Perspectives in human occupation: Participation in life* (pp. 278–296). Philadelphia: Lippincott Willams & Wilkins.

ldhe, D. (1991). *Instrumental realism: The interface between philosophy of science and philosophy of technology.* Bloomington: Indiana University Press.

Individuals With Disabilities Education Act of 1997, Pub. L. 105–117.

Jackson, J., Carlson, M., Mandel, D., Zemke, R., & Clark, F. (1998). Occupation in lifestyle redesign: The Well Elderly Study occupational therapy program. *American Journal of Occupational Therapy, 52,* 326–336.

Johnson, J. (1996). School-based occupational therapy. In J. Case-Smith, A. S. Allen, & P. N. Pratt (Eds.), *Occupational therapy for children* (3rd ed., pp. 693–716). St. Louis, MO: Mosby.

Knussen, C., & Cunningham, C. C. (1988). Stress, disability, and handicap. In S. Fisher & J. Reason (Eds.), *Handbook of life stress, cognition, and health* (pp. 335–350) Chichester, UK: John Wiley.

Law, M., Baum, M. C., & Dunn, W. (2005). *Measuring occupational performance: Supporting best practice in occupational therapy* (2nd ed.). Thorofare, NJ: Slack.

Lazarus, R. S., & Folkman, S. (1991). The concept of coping. In A. Monat & R. S. Lazarus (Eds.), *Stress and coping: An anthology* (3rd ed., pp. 189–206). New York: Columbia University Press.

Lollar, D. J. (2003). Foreword. In P. Kramer, J. Hinojosa, & C. B. Royeen (Eds.), *Perspectives in human occupation: Participation in life* (pp. vii–viii). Philadelphia: Lippincott Williams & Wilkins.

Luebben, A. J. (2003). Ethical concerns: Human occupation. In P. Kramer, J. Hinojosa, & C. B. Royeen (Eds.), *Perspectives in human occupation: Participation in life* (pp. 297–311). Philadelphia: Lippincott Willams & Wilkins.

Metzler, C. (1997, July). A better idea. *OT Week, 11,* 14–15.

Metzler, C. (1998, February). Key issues in IDEA. *OT Week, 12,* 10.

Mosey, A. C. (1996). *Applied scientific inquiry in the health professions: An epistemological orientation* (2nd ed.). Bethesda, MD: American Occupational Therapy Association.

Murphy, R. F. (1990). *The body silent.* New York: W. W. Norton.

Nagi, S. Z. (1965). Some conceptual issues in disability and rehabilitation. In M. B. Sussman (Ed.), *Sociology and rehabilitation* (pp. 104–113). Washington, DC: American Sociological Association.

Nagi, S. Z. (1991). Disability concepts revisited: Implications for prevention. In A. M. Pope & A. R. Tarlov (Eds.), *Disability in America* (pp. 309–327). Washington, DC: National Academies Press.

Padilla, R. (2003). Clara: A phenomenology of disability. *American Journal of Occupational Therapy, 57,* 413–423.

Parkes, C. M. (1998). *Bereavement: Studies of grief in adult life.* Madison, CT: International Universities Press.

Parkes, C. M., & Weiss, R. S. (1983). The recovery process. In *Recovery from bereavement* (pp. 155–168). New York: Basic Books.

Perkinson, H. J. (1984). *Learning from our mistakes: A reinterpretation of twentieth-century educational theory.* Westport, CT: Greenwood Press.

Perkinson, H. J. (1993). *Teachers without goals, students without purposes.* New York: McGraw-Hill.

Popper, K. R. (1985). *Popper selections* (D. Miller, Ed.). Princeton, NJ: Princeton University Press.

Popper, K. R. (1992). Emancipation through knowledge. In L. J. Bennett (Trans.), *In search of a better world: Lectures and essays from thirty years* (pp. 137–150*).* London: Routledge.

Price-Lackey, P., & Cashman, J. (1996). Jenny's story: Reinventing oneself through occupation and narrative configuration. *American Journal of Occupational Therapy, 50,* 306–314.

Rogers, J. C., & Holm, M. B. (1994). Nationally Speaking—Accepting the challenge of outcome research: Examining the effectiveness of occupational therapy practice. *American Journal of Occupational Therapy, 48,* 871–876.

Schön, D. A. (1983). *The reflective practitioner: How professionals think in action.* New York: Basic.

Tham, K., & Kielhofner, G. (2003). Impact of the social environment on occupational experience and performance among persons with unilateral neglect. *American Journal of Occupational Therapy, 57,* 403–412.

Trombly, C. A. (1993). The Issue Is—Anticipating the future: Assessment of occupational function. *American Journal of Occupational Therapy, 47,* 253–257.

Trombly, C. A. (1995). Occupation: Purposefulness and meaningfulness as therapeutic mechanisms [Eleanor Clarke Slagle Lecture]. *American Journal of Occupational Therapy, 49,* 960–972.

Wilbarger, P., & Wilbarger, J. L. (1991). *Sensory defensiveness in children aged 2–12: An intervention guide for parents and other caretakers.* Santa Barbara, CA: Avanti Educational Programs.

Wilbarger, P., & Wilbarger, J. L. (1997). *Sensory defensiveness and related social/emotional and neurological problems* (Course syllabus). Oak Park Heights, MN: Professional Development Programs.

Wood, P. H. N. (1980). Appreciating the consequences of disease: The international classification of impairments, disabilities, and handicaps. *WHO Chronicle, 34,* 376–380.

Wood, W. (1998). Nationally Speaking—It is jump time for occupational therapy. *American Journal of Occupational Therapy, 52,* 403–411.

World Health Organization. (1980). *International classification of impairments, disabilities and handicaps.* Geneva, Switzerland: Author.

World Health Organization. (1990). *International classification of diseases* (10th rev.). Geneva, Switzerland: Author.

World Health Organization. (2001). *International classification of functioning, disability and health—Short version.* Geneva, Switzerland: Author.

Youngstrom, M. J. (2002). *Report of the chairperson of the commission on practice, III.C. to the representative assembly* (RA Charge No. 2002M29). Bethesda, MD: AOTA Press.

Appendix 10.A

Constructing and Reconstructing Lifestyles Using Activities: The Occupational Therapy Reflective Staircase Worksheet

Name of the person:

Age:

Brief activity history:

Concerns, needs, wants, and priorities of the person that could guide evaluation, treatment, and possible outcomes related to activity performance:

Concerns, needs, wants, and priorities of the caregiver or significant other involved, which could guide evaluation, treatment, and possible outcomes related to activity performance:

Additional notes (e.g., you may want to include medical precautions, disposition plans, contexts in which activities are usually performed, other factors that may affect activity performance):

Note. "Constructing and Reconstructing Lifestyles Using Activities: The Occupational Therapy Reflective Staircase Worksheet" was created by the author.

Problem (related to activity chosen together with the person):

Guess:

Performance of the activity–address the problem:

Criticize the guess:

Make a better guess:

Reframe the problem, if needed:

11

◈

Using Activities as Challenges to Facilitate Development of Occupational Performance

Margaret Kaplan, PhD, OTR/L

Previous chapters of this text have discussed how activities are used in occupational therapy as an end goal. Occupational therapists determine which areas of occupation are meaningful to a client and have become difficult to perform. Interventions include the development of compensatory strategies, selection and modification of available assistive devices, design and fabrication of unique assistive devices, modification of the context, and focused practice of relevant tasks.

Critical interventions exist to enable clients to improve their performance in selected activities. If underlying impairments remain unchanged, however, these improvements are not likely to generalize and make their way into the performance of other occupations. When a therapist determines that a client demonstrates the potential to improve underlying factors or performance skills, the client deserves the opportunity to work toward such restoration of foundational motor, cognitive, or interactive capacities.

Think about the goals you would set for yourself, or a loved one, if faced with limitations in activity performance. Suppose your friend is unable to perform instrumental activities of daily living because his organizational and problem-solving skills have been affected by a traumatic brain injury (TBI). If he exhibits the potential to improve these underlying cognitive skills, would an occupational therapy program consisting only of specific task practice be sufficient? What if your younger sister demonstrates impairments in hand coordination that limit her ability to learn handwriting skills? You would want occupational therapy to offer her the opportunity to improve her underlying limitations in addition to specific handwriting practice or the provision of adapted writing utensils. Suppose your grandfather has survived a stroke with intact cognition. He demonstrates some movement throughout his paretic left arm but is unable to use the arm for task performance. Would you be satisfied with an occupational therapy program that is limited to teaching one-handed self-care techniques?

Occupational therapists and occupational therapy assistants provide interventions that improve performance in areas of occupation through balanced interventions that maximize the client's potential to improve client factors and performance skills (factors internal to the client) and minimize activity limitation through compensatory approaches (factors external to the client). Figure 11.1 illustrates the fact that practitioners balance these internally and externally directed interventions to promote performance of occupations that will enhance participation in family and community situations.

Improvements in internal factors are critical to the occupational therapy process because they enable clients to perform an infinite number of tasks in a variety of situations. Such improvements empower them to create and discover unanticipated occupations and roles. Practitioners who work with children often use play activities as a means to facilitate and encourage the development of more mature performance skills (internal factors). A careful balance is planned to present a client with the "just-right challenge"—one that is neither so far above the client's present abilities that it is frustrating nor so far below that new learning does not occur.

In this chapter, I describe the use of occupation as means (Case-Smith, 2005; Trombly Latham, 2008), in which practitioners design activities to provide structured challenges to reduce specific impairments in client factors and improve specific performance skills (see Figure 11.1). Practitioners use activities in three major ways to promote improvements in internal factors:

1. They present an activity to provide the interest level that enables clients to exert more effort, complete more repetitions of a desired behavior, or sustain performance for a longer duration.
2. They manipulate a select activity and environmental conditions to present graded challenges to specific skills.

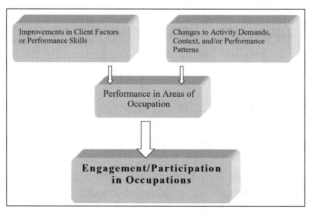

Figure 11.1. Activity-based intervention in occupational therapy is a balance between internally and externally directed interventions to improve performance in areas of occupation and, ultimately, participation in valued roles.

3. They select activities that will provide problems that challenge a client to develop effective cognitive or motor strategies that can be generalized to an unlimited variety of future situations.

Although categories overlap somewhat, occupational therapy students must understand when each type of occupation means may be most appropriate and which concepts are most relevant to apply when using occupation as means in each of these three ways.

Using Activities to Elicit Greater Effort, Repetition, or Duration Than Traditional Exercise

Historically, the earliest use of activities in occupational therapy may have been as a medium to facilitate improvement in underlying client factors and performance skills (Taylor, 1929). Research findings (Bloch, Smith, & Nelson, 1989; Kircher, 1984; Steinbeck, 1986) have indicated that healthy adults exert greater cardiovascular and muscular effort, as evidenced by faster heart rate and increased electromyographic activity in selected muscles, when performing activities that they perceive to be fun (e.g., jumping rope) compared with exercises with similar motor components (e.g., jumping in place). Using activities as interventions is relevant when treatment goals are to improve cardiopulmonary and specific muscle endurance.

Performance of interesting or personally meaningful activity also promotes greater repetition and prolonged duration of physical output than performance of routine exercise programs (DeKuiper, Nelson, & White, 1993; Hsieh, Nelson, Smith, & Peterson, 1996; Lang, Nelson, & Bush, 1992; Miller & Nelson, 1987; Nelson et al., 1996; Riccio, Nelson, & Bush, 1990; Steinbeck, 1986; Yoder, Nelson, & Smith, 1989). This fact is well understood in current popular culture, as evidenced by the use of dance routines and embedded games during aerobic exercise and muscle-toning sessions at community fitness centers. When muscle endurance or joint flexibility are treatment goals, it is advantageous for the client to produce more repetitions over a longer duration of actions that demand optimal levels of muscle output or soft tissue elongation (Downey & Darling, 1994). When seeking to decrease distal limb edema, repetitive isotonic contractions of muscles in the targeted body segment are a recognized complement to medical and positioning interventions (Burkhardt, 2004; Cooper, 2008). For example, to improve range for overhead reach and to stretch painful muscles, one client found that putting dishes away on high shelves provided repetitive reaching during a task that was necessary and important to that client. This client found that a Pilates exercise routine enabled her to engage in the exercises recommended by the therapist more regularly and for longer periods than did a standard exercise regime (Earley & Shannon, 2006).

Research findings have provided evidence that people with disabilities exhibit greater range of motion (i.e., perform closer to their maximum potential) when engaged in interesting activities than when performing under conventional exercise conditions. In one study, Van der Weel, van der Meer, and Lee (1991) encouraged children with cerebral palsy who exhibited right hemiparesis to actively perform the forearm movements of pronation and supination. While performing in the experimental condition, the children were instructed to use a drumstick to bang on drums that were positioned to require full forearm range of motion. During the control condition, the same children were instructed to move the drumstick back and forth as far as they could in the frontal plane. Range of movement was significantly greater when banging the drums than during the abstract exercise condition.

Sietsema, Nelson, Mulder, Mervau-Scheidel, and White (1993) produced similar findings in their study of forward reach in adults with hemiparesis caused by TBI. Neurodevelopmental treatment strategies were used to prepare study participants for forward reach from the sitting position. In the exercise condition, participants reached out their hands as far as they could in a rote manner. In the activity condition, they reached forward to control Simon®, a popular computer-controlled game that challenges players to repeat its sequences of flashing lights and sounds by pressing colored panels. Data collected through computerized motion analysis revealed that participants displayed significantly greater mobility when engaged in the activity than when they attempted to reach forward in a purely exercise context.

In pediatric intervention, the use of playful, inviting sensory integration equipment serves, in part, to pique children's interest in and sustain their performance of activities that provide vestibular, tactile, or proprioceptive stimuli that they might otherwise avoid. The introduction of imaginative play may engage the child still further, thus encouraging longer duration of involvement and expenditure of greater effort during treatment sessions. Increased practice of gross motor developmental actions within the context of a nontherapy, gamelike group event resulted in greater improvements in skill acquisition for young children with Down syndrome than for those who received only physical therapy (Fiss & Effgen, 2008).

What makes an activity engaging enough that it will entice a person to continue a performance while repetitively performing a prescribed exercise or practicing a new skill? The answer depends on each person. A person's interest in specific activities is influenced by a complex array of factors, including his or her cultural background, age, prior experiences, and current abilities. In addition to these factors, developmental level must be taken into account when providing choices of activities to children. Usually, the therapist engages the child by making the purpose of the activity clear, for example, "Let's build a garage for your car," "Let's make a valentine's card for Mom," and "Stay on the boat [bolster], here come some waves, don't fall in the water." Depending on developmental level, the introduction of pretend play and social play can provide an additional level of interest and motivation that increases the effort or duration of the activity engagement (Humphry, 2002; Humphry & Wakeford, 2006). As children get older, the judicious use of small groups can be extremely effective in modeling behavior and motivating children to participate with peers.

In their attempt to create activities that will entice clients to perform repetitive practice of specific movements or skills, occupational therapists may be tempted to present tasks that are so contrived that they hold little meaning for their clients (Fisher, 1998). If an occupational therapy activity does little to engage the client, no advantage exists in choosing such an activity over exercise as an intervention.

The occupational therapist must learn as much as possible about each client's previous skills, interests, and activity background. This information, combined with knowledge of the person's current strengths and limitations, is critical to setting feasible treatment goals. Parents and family members can be invaluable in providing insight into what engages a child who appears to have little interest in his or her environment. A favorite object from the home or classroom can be used to develop an activity: "Let's put your doll to sleep" or "Can you help your teddy bear to draw a picture?" Although this background information may also be helpful when selecting therapeutic activities, activities that engage the client do not necessarily need to be related to a client's prior repertoire of activity interests. "It does not matter whether one originally wanted to do the activity, whether one expected to enjoy it, or not. Even a frustrating job may suddenly become exciting if one hits upon the right balance" (Csikszentmihalyi & Csikszentmihalyi, 1988, p. 32).

For many adults, an enabling activity need not have been a favorite prior pastime. In fact, sometimes a well-meaning practitioner is disappointed to learn that selecting a favorite task as a therapeutic interventions frustrates clients rather than bringing them pleasure. The client who worked as an electrician may become disheartened to see that simple wiring tasks are now excessively challenging. The avid puzzle solver may be dismayed to be practicing crossword puzzles designed for children. The match between an activity's intrinsic interest level and the person's understanding of why the practice is important is key in determining how successful an activity will be in eliciting pleasure during sustained performance. As in all other aspects of occupational therapy, active involvement in the total therapeutic process enhances a client's motivation to participate.

Occupational therapists and occupational therapy assistants must consider a few critical words of caution when using activities to elicit repetitive performance of prescribed movement sequences. First, repetitive movements must be performed only from a position of optimal alignment. The practitioner must avoid activities that are ergonomically unsound while providing appropriate therapeutic positioning and handling to enhance the client's performance and comfort. Second, therapeutic activities should not be introduced unless the client demonstrates adequate prerequisite factors and skills. For example, introducing a task that requires repetitive active reaching has no therapeutic value unless the client exhibits the necessary joint play and muscle distensibility that will allow adequate passive range of motion at all the joints of the shoulder complex. Finally, practitioners need to remember that repetition must occur naturally within the activity performance (Figure 11.2). Setting up a checkerboard affords the opportunity for repetitive practice of reach, grasp, and release. The activity component, however, is maintained only if this initial placement of game pieces is followed by an actual game of checkers (with a family member, a volunteer, or another client). In an effort to foster even more repetition, a practitioner may be tempted to ask a client to remove the check-

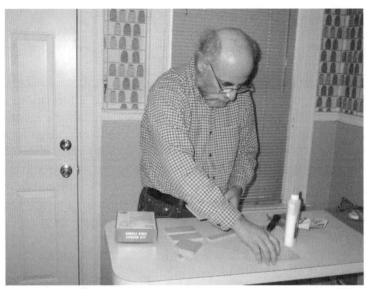

Figure 11.2. Client engaging in assembling a wood kit using repetitive reach, grasp, and manipulation while increasing standing balance and tolerance.

ers and begin the task again. Although this contrivance may be effective once or twice, it quickly reduces what may have begun as an interesting activity to a rote exercise that is unlikely to maintain the client's interest over time.

CASE SCENARIO 11.1: JACK

Jack is a 75-year-old man who sustained a stroke with resulting left-side hemiparesis and is now receiving occupational therapy on an inpatient rehabilitation unit. Goals were to increase standing balance, sustained visual attention to both right and left fields, and fine motor coordination, especially during bilateral tasks. Jack was able to stand for less than 5 min during manipulation tasks, then needed to stop and sit down to rest. He needed frequent verbal cues to attend to the left visual field. The occupational therapist learned from Jack that he liked to work with wood and would be interested in building something. The occupational therapist asked Jack about building a bird house for his small backyard at home, and Jack seemed quite excited about the idea. The occupational therapist chose a precut, eight-piece wood birdhouse kit and set up the pieces and directions at a standing-height table with pieces on both the right and the left sides of the table. Jack was able to stand and work on the birdhouse for 20–25 min without asking for a rest break, and he maintained visual attention to both sides of the visual field to read directions, find the correct part, match it up with another part, and compare it with the diagram. Jack continued work on the birdhouse and was able to maintain his standing balance for 20–30 min at a time. He required much less cuing to search both sides of the visual field for the pieces and supplies he needed.

Using Activities to Provide Graded Challenges

Repetition alone will not promote improvement in all client factors and performance skills. When client goals are to enhance muscle strength, range of motion, balance, coordination, manipulation, social skills, or other skills that have the capacity to improve on a continuum, practice sessions must afford opportunities for incremental increases in appropriate demands. The key to effectively using activities to provide graded challenges is the therapist's identification of a specific, relevant continuum on which gradations will be introduced. For example, if the client's goal is to improve active hip and pelvic mobility when sitting, placement of activity objects in relation to the client will represent a relevant continuum. Because the weight or size of activity objects will essentially be irrelevant to the specific performance of active hip motion, these factors will not be manipulated when making incremental changes to the activity demands. Gentile's (1972, 1987) concept of *regulatory conditions* refers to those environmental features that directly influence a person's choice of strategies for performing a selected task. When designing activities to present graded challenges, practitioners determine which features in the environment and the selected task are regulatory to the skills they seek to challenge (Sabari, 1991). Figure 11.3 illustrates the variety of regulatory conditions that can be manipulated to influence the performance requirements for engaging in therapeutic tasks.

GOAL OBJECTS AND TOOLS

Goal objects and tools are those items that a person must act on or manipulate within the course of task performance. These objects and tools can be adapted according to size, shape, weight, and texture (American Occupational Therapy Association, 1993; Trombly Latham, 2008). In addition, their position in relation to the person will significantly influence which movements and balance adjustments will be required for task performance. Goal objects may also vary between being static, such as a jar of paint placed next to an easel, and in motion, such as a ball during a game of catch or the action figures in a computer game. When goal objects are moving, their trajectories may be either

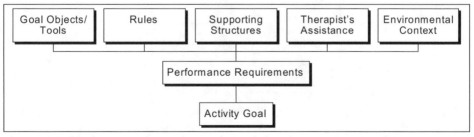

Figure 11.3. Regulatory conditions that can be graded to alter an activity's performance requirements.

predictable or unpredictable. Each variation places different demands on the person's requirements to use perceptual–motor skills and timing.

RULES

Rules guide the performance of hobbies, crafts, games, and sports. Creative adaptations to rules can tailor an activity to allow for grading along dimensions as varied as turn-taking, cognitive complexity, social interaction, use of imagination, and specific motor skills.

SUPPORTING STRUCTURES

Supporting structures can be graded to provide incremental challenges to balance and dynamic motor performance. Whether a supporting structure is a chair, a bolster, a floor surface on which the client stands, or a piece of suspended play equipment, the occupational therapist or occupational therapy assistant can create variations in shape, weight, texture, base of support, and degree of external support. In addition, supporting structures can be graded along a continuum, beginning with stationary support to increasingly unstable or dynamic surfaces.

PRACTITIONER

The practitioner may also be viewed as a regulatory condition that influences the client's performance requirements. Practitioners can vary the ways in which they provide instructions and feedback and the ways in which they provide physical handling to support or assist a client in task performance. Such assistance is graded down incrementally to provide clients with opportunities to develop increasing ability in the skill toward which their intervention is focused (see Figure 11.4).

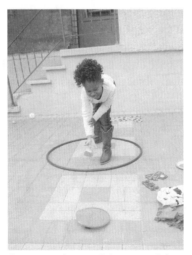

Figure 11.4. Grading the regulatory condition of distance of the target from the child. The ring gives enhanced visual cues about distance.

Environmental Context

Finally, the environmental context introduces a variety of additional regulatory conditions. Competitive noises or visual distractions place higher demands on attentional skills and can be graded through adaptations to the setting in which therapeutic intervention is provided. Physical obstacles, even when they are not central to the actual activity, can be used to pose graded cognitive, perceptual, and motor challenges. Table 11.1 offers examples of selected factors and corresponding regulatory features that would be appropriate to adjust when the intervention is designed to present relevant, graded challenges.

The next case scenario provides a clinical example of how one occupational therapist uses activity grading within a group setting to assist clients in achieving specific goals related to trusting others and developing a repertoire of wellness behaviors.

Table 11.1. Regulatory Features of Tasks That Correspond With Grading to Challenge Specific Client Factors or Skills

Factor	Intervention Strategies
Figure–ground perception	• Complexity of the visual background, similarity between the visual background and the key foreground object (provided in real-life hide-and-seek games or paper-and-pencil puzzles)
Active ROM: shoulder flexion	• Height of object placement
Active ROM: finger flexion	• Size of handles to grasp
Strength of specific muscles	• Placement of objects in relation to gravity (gravity eliminated to lightweight objects to be moved against gravity) • Increased weight (resistance) against gravity • Length of lever arm (short resistance arm to progressively longer resistance arm)
Praxis	• Complexity of a novel motor task
Fine motor coordination and dexterity	• Size and shape of tool (gross to fine grasp) • Size, texture, and shape of objects to be manipulated • Increased demands on speed of performance • Increased demands on manipulation of objects
Standing balance	• Size and stability of base of support (progress from larger, most stable base to smaller, less stable base) • Amount of weight shift required in all planes of motion (achieved through placement of goal objects in relation to the person)
Attention span	• Increased time necessary to complete a task
Social interaction	• The interactive nature of tasks, which may progress from parallel task performance alongside another person, to activities requiring dyadic interaction, to activities requiring increasing amounts of sharing views and feelings with one or more persons

Note. ROM = range of motion.

CASE SCENARIO 11.2: CYNTHIA

Cynthia is coordinating a relaxation group for six members who attend an outpatient community mental health day program. All clients are considered to have serious mental illness. This group is part of a larger wellness program in which participants are learning to manage their psychiatric symptoms and develop healthier lifestyles. Group members exhibit difficulty committing themselves to new styles of behavior and to exposing their vulnerabilities to others. Cynthia will grade the group's activities along a continuum of increasing trust within a group framework and use the clients' strengths and interests in maintaining good health to motivate interest.

At the first session, the group members are required to take off their coats (hanging them on wall hooks that are clearly visible in the same room) and sit in a circle on wooden chairs. Initial activities include practicing deep-breathing strategies and performing active stretching of neck muscles. At subsequent sessions, clients also remove their shoes to practice foot and ankle stretches, then progress to facial exercises with eyeglasses removed. Cynthia encourages group members to appreciate the humor in their facial expressions of frowning, grinning, and pouting to enhance their level of trust and comfort in doing awkward and unfamiliar movements. Gradually, larger body movements are added to the group repertoire. Eventually, Cynthia demonstrates relaxation activities performed supine on a floor mat and encourages group members to try these in private at home as well. Cynthia is alert to the discomfort that her clients might feel, especially when a new activity is added. She is mindful that it takes time to learn to relax and extends the time for each relaxation technique in response to the group's behaviors. An ultimate goal of this grading process is for clients to reach a level of comfort at which they are able to sufficiently trust the group to engage in a full repertoire of relaxation exercises considered to be popular and healthful in society at large and to use these techniques to relieve stress or symptoms in their daily lives.

Precautions similar to those described when using activities to promote repetitive, sustained performance also hold true when practitioners present activities as a series of graded challenges. The practitioner must ensure that in any activity requiring movement, the client is performing from a position of optimal body alignment. Particularly when grading is achieved by altering a support surface or by introducing objects that have been strategically placed in increasingly more challenging locations, the practitioner must pay close attention to the client's general body posture and to maintaining appropriate alignment at specific body segments. If the practitioner does not, what he or she planned as a therapeutic intervention may promote inefficient and potentially harmful motor strategies.

Before selecting a treatment sequence that is based on graded activity performance, the therapist must determine whether the client demonstrates the potential to benefit from this type of intervention. Simply providing increasingly difficult challenges does not always result in functional improvements. Occupational therapists must collaborate with other team members to determine what combination of medical, orthotic, physical, and educational measures should precede or accompany graded activity performance.

Practitioners should strive to avoid two common mistakes when using activity grading as a therapeutic intervention. First, activity grading becomes counterproductive when the client perceives it as an unfair "tease." In this situation, a well-meaning but overzealous practitioner constantly upgrades the challenge of therapeutic tasks so that the client never achieves the satisfaction of performing activities more easily. For example, after struggling to achieve improved reach in the context of making a macramé rug, the client deserves an opportunity to work with the materials positioned within reasonable distance. The practitioner, however, in an attempt to continually challenge the client's improving abilities, constantly repositions the wall-mounted rug so that it is always just out of comfortable reach. Blanche (2008) has warned practitioners who use toys as lures to motivate young children to reach or ambulate that the practice becomes misguided if, in an attempt to upgrade the child's efforts, the practitioner constantly moves the toy farther and farther away as the child approaches.

A second problem occurs when a client is participating in an occupational therapy program designed to promote improvements in multiple areas. For example, a child may be working to improve cognitive and gross mobility skills. It would be a mistake to grade treatment activities so that cognitive and gross mobility challenges are simultaneously increased. Rather, the practitioner should account for the likelihood that increased demands in one skill domain might have a negative effect on the child's demonstrated skills in other domains.

Consider how you might function if you were challenged to your ultimate limits in trying to perform a triple-axel ice skating jump. Would that be the best moment for you to grapple with a difficult mathematics problem? Similarly, a woman who demonstrates dual problems with balance and fine hand coordination may recently have achieved the ability to sit unsupported in a standard chair. When confronted with a challenging task in which she must manipulate objects with both hands, however, her ability to function at her highest level in maintaining sitting balance may be temporarily diminished. In another example, a young woman who has survived a TBI may demonstrate problems related to socially appropriate behavior and cognitive processing and motor control. When the treatment emphasis is on upgrading demands for social interaction, the intellectual and motor challenges of a group activity must be kept as simple as possible. The skillful practitioner knows how to alter a task's regulatory conditions so that when grading up on one dimension, demands to other domains will be kept at manageable levels. In many cases, the practitioner will structure the activity so that competing demands are temporarily graded down.

Using Activities to Promote Development of Effective Strategies for Performance Skills

For many people, the essential occupational therapy goal is to develop performance skills through a process of learning. Teaching and learning as part of occupational therapy intervention are necessary for clients of all ages whose goals are to improve postural control, motor control, cognitive abilities, interpersonal skills, and coping mechanisms. Neither activity repetition nor activity grading may be a sufficient intervention when the therapeutic goal is to assist clients in learning and generalizing effective strategies for their performance of daily tasks.

Strategies are organized plans or sets of rules that guide action in a variety of situations (Sabari, 2004). Everyone has developed a variety of strategies that serve as foundational guidelines for effective participation in daily activities. Many of these strategies have been so well learned that they seem to be automatic. Without them, however, the challenges of performing occupations would be overwhelming. Children learn strategies by experimenting with movement and manipulation of objects and by using verbal and nonverbal communication to perform actions and obtain desired results. Most children learn effective strategies over time with practice and support from adults. Children with motor and cognitive impairments often have difficulty in learning new strategies and may need specific help to consider and try new ways of doing things.

MOTOR STRATEGIES

Motor strategies include the vast repertoire of kinematic and kinetic linkages that underlie performance of skilled, efficient movement. For example, when reaching forward to turn on the computer, the strategy of anteriorly tilting the pelvis ensures sufficient mobility of the trunk and scapula. The strategy of abducting and upwardly rotating the scapula enhances the smooth mobility of the arm's trajectory (Neumann, 2002). Specific hand-shaping (Jeannerod, 1990) and visual guidance (Shumway-Cook & Woollacott, 2007; Wing & Frazer, 1983) strategies enable the index finger to reach the start button with minimal effort. Other motor strategies include those automatic plans of action that enable people to maintain their balance throughout infinite varieties of environmental support and challenges to their centers of mass. In addition, people routinely implement strategies that will ensure their "postural readiness" (Zhang et al., 2002) to perform desired tasks. Think about the task of turning on the computer. What strategies do you use for establishing a base of support and alignment of body segments that ultimately make it easier and more efficient to accomplish your goal?

COGNITIVE STRATEGIES

Cognitive strategies include the multiple and varied tactics people use to facilitate processing, storage, retrieval, and manipulation of information. What cognitive strategies have you found to be useful in negotiating the academic demands of being a college or graduate student? Sitting close to a lecturer and jotting down questions to ask after class may be effective strategies that enable one to process information in a large, noninteractive class setting. Regularly reorganizing and rewording class notes aids in storing course information. Categorizing and drawing one's own visual models may be helpful in storing, retrieving, and manipulating information. Cognitive strategies influence people's performance of all activities, whether they be simple or complex. Grocery shopping can be achieved more efficiently if one uses the strategies of taking a kitchen inventory, generating a shopping list, organizing the list according to the supermarket layout, and assembling appropriate discount coupons. When basic self-care tasks are challenging to people because of brain injury or developmental disabilities, selection and use of appropriate cognitive strategies make it possible to achieve independence and autonomy.

INTERPERSONAL STRATEGIES

Interpersonal strategies assist people in their social interactions with other people. During childhood and adolescent development, and every time people join a new group, people learn the normative practices of social engagement in a given context. Interpersonal strategies are required for forming and maintaining friendships, for expressing one's opinions in various situations, for enlisting assistance from strangers or family members, and for conducting routine transactions within one's communities. Many people requiring occupational therapy intervention can benefit from the opportunity to develop more effective interpersonal strategies.

SENSORY STRATEGIES

Sensory strategies include the methods everyone uses to modulate their awareness of the myriad sensory stimulations and input in their surroundings. At times, a person may need to habituate or screen out, for example, the light touch of his or her shirt sleeve on the skin or the birds chirping outside the classroom window. At other times, it is important to attend carefully to certain sensory aspects of the environment such as the teacher giving out instructions for homework or the status of the walk–don't walk light at the corner. If people have difficulty in processing and regulating sensory input, practitioners want to help them to find the type and pattern of sensory input that helps them to pay attention to necessary stimuli and screen out those that may be distracting. Practitioners can practice methods of regulating arousal by using deep touch pressure and proprioceptive input to calm and focus a person or by using some movement activities to alert the person. One program that has been developed to help children recognize their arousal states and teach self-regulatory sensory strategies is the Alert Program (Williams & Shellenberger, 1996). This program uses cognitive and sensory strategies to improve a child's ability to match level of alertness to the demands of the situation or task.

Strategies should be viewed as frameworks rather than as recipes. They provide practitioners with foundational skills that are meant to be adapted to the ever-changing demands of the occupations in which they engage and the infinite variations of multiple environments. Although there is never just one effective strategy, some strategies may have a more negative effect on a person's future success or well-being. The practitioner must guide clients toward developing strategies that are likely to have long-term positive implications.

People develop strategies through a process of encountering problems, implementing solutions, and monitoring the effects of the solutions. "In child development, an experienced adult guides the child through problem-solving activities and structures the child's learning environment by selecting, focusing, and organizing incoming stimuli" (Toglia, 2005, p. 30). During development, both practice and assistance in developing neuromotor strategies for postural control are important to the child's ability to develop reach and grasp (Duff & Charles, 2004). When children have difficulty with postural control, they tend to move less; explore the environment less; and therefore have less practice with postural control, reaching, and manipulation.

In therapy, practitioners set up the environment and use feedback to facilitate the child's search for a solution to what he or she wants to do (Kaplan, 2010). Children with neuromotor problems often have particular difficulty in developing anticipatory postural control and require encouragement to practice developing strategies in multiple contexts (Valvano, 2004). The importance of practicing postural control strategies as part of goal-directed tasks requiring movement has been documented in children with cerebral palsy (Palisano, Snider, & Orlin, 2004; Westcott & Burtner, 2004). Children with Asperger syndrome (Gillberg, 2003), developmental coordination disorder, and learning disabilities (Taylor, Fayed, & Mandich, 2007) have been described as having difficulty in modifying ineffective strategies during motor tasks and handwriting. Cognitive–behavioral strategies can be used to help children state the goal of the action explicitly, make a plan, and evaluate their own performance. The child is taught to evaluate the result, to think of a different method, or to modify his or her technique during the next attempt (Sangster, Beninger, Polatajko, & Mandich, 2005).

Strategy development continues throughout people's lives. New jobs, new relationships, and new hobbies present people with new sets of problems to be solved. Changes in their physical status, concomitant with normal aging, disease, or disability, create the need for altered strategies when performing familiar tasks.

Sometimes people are lucky enough to get advice or instruction to guide them in the formation of new strategies. One's success in tennis will be enhanced if one learns, early on, some basic rules about postural set, kinematic linkages, and offensive and defensive tactics. Facility at the computer keyboard will be promoted if one practices touch-typing techniques. Ergonomic strategies for the positioning of workstation materials will have a positive impact on one's long-term visual and musculoskeletal health. A coworker's advice about how to interact with a particular administrator will guide one in developing effective on-the-job strategies.

Vygotsky (1978) believed that children learn through social interactions. Parents and others intuitively understand and provide the just-right challenge (Case-Smith, 2005) for their child and encourage a new skill by providing enough support for the child to try it. The adult withdraws the support or grades down the level of support as the child no longer needs it. For example, Gina's parents see that she can stand by the furniture and take steps sideways. She is starting to let go with one hand and turn to look around the room. They encourage her to let go with both hands and take a step toward them. At first, they stay barely one step away with arms outstretched to catch her. As she gains confidence in taking one step without support, they move further and further away. If Gina was not ready to take a step on her own, this would not be a just-right challenge. If her parents asked her to take 10 steps rather than 1 on the first attempt, the challenge would be far beyond her capabilities.

How do practitioners use activities to assist clients in developing useful strategies? They structure tasks in a safe environment that provides clients with opportunities to try out different solutions to actual problems. The occupational therapist or occupational therapy assistant selects the problems in accordance with each client's goals. For example, for Trina, a preschool child with balance dysfunction, the problem might be to figure out how to stay upright while pushing a doll carriage. Instead of providing solutions, the practitioner offers Trina suggestions through physical handling and artful structuring of the play situation (Pierce, 1997). For Scott, a young adult with schizophrenia, a set of problems might be presented within the context of working as a salesperson in the hospital-run thrift shop. Potential problems could include the challenge of interacting appropriately with customers or maintaining interest in the work when business is slow. The practitioner would assist Scott in reflecting on the efficacy of the solutions he has chosen and help him to determine strategies that might guide his future performance in this and other work experiences. The ultimate goal in this type of activity intervention is for the client to develop strategies that can perhaps be generalized to a wide variety of occupations and environments.

Self-awareness and self-monitoring skills are critical prerequisites to a person's ability to generate and apply appropriate strategies. *Metacognition* (Katz & Hartman-Maier, 1998) is the knowledge and regulation of personal cognitive processes and capacities. It includes an awareness of personal strengths and limitations and the ability to evaluate task difficulty, plan ahead, choose appropriate strategies, and shift strategies in response to environmental cues. The Alert Program (Williams & Shellenberg, 1996) has been successfully used to help children with emotional and sensory-processing disturbances recognize their own need for self-regulation and generate effective cognitive and sensory strategies that help them match their own alertness to the demands of the situation or task (Barnes, Vogel, Beck, Schoenfeld, & Owen, 2008).

Toglia's (2005) Dynamic Interactional Model for people with cognitive impairments caused by brain injury emphasizes the importance of metacognition. In this treatment approach, occupational therapy intervention begins by helping clients to develop insight about personal strengths and deficits through a program that challenges them to estimate task difficulty, predict outcomes, and evaluate personal performance. The practitioner then presents tasks that have been synthesized to present selected challenges and that guide the client in selecting appropriate strategies for meeting these challenges. Self-review of one's own performance and guided planning for tackling the challenges of future tasks are key factors in the therapeutic process.

The Cognitive Orientation to Daily Occupational Performance is a strategy-based skill acquisition approach. This approach is based on the cognitive–behavioral work of Meichenbaum (1977) and Feuerstein, Haywood, Rand, Hoffman, and Jensen (1986) and has been studied with children with developmental coordination disorder. The three objectives are skill acquisition, cognitive strategy development, and generalization and transfer. The child sets the goals with help from the therapist, using the Canadian Occupational Performance Measure (Law et al., 2005). The therapist engages in ongoing performance analysis to ensure that the child's motivation is maintained; he or she understands the task requirements, and there is a balance of child ability, task demands, and environmental conditions to support occupational performance. The child is taught to use a line of self-talk that includes questions such as "What do I want to do?" "How am I going to do it?" and "How well did my plan work?" This approach has been used to address motor problems (Taylor et al., 2007) and handwriting problems (Banks, Rodger, & Polatajko, 2008).

The use of activities to stimulate strategy development requires extensive knowledge and creativity. Whether the intervention is directed toward developing motor, cognitive, interpersonal, or coping strategies, the practitioner must be an expert about that area of function. A thorough knowledge base, skill in analyzing performance, and the ability to anticipate how environmental and task demands are likely to affect function are required for effective intervention.

CASE SCENARIO 11.3: JOEY

Joey is a 6-year-old boy who has been referred to occupational therapy because his excessive activity level, impulsiveness, and motor uncoordination are affecting his ability to function successfully in his first-grade classroom. The occupational therapist has determined that Joey has difficulty identifying environmental cues that are important to successful activity outcomes. Therefore, one occupational therapy goal is to help him develop strategies to improve his ability to match his motor acts to the requirements of the task.

Because Joey demonstrates great interest in the suspended bolster swing, the occupational therapist presents a problem. She informs Joey that the clown has not eaten today and is very hungry. A bucket of "chocolate-flavored" beanbags that are the clown's favorite food is placed at a distance that the therapist judges to be challenging but still close enough for Joey to be able to throw the food through the clown's mouth. The therapist asks Joey, "What shall we do?" By asking Joey to tell her what he intends to do before he does it, the therapist ensures that he focuses on the relevant characteristics of distance, size, and position of the clown's mouth and the size and weight of the beanbags. His interest level in the activity will help him learn to screen out extraneous environmental stimuli. After Joey throws the food, he must tell the occupational therapist what happened. To help him learn to assess his own performance, the therapist gives such feedback as "You threw the food too hard" or "Look at the mouth when you throw." The therapist can also help Joey learn to modify his strategies as needed by encouraging him to try another way or asking him "What can you do differently?"

The occupational therapist creates a safe environment with a playful atmosphere in which Joey can feel comfortable experimenting and making mistakes (Figure 11.5). In this way, Joey will learn to engage in these strategies:

- Focus on characteristics that are relevant to the task;
- Assess his own behavior and actions about outcome and performance; and
- Implement changes in his behavior and actions on the basis of the assessment.

In addition, the occupational therapist has collaborated with Joey's teacher to develop ways of encouraging Joey to use these strategies during classroom activities.

A key component is that the activity challenges must be presented in a safe environment that allows for mistakes, self-reflection, and dynamic interaction with the practitioner. Although providing this type of activity intervention in a naturalistic environment has value, the practitioner must consider

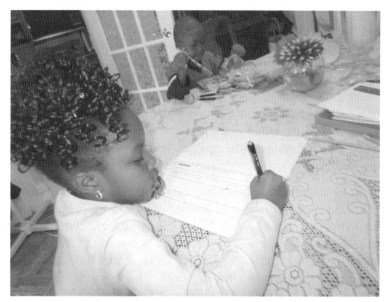

Figure 11.5. Child evaluating her own performance.

that public spaces may be embarrassing places for clients to be developing basic strategies. For example, a supermarket or public library may not be an appropriate place to try new motor or cognitive strategies. Rather, the practitioner can simulate challenges in the client's home or in the therapy setting, where it may be emotionally and physically safer to begin the process of strategy development. Once the client has sufficiently mastered the necessary strategies, it is then advisable to provide opportunities to practice in real-world environments.

Summary

The use of activities as interventions to improve client factors or develop performance skills is an important component of occupational therapy intervention. On the basis of a client's goals, the practitioner determines whether the activity program will be structured to elicit repetition or longer duration of a desired behavior, present graded challenges to specific skills, or provide problems that challenge the client to develop appropriate strategies.

Regardless of the treatment setting, client background, or type of activity intervention, several criteria must be met. First, the client must be ready to participate in the selected activity. Prerequisite skills for performance must be assessed and interventions instituted to reduce physical, cognitive, or emotional factors that might hinder performance. Such constraints to performance can render an activity intervention useless or even harmful to a client. Second, the activity must be synthesized for each person. This synthesis is necessary to ensure that the activity will be useful in developing skills that are specifically relevant to that person and will meet the third criterion, which is that the activity must provide some level of inherent interest to the person. In addition, the client must understand the dual purpose of the activity. Many clients are confused by the occupational therapy process. When an occupational therapy intervention is designed to promote improvements in underlying client factors or performance skills, clients need to be able to differentiate the underlying therapeutic purposes from the activity itself. Finally, occupational therapy intervention to improve client factors or performance skills is never isolated from the projected impact on a client's ability to perform meaningful tasks. The ultimate goal is always to facilitate performance of activities and roles that are meaningful to the person in the context of his or her life.

Acknowledgments

I acknowledge Suzanne White and Richard Sabel, both clinical assistant professors, SUNY Downstate Medical Center, Brooklyn, New York, for providing the case scenarios about Cynthia and Jack, respectively. I especially want to acknowledge Joyce Sabari, who provided the bedrock and support for this chapter through previous editions of this book.

References

American Occupational Therapy Association. (1993). Position Paper—Purposeful activity. *American Journal of Occupational Therapy, 47,* 1081–1082.

Banks, R., Rodger, S., & Polatajko, H. J. (2008). Mastering handwriting: How children with developmental coordination disorder succeed with CO-OP. *OTJR: Occupation, Participation and Health, 28,* 100–109.

Barnes, K. J., Vogel, K. A., Beck, A. J., Schoenfeld, H. B., & Owen, S. V. (2008). Self-regulation strategies of children with emotional disturbance. *Physical and Occupational Therapy in Pediatrics, 28*(4), 369–387.

Blanche, E. I. (2008). Play in children with cerebral palsy. In L. D. Parham & L. S. Fazio (Eds.), *Play in occupational therapy for children* (2nd ed., pp. 375–393). St. Louis, MO: Mosby.

Bloch, M. W., Smith, D. A., & Nelson, D. L. (1989). Heart rate, activity, duration, and affect in added-purpose versus single-purpose jumping activities. *American Journal of Occupational Therapy, 43,* 25–30.

Burkhardt, A. (2004). Edema control. In G. Gillen & A. Burkhardt (Eds.), *Stroke rehabilitation: A function-based approach* (2nd ed., pp. 219–228). St. Louis, MO: Mosby.

Case-Smith, J. (2005). Development of childhood occupations. In J. Case-Smith (Ed.), *Occupational therapy for children* (pp. 88–116). St. Louis, MO: Mosby.

Cooper, C. (2008). Hand impairments. In M. V. Radomski & C. A. Trombly Latham (Eds.), *Occupational therapy for physical dysfunction* (6th ed., pp. 1132–1170). Baltimore: Lippincott Williams & Wilkins.

Csikszentmihalyi, M., & Csikszentmihalyi, I. S. (Eds.). (1988). *Optimal experience: Psychological studies of flow in consciousness*. New York: Cambridge University Press.

DeKuiper, W. P., Nelson, D. L., & White, B. E. (1993). Materials-based occupation versus rote exercise: A replication and extension. *Occupational Therapy Journal of Research, 13,* 183–197.

Downey, J., & Darling, R. (Eds.). (1994). *Physiological basis of rehabilitation medicine* (2nd ed.). Boston: Butterworth-Heinemann.

Duff, S. V., & Charles, J. (2004). Enhancing prehension in infants and children: Fostering neuromotor strategies. *Physical and Occupational Therapy in Pediatrics, 24*(1/2), 129–172.

Earley, D., & Shannon, M. (2006). The use of occupation-based treatment with a person who has shoulder adhesive capsulitis: A case report. *American Journal of Occupational Therapy, 60,* 397–403.

Feuerstein, R., Haywood, H. C., Rand, Y., Hoffman, M. B., & Jensen, M.R. (1986). *Learning Potential assessment device manual*. Jerusalem: Hadassah–Wizo–Canada Research Institute.

Fisher, A. G. (1998). Uniting practice and theory in an occupational framework [Eleanor Clarke Slagle Lecture]. *American Journal of Occupational Therapy, 52,* 509–519.

Fiss, A. C., & Effgen, S. K. (2008). Effect of increased practice using sensorimotor groups on gross motor skill acquisition for children with Down syndrome. *Pediatric Physical Therapy, 20*(1), 112–113.

Gentile, A. M. (1972). A working model of skill acquisition with application to teaching. *Quest, 17,* 3–23.

Gentile, A. M. (1987). Skill acquisition: Action, movement, and neuromotor processes. In J. H. Carr, R. B. Shepherd, J. Gordon, A. M. Gentile, & J. N. Held (Eds.), *Movement science: Foundations for physical therapy in rehabilitation* (pp. 111–187). Rockville, MD: Aspen.

Gillberg, C. (2003). Deficits in attention, motor control, and perception: A brief review. *Archives of Disease in Childhood, 88*(10), 904–910.

Hsieh, C. L., Nelson, D. L., Smith, D. A., & Peterson, C. Q. (1996). A comparison of performance in added-purpose occupations and rote exercise for dynamic standing balance in persons with hemiplegia. *American Journal of Occupational Therapy, 50,* 10–16.

Humphry, R. (2002). Young children's occupations: Explicating the dynamics of developmental processes. *American Journal of Occupational Therapy, 56,* 171–179.

Humphry, R., & Wakeford, L. (2006). An occupation-centered discussion of development and implications for practice. *American Journal of Occupational Therapy, 60,* 258–267.

Jeannerod, M. (1990). *The neural and behavioral organization of goal-directed movements*. Oxford, ON: Clarendon.

Kaplan, M. (2010). A frame of reference for motor skill acquisition. In P. Kramer & J. Hinojosa (Eds.), *Frames of reference for pediatric occupational therapy* (pp. 390–424). Baltimore: Lippincott Williams & Wilkins.

Katz, N., & Hartman-Maier, A. (1998). Metacognition: The relationships of awareness and executive functions to occupational performance. In N. Katz (Ed.), *Cognition and occupation in rehabilitation: Cognitive models for intervention in occupational therapy* (pp. 323–342). Bethesda, MD: American Occupational Therapy Association.

Kircher, M. A. (1984). Motivation as a factor of perceived exertion in purposeful versus nonpurposeful activity. *American Journal of Occupational Therapy, 38,* 165–170.

Lang, E. M., Nelson, D. L., & Bush, M. A. (1992). Comparison of performance in materials-based occupation, imagery-based occupation, and rote exercise in nursing home residents. *American Journal of Occupational Therapy, 46,* 607–611.

Law, M., Baptiste, S., Carswell, A., McColl, M. A., Polatajko, H., & Pollock, N. (2005). *The Canadian Occupational Performance Measure* (4th ed.). Ottawa, Ontario: CAOT Publications.

Meichenbaum, D. (1977). *Cognitive–behavioral modification: An integrative approach.* New York: Plenum Press.

Miller, L., & Nelson, D. L. (1987). Dual-purpose activity versus single-purpose activity in terms of duration of task, exertion level, and affect. *Occupational Therapy in Mental Health, 7*(1), 55–67.

Nelson, D. L., Konosky, K., Fleharty, K., Webb, R., Newer, K., Hazboun, V. P., et al. (1996). The effects of an occupationally embedded exercise on bilaterally assisted supination in persons with hemiplegia. *American Journal of Occupational Therapy, 50,* 639–646.

Neumann, D. A. (2002). *Kinesiology of the musculoskeletal system: Foundations for physical rehabilitation.* St. Louis, MO: Mosby.

Palisano, R. J., Snider, L. M., & Orlin, M. N. (2004). Recent advances in physical and occupational therapy for children with cerebral palsy. *Seminars in Pediatric Neurology, 11,* 66–77.

Pierce, D. (1997). The power of object play for infants and toddlers at risk for developmental delays. In L. D. Parham & L. S. Fazio (Eds.), *Play in occupational therapy for children* (pp. 86–111). St. Louis, MO: Mosby.

Riccio, C. M., Nelson, D. L., & Bush, M. A. (1990). Adding purpose to the repetitive exercise of elderly women through imagery. *American Journal of Occupational Therapy, 44,* 714–719.

Sabari, J. (1991). Motor learning concepts applied to activity-based intervention with adults with hemiplegia. *American Journal of Occupational Therapy, 45,* 523–530.

Sabari, J. (2004). Activity-based intervention in stroke rehabilitation. In G. Gillen & A. Burkhardt (Eds.), *Stroke rehabilitation: A function-based approach* (2nd ed., pp. 75–92). St. Louis, MO: Mosby.

Sangster, C. A., Beninger, C., Polatajko, H. J., & Mandich, A. (2005). Cognitive strategy generation in children with developmental coordination disorder. *Canadian Journal of Occupational Therapy, 72,* 67–77.

Shumway-Cook, A., & Woollacott, M. (2007). *Motor control: Translating research into clinical practice* (3rd ed.). Baltimore: Lippincott Williams & Wilkins.

Sietsema, J. M., Nelson, D. L., Mulder, R. M., Mervau-Scheidel, D., & White, B. E. (1993). The use of a game to promote arm reach in persons with traumatic brain injury. *American Journal of Occupational Therapy, 47,* 19–24.

Steinbeck, T. M. (1986). Purposeful activity and performance. *American Journal of Occupational Therapy, 40,* 529–534.

Taylor, M. (1929). Occupational therapy in industrial inquiries. *Occupational Therapy and Rehabilitation, 8,* 335–338.

Taylor, S., Fayed, N., & Mandich, A. (2007). CO-OP intervention for young children with developmental coordination disorder. *OTJR: Occupation, Participation and Health, 27,* 124–130.

Toglia, J. P. (2005). A dynamic interactional approach to cognitive rehabilitation. In N. Katz (Ed.), *Cognition and occupation across the life span* (pp. 29–72). Bethesda, MD: AOTA Press.

Trombly Latham, C. (2008). Occupation: Philosophy and concepts. In M. V. Radomski & C. Trombly Latham (Eds.), *Occupational therapy for physical dysfunction* (6th ed., pp. 339–357). Baltimore: Lippincott Williams & Wilkins.

Valvano, J. (2004). Activity-focused motor interventions for children with neurological conditions. *Physical and Occupational Therapy in Pediatrics, 24*(1), 79–107.

Van der Weel, F. R., van der Meer, A. L. H., & Lee, D. N. (1991). Effect of task on movement control in cerebral palsy: Implications for assessment and therapy. *Developmental Medicine and Child Neurology, 33,* 419–426.

Vygotsky, L. S. (1978). *Mind in society: The development of higher psychological processes.* Cambridge, MA: Harvard University Press.

Westcott, S. L., & Burtner, P. (2004). Postural control in children: Implications for pediatric practice. *Physical and Occupational Therapy in Pediatrics, 24*(1), 5–55.

Williams, M., & Shellenberger, S. (1996). *How does your engine run? A leader's guide to the Alert Program for Self-Regulation.* Albuquerque, NM: Therapy Works.

Wing, A. M., & Frazer, C. (1983). The contribution of the thumb to reaching movements. *Quarterly Journal of Experimental Psychology: Human Experimental Psychology, 35*(A), 297–309.

Yoder, R. M., Nelson, D. L., & Smith, D. A. (1989). Added-purpose versus rote exercise in female nursing home residents. *American Journal of Occupational Therapy, 43,* 581–586.

Zhang, L., Abreu, B. C., Gonzales, V., Huddleston, N., & Ottenbacher, K. J. (2002). The effect of predictable and unpredictable motor tasks on postural control after traumatic brain injury. *Neurorehabilitation, 17*(3), 225–230.

12

Moving From Simulation to Real-Life Activity and Human Occupation

Anita Perr, MA, OT, ATP, FAOTA
Paulette Bell, MA, OTR

The subject of this chapter is the significance of activities in the last steps of the habilitation or rehabilitation process and in preparation for real-life human occupation. Although many textbooks concentrate on occupational therapy and its use of purposeful activities in controlled environments such as an occupational therapy clinic or lab or in a patient's room or home, in this chapter we address the value of client-centered activities as part of the end goal of occupational therapy, namely, a client's return to real life. *Real life* involves participation in activities or occupations outside the controlled therapeutic environment. It often requires that a client engage in activities that he or she commonly performed in specific contexts and settings before his or her illness or injury. Often, real life for a client with disabilities also requires that he or she engage in new occupations and perform activities in new ways. Such new activities may be necessary to address changes in the client's ability to participate in activities of daily living, home care, hobbies, and work.

The occupational therapist and occupational therapy assistant assume a critical role in the integration of a client into his or her natural contexts. Using the therapeutic value of active participation in purposeful activities, occupational therapists work in collaboration with the client, caregivers, significant others, and other professionals to match the client's engagement in an activity with particular therapeutic goals. The process by which a client is reintegrated into his or her environment involves transition along a continuum from performance of contrived activities in a clinical or controlled environment (e.g., stacking blocks) to performance of simulated activities in a clinical environment (e.g., role playing a job interview with other clients), performance of simulated activities in a real environment (e.g., pretending to brush one's teeth at the bathroom sink), performance of real activities in a simulated environment (e.g., shaving at the sink in the occupational

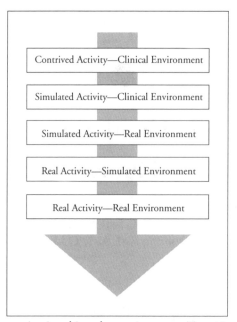

Figure 12.1. Client reintegration into his or her environment. Transitions along a continuum of activities are from contrived simulations to real-life occupations.

therapy clinic), and finally to performance of real activities in a real environment (e.g., taking a bus to school or making a meal at home). This process is depicted in Figure 12.1, which illustrates the client's reintegration into his or her environment. Simulation is a central concept in this transition and is discussed in the course of this chapter.

Participation in Real-Life Activity and Occupation as the Goal of Occupational Therapy Intervention

The ability to participate in real life is the ultimate goal for clients receiving occupational therapy. Through a collaborative process, the client and occupational therapist identify and develop client-centered goals, which means that occupational therapy goals are developed in conjunction with the client and his or her significant others to meet the client's needs and address his or her specific environmental and personal factors.

One must consider the idea that real-life functioning assumes that the client is able to function independently. Occupational therapists are often concerned with their clients being independent and able to complete tasks by themselves. This goal, however, is only relevant if it is acceptable to and appropriate for the client. The client's culture, support systems, and values should be considered when defining *optimal participation*. The concept of *independence* is of major importance itself because many people associate independence with the ability to perform or complete specific tasks, activities, or occupations. For occupational therapists and occupational therapy assistants, however, the concept of independence is defined from the client's perspective. In other words, what is important is the client's ability to direct his or her life.

Independence is not necessarily based on the performance of the various tasks; rather, independence is the ability to execute the task in a manner that is acceptable to the client. Thus, independence for one client may be very different from independence for another client. For example, a person who needs or wishes to prepare food should be able to complete certain tasks to be considered independent in food preparation. Yet another client who has never cooked a meal and can afford to eat in restaurants may not wish to prepare meals. Such a client may remain independent by being able to acquire food and feed himself or herself.

This understanding of independence becomes increasingly complex when one begins to adapt an activity or use assistive devices. Society often views people with disabilities differently from people without disabilities, judging people with disabilities according to different standards. Many people view those with disabilities as limited in their participation because they use an adaptation or assistive device. For instance, a person who had a brain injury may need to use a piece of assistive technology to track appointments and keep lists of instructions for completing daily tasks. A person without a disability may use a personal digital assistant with a very similar scheduling and reminder program, yet the person with the disability might be the one labeled negatively as requiring assistance. Such double standards illustrate how society may judge people with disabilities (and perceive their level of independence) unfairly.

When independence is a goal, occupational therapists and occupational therapy assistants may modify environmental factors, use assistive technology, or integrate compensatory strategies to facilitate the client's participation in an activity. For instance, one goal for a person paralyzed after a cervical spinal cord injury may be to navigate his or her environment using a manual or power wheelchair. In this situation, independence requires the use of a wheelchair (assistive technology). Ultimately, from a practitioner's point of view, the client is independent in mobility when the wheelchair is fully integrated into his or her real-life routine and when he or she can independently move around in his or her environments. The use of a compensatory strategy or device, then, does not negate a person's independence; rather, such strategies are simply the means that allow the person to be independent.

Some clients may not be capable of full independence or may not desire full independence. With a client who does not believe he or she is capable of full independence in a particular activity, the occupational therapist must first evaluate the client to identify the obstacles. Do cognitive, psychological, or physical impairments limit independence? Is partial independence feasible? The therapist may intervene by simplifying the activity to match the client's level of function and thus encourage his or her participation. In addition, the occupational therapist or occupational therapy assistant may adapt the activity, manipulate the contextual factors, or teach the client to use assistive devices and compensatory techniques to facilitate task performance. The practitioner may also train the client to instruct others to help meet his or her needs.

In the following example, the occupational therapist and the client determine the client's potential for partial independence, and they select activities that lead to this goal. Although the client wants to dress independently, she is unable to do so fully because of paralysis in the dominant right upper extremity, decreased dexterity in the nondominant left hand, and difficulty sequencing the dressing activity. The therapist's initial intervention may include a simulated activity in the clinic such as having the client manipulate various clothing fasteners on a dressing board to improve dexterity in the left hand. Next, the client may learn compensatory one-handed dressing techniques with the use of assistive devices, such as buttonhooks and elastic shoelaces, during dressing at the bedside. In addition, the occupational therapist may set up a contrived or simulated activity in the clinic to improve the client's ability to sequence the steps in dressing. The client may then progress to applying sequencing strategies so that he or she can dress during the morning routine. After the client has maximized the ability to dress, he or she may still be only partially independent in this area. The client may then need to think about when and how to ask for assistance appropriately.

As another example, a young man (Figure 12.2) practices a sliding transfer with an occupational therapist in an occupational therapy clinic. The eventual goal is for him to transfer independently to and from all surfaces,

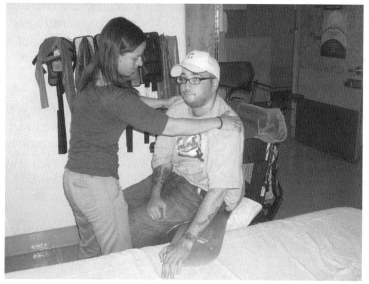

Figure 12.2. Young man with sitting balance and coordination problems works on integrating upper and lower body movements while practicing a sliding-board transfer with his outpatient occupational therapist.

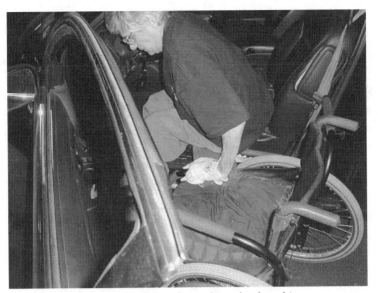

Figure 12.3. Man transfers independently to his car.

the hardest of which is the transfer to and from a car. Figure 12.3 shows another man who has mastered the transfer to and from his car. He is pictured performing this activity in the parking area of his apartment building. As you can see, he uses a wheelchair, protective gloves, and a sliding board. When he has these devices, he is independent.

A client who does not wish to perform all aspects of his or her daily activities personally may still exert control over his or her routine by determining which activities to delegate to others. The practitioner's intervention may include activities that help the client improve the clarity and the manner in which he or she gives instructions to caregivers. The practitioner and client may engage in role play to optimize client–caregiver interactions. Activities that begin as simulations, such as role-playing in a controlled environment, then transition into real life as the client directs the caregiver at home.

The goal of many clients, however, is to become as independent as possible. Let us examine a client who was paralyzed after a spinal cord injury. Case scenario 12.1 illustrates real-life activities that require assistance and how the client defines independence.

This case illustrates three crucial points. First, Daphne actively participates in some tasks and delegates others to her roommate. Second, Daphne's delegation does not diminish her sense of independence because she retains control over which tasks she delegates. Third, Daphne continues to strive for even greater independence for the future. Daphne is not independent in performing the task of wheelchair maintenance. Although she requires help in managing the maintenance of her wheelchair, she is independent in managing her routine in this area.

CASE SCENARIO 12.1: DAPHNE

During the rehabilitation process, Daphne participates in a seating and wheeled mobility evaluation and eventually receives a power wheelchair and seating system that enable her to negotiate smooth and uneven terrain both indoors and outside. She is able to transfer independently to and from her wheelchair. Daphne has not been able to position her wheelchair for charging, to connect her wheelchair to the battery charger in the evening, or to unplug the charger and position the wheelchair for her transfer in the mornings. Daphne lives with a roommate who is able to assist her with these activities. Daphne considers herself an independent person and hopes that she will be able to devise a method to charge her wheelchair herself. For now, she is satisfied with her roommate assisting her, which allows her to spend her time on other tasks. Currently, this aspect of her real life is one in which she uses assistance. Her independence hinges on her ability to instruct others in the appropriate care or assistance that she requires.

EXERCISE 12.1: LIFE AS A STUDENT

Consider life as a student away from home and answer the questions that follow. The context in which you perform activities has changed; the human environment no longer includes your parents. How do you define your new level of independence? Does this independence differ from the independence you had living at home with your family? If so, in what ways? Consider your level of freedom. Who controls or directs your activities and your occupations? Consider the different ways in which people with disabilities may experience independence.

You may consider yourself independent because you have the freedom and the responsibility to make your own decisions, prioritize your activities, and accept the consequences of your decisions. In the same manner, a person with a disability may experience independence through personal performance, through the decision to delegate a time-consuming or difficult task, and by directing others to meet his or her needs.

DEPENDENT OR INDEPENDENT?

Independence is a simple word and yet the more one explores it, the more complex it becomes. Try answering the following series of questions in Exercise 12.2. Be open minded, and take the time to think carefully about your answers.

EXERCISE 12.2: INDEPENDENT MEAL PREPARATION

Answer the following questions on the basis of your experience:

- What is independent meal preparation?
- Does independent meal preparation require cooking? Using a microwave oven? Using the stove top or range? Following a recipe? Does preparation of a cold meal count?
- Does independent meal preparation include getting packages from cabinets and the refrigerator and opening them, or is it still independent meal preparation if someone else cooks and puts together the meals and you merely put them on the table?
- Does independent meal preparation require independently obtaining the food? Does it require shopping? Making a shopping list? Carrying food home?
- Is it independent meal preparation if you order a meal from a restaurant or from a local delivery service? Does money management matter, or can a personal assistant leave the money? Can you run a tab that someone else pays and still be independent?
- Select one of the following clients with a disability and answer the preceding questions for him or her: a woman who has had a stroke resulting in left hemiparesis, a young man who has been diagnosed with depression, or a young woman with cerebral palsy resulting in spastic diplegia.

Are the answers different for the client than for you? Why would we hold a person with a disability to a different standard than we do for ourselves? Does this mean that planning for your client to order food or for the client to organize having someone else prepare meals is an appropriate activity? Absolutely! You have to know your client, his or her family members and support system, and his or her needs, and then plan treatment accordingly.

EXERCISE 12.3: INDEPENDENT HOME MANAGEMENT

Answer the following questions on the basis of your experience:

- What is independent home management?
- Do you have to be able to mow a lawn?
- What if you live in an apartment and have no lawn?
- What if you hire someone else to do it?

Do your answers change for a client? The client's neighbor may have a lawn care service, or an adolescent in the neighborhood may do the work. If this choice is acceptable for the neighbor, is it acceptable for your client? What if no one else in the neighborhood receives this service? Similar questions can be asked for every activity. Why is it acceptable for people without disabilities to hire a maid, but so important for clients to be able to make a bed or iron a shirt?

What is really important actually depends on the client and his or her own situation. As occupational therapists or occupational therapy assistants, we should not force our values on our clients. Our role is to help our clients meet their needs as they define them, so if the ability to manage household help is what is important to the client, then *that* is what is important for the therapist to consider.

Habilitation and Rehabilitation: A Collection of Transitions and Activity Simulations

When discussing habilitation and rehabilitation, we are concerned with independence and participation in real life. Many changes occur during the transition to real life. Most people like to organize these events in some sort of order. Thinking of the process of habilitation or rehabilitation as a series of transitions may be helpful. The chronology of these transitions generally moves a person from dependence (difficulty in performing or inability to perform life skills) to independence (or the ability to perform the life skills without assistance). Each step along the way involves a transition, and at the completion of each transition, the person is closer to independent participation. At each transition, the client actively participates in selecting and performing activities specifically chosen to promote the acquisition of skills toward a goal.

Although people try to place events in a sensible order, the process of habilitation or rehabilitation often does not occur in an orderly and predetermined fashion. For example, some people start the process with total dependence and may require contrived activities in the clinic or other externally structured environments to master initial subskills. Contrived activities can be meaningful to the client if he or she understands their place in the overall treatment plan. The client should understand that these activities are temporary and transitional in nature and provide an opportunity for him or her to learn skills that he or she will later integrate into performance of the real-life occupations.

Other people may start somewhere further along the continuum and focus on learning or relearning actual skills in a simulated environment. Still others start at different points in different performance areas. For example, one client may be dependent in one area such as dressing and be further along the continuum in another area such as work activities and computer

CASE SCENARIO 12.2: DANA

Dana experiences severe anxiety when he takes the elevator to his job on the 15th floor of a high-rise office building. Dana's goal is to become independent in taking the elevator by himself without feeling anxious. Presently, however, he becomes physically ill when simply contemplating the idea. Because of his dependence in this activity, the occupational therapist has decided to initiate intervention by engaging Dana in simple, nonthreatening activities that involve the elevator. Dana and his therapist discuss the activities, and with Dana's input, they make slight modifications. They decide on the following: Dana will watch the elevator doors open and close, watch people get on and off, push the button to summon the elevator, and quickly walk on and off the stationary elevator. During these activities, the therapist encourages Dana to discuss his level of comfort or discomfort, and the therapist in turn provides support and encouragement. Although contrived, these activities are meaningful to Dana and actively engage him.

use. Here, the difference in performance level may be because the person has relatively intact fine motor coordination for computer use but impaired balance and gross motor performance, which are needed for dressing while sitting on the edge of the bed.

The process, or movement through the transitions, varies among clients. Moreover, discrepancies also occur between the expectations and the actual process for an individual client. No one can say exactly how long a person will stay in any stage of the process or whether he or she will move forward and backward several times during the progression. Some people never make the journey all the way to full independence. They may achieve a certain level of independence but not total independence, or perhaps not the level of independence that they or their family members expected or desired. In addition, a client may choose to use assistance for a tiring or time-consuming task to save his or her energy for another task in which independent performance is a higher priority.

Occupational therapy should continue by teaching John in Exercise 12.4 how to position himself and how to move to put on his socks and shoes. He is a bright boy and has already mastered the concepts of "on" and "off." Now that his dynamic balance in long sitting is good, he can build on this ability by performing the actual task. Dressing the doll would be an unnecessary detour because he is moving toward his goal.

Instead of following a neat, linear, and predictable timetable, the process of habilitation or rehabilitation sometimes winds forward, sometimes backward, and sometimes in a circular pattern. Occupational therapists set goals and expectations in conjunction with their clients on the basis of a wealth of information, including the occupational therapists' previous experiences,

---

Exercise 12.4: John

John is a bright 6-year-old who, after months of therapy, is now able to maintain good dynamic balance in long sitting. John's goal is to learn to put on his socks and shoes by himself. Where along the continuum would you begin your occupational therapy intervention, and why? Which activities would you select? How would you grade the activity you select? How would you teach John the concepts of "on" and "off" as he places and removes large plastic rings on a pole as he sits on the clinic floor? How would you teach him how to put the socks and shoes on the Raggedy Andy doll? How would you teach him how to position himself so he can put the socks on his own feet?

---

the client's current level of functioning, the context, and the occupational therapists' knowledge of body structures and body functions. The therapist adjusts treatment sessions and revises goals when necessary in response to the winding trail of progress.

Although most people would prefer a more predictable process, it is not possible because of the unpredictable nature of habilitation and rehabilitation. People are not machines, and many factors such as attitudes, values, mental functions, and physical geography affect their ability to participate in therapy programs and to perform activities. This unpredictability is sometimes unsettling for occupational therapy students. Clients and family members may have difficulty accepting this unpredictability as well. Clients and family members often view the repetition of previously learned skills as a step backward. Occupational therapists and occupational therapy assistants must reassure clients, families, and others involved that the process is complex and somewhat unpredictable and that repetition or movement to a previous step does not signify failure. As new practitioners gain more experience, their expectations may match the actual outcome more closely, but the expected procedure may still require some modification. Practitioners and clients must accept these facts and adjust the program and expectations to meet the clients' current needs and abilities. Occupational therapy will otherwise be less meaningful and less effective.

Although the exact process is unpredictable, some trends are evident in the timing and order of the transitions and stages (see Figure 12.4). The first transition is one that occurs when someone detects a problem in body function or structure or a problem with participation. At that instant, the client changes (or transitions) from being a person without a disability to a person with a disability.

As we now discuss, simulation of real-life activity plays a role in occupational therapy at each level of transition. After a traumatic injury or illness, the client has a period of medical recovery. During this period, the client's

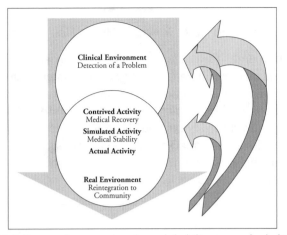

Figure 12.4. Stages of progression through habilitation and rehabilitation.

primary focus is survival. Initiating occupational therapy may be possible at this point. As a result of the client's condition, occupational therapists and occupational therapy assistants often limit sessions to activities that do not closely resemble real life. For example, the practitioner may ask the client to grasp objects of various shapes and sizes, place and release these objects on various planes, and perform certain movement patterns while sitting or lying in bed. These activities, although contrived, are crucial to promote joint range of motion and muscle flexibility throughout the upper extremities. The client may not associate these actions with the accomplishment of an activity (such as self-feeding) that he or she will perform in the future. At this stage, the client performs contrived activities in a clinical environment (see Figure 12.1).

As the person becomes more medically stable, he or she may be better able to participate in therapy. During this stage of transition, learning various skills becomes the focus of occupational therapy. The practitioner may teach the skills individually, and the skills may or may not be related to each other and are sometimes referred to as *subskills*. After the client masters the subskills to some degree, the practitioner combines them in certain groupings to simulate various real-life activities. In this case, the client performs simulated activities in a clinical environment (see Figure 12.1).

As therapy progresses, activities resemble real life more closely. Simulation of activities varies greatly and is addressed in greater detail later in this chapter. Initially, activities in a client's treatment session may seem quite different from the expected, eventual activity performance. The client sometimes has difficulty identifying the usefulness of a given task in relation to his or her own needs and may perform individual skills out of sequence or in awkward ways. The client may skip some steps or skills altogether at this point. The treatment sessions seem to be an abstract representation of real life, which can be frustrating for the client and for others involved in the client's progres-

---

CASE SCENARIO 12.3: OUTPATIENT MENTAL HEALTH CLINIC

In an outpatient mental health clinic, a client has learned, at different times, strategies to control impulsive behavior and to foster taking turns, basic money management skills, and how to be appropriately assertive. The client eagerly participated in the activities to learn these skills and was able to master them individually. Next, the client and the occupational therapist plan a trip to the local supermarket to shop for an upcoming holiday party. In this situation, the client has the opportunity to integrate learned skills into a successful shopping experience.

---

sion. For this reason, the occupational therapist and occupational therapy assistant must reassure the client and family that the simulations reflect real-life situations and that the actual activities will be brought into the clinical environment. Simulations are crucial to treatment, and they become increasingly more realistic. At the end of this phase, the client performs simulations in real environments to prepare for real occupational performance in the real environment. As discussed previously, practitioners may skip steps along this continuum or revisit them until the client achieves maximal performance of the activity in the real environment. The following example demonstrates that a person may learn skills out of sequence and then later integrate them into a real-life activity or occupation.

SIMULATION

Simulation is "[t]he imitative representation of the functioning of one system or process by means of the functioning of another" (*Merriam-Webster's Online Dictionary,* 2009). A synonym for *simulated* is *virtual,* which refers to an entity (e.g., object, issue, circumstance, situation) that gives the appearance of being real but is not real in actuality.

The use of simulation to develop expertise for the improvement of human performance is not unique to habilitation or rehabilitation. Everyone can remember practicing each component of a certain skill before putting them together and practicing the entire skill in a protected environment and then performing it successfully in the real environment. Learning a balance beam routine is one example of this process. A gymnast may begin by practicing each jump and flip on a mat. She may also practice walking on a straight line marked on the floor. For the gymnast, these are subskills, which only distantly resemble the final routine. Once the gymnast masters the individual subskills, she then combines them. However, the routine is still not exactly the same as the real-life routine; it is a simulation. For example, the gymnast may perform the routine more slowly or on a low or wide beam. Finally, the gymnast performs the routine in its appropriate context, completing the mastery phase of simulation. For the gymnast, real-life performance of the routine occurs during a competition or exhibition. At any time, however, the gymnast may return to simulation to refine and practice the individual skills.

Simulation is commonplace in many areas such as engineering, product design, development, testing and marketing, industry, and health care. Mechanical simulations or mock-ups, computer-driven simulations, virtual reality, and interactive simulations can provide an accurate representation of the real world. People can analyze product testing, efficiency, and worker and consumer behaviors via simulations. In marketing, the process of testing a concept, then building and testing a prototype, can measure the viability of ideas long before the product is actually manufactured, thus saving valuable time, effort, and money (Eastlack, 1968). The value of rigorous testing simulations to determine the durability, effectiveness, and viability of various products and processes cannot be overstated.

Physical interactive simulation is a dynamic technique that goes beyond computer simulation or visual interactive simulation to provide a highly accurate representation of the real world (Winarchick & Caldwell, 1997). Through physical interactive simulation, human performance of a task can be simulated and evaluated in a three-dimensional physical model. For example, Delphi Chassis Systems and Sinclair Community College, both of Dayton, Ohio, worked together to establish a workplace prototype lab in which analysis of an entire production model saved Delphi Chassis Systems millions of dollars. Users of physical interactive simulation are able to interact with models before determining their work site setups to maximize productivity and save wasted time and money in development. The models are easy to construct, rearrange, and modify to provide a variety of analyses including motion economy and ergonomics (Winarchick & Caldwell, 1997).

In the United Kingdom, the National Metals Technology Centre (Namtec) launched an advanced computer design, modeling, and simulation center in 2006 to serve a wide cross-section of manufacturing businesses, metal producers, and engineering firms. Working environments, assembly processes, and product designs are simulated in three-dimensional cinematographic style that allows in-depth scrutiny, thus helping to limit errors early and reduce or eliminate the need for physical prototypes (Barrett, 2007). In this way, the running of a new manufacturing plant can be simulated in its entirety before it is built. Also, Namtec's virtual reality suite can project computer-generated three-dimensional images of processes and products and allow them to be rotated, zoomed in or out on, and modified. As a result, users are able to refine their designs and optimize manufacturing methods and plans before making substantial capital investments to implement them.

Virtual online worlds such as Second Life (www.second life.com) exist entirely on the Internet as computer-based, simulated environments in which users interact and live via personally customized human representations of themselves, known as *avatars* (Howarth, 2009). Second Life, the most popular virtual world used by the public, was launched by Linden Lab in 2003. In 2008, it had an estimated 13 million residents from more than 100 countries. Second Life is an elaborate simulated world, and its program is voice enabled to allow the user to hear and see other avatars, providing real-time social interaction (Hansen, 2008). Included in this virtual three-dimensional universe are universities; libraries; tourist attractions and destinations; social interactive venues for educational, entertainment, and cultural opportunities; and even discussion and support groups.

In one example, a large hospital in California previewed its proposed multimillion-dollar health care complex on Second Life many years before the facility's expected completion. As avatars, staff, patients, and other visitors could tour, experience, and interact with the new technology and with the cutting-edge health care innovation of the (virtual) hospital, including patients' rooms, bedside environmental controls, and surgical suites (Bruck, 2008). This virtual project preview was initially intended as a marketing and staff recruitment tool but could also provide valuable "product testing" and useful feedback to inform the design and use of space in the facility.

Many people are attracted to Second Life to access and disseminate health care information. Academicians, businesses, not-for-profit organizations, and self-help groups all flock to Second Life to explore ways in which to leverage their influence (Bruck, 2008). U.S. agencies such as the Centers for Disease Control and Prevention and the National Institutes of Health are active in Second Life. The Centers for Disease Control and Prevention offer virtual health fairs and podcasts and hold virtual meetings on a variety of health topics, with the goal of influencing the real-world health decisions of visitors.

Second Life is a boon for many people, including those with social anxiety and autism, who can use the virtual world to socialize, reduce fear, reduce stress, and develop social skills (Bruck, 2008). Avatar dating is popular because it is less threatening to the ego and self-esteem while allowing for personal and physical safety. Some avatar couples in Second Life are getting married in the real world (Fiorino, 2009). Many use time spent in the virtual world as a temporary escape from a stressful reality.

Some universities are using Second Life as a virtual teaching and learning location in which problem-based learning and self-teaching groups can meet and actively interact. By giving students enough time to interact with other avatars (e.g., patients, staff members, other professionals) in a safe, simulated environment, it is possible to decrease student anxiety and perhaps increase competence in learning a new skill (Hansen, 2008). Education in the virtual world is not a replacement for face-to-face real-life teacher–student interaction but rather an adjunct learning tool—especially in health care education, where the real-life human experience in the natural environment is critical and cannot be simulated.

Virtual worlds such as Second Life are a part of our present reality. On-line users of all ages can benefit from this technology that offers immersion, simulation, role playing, and socialization and provides opportunities for creative expression, fun, forming relationships, and learning from and collaborating with others all over the world.

Industries such as aeronautics and medicine, in which the risk of real-life practice is very high, have long used simulation and virtual gaming technologies to train new employees and help veterans hone their skills. Simulation is a powerful training tool, allowing for multiple practice opportunities, provision of feedback and assessment, and adjustment of environmental demands, all in a safe and controlled learning environment (Brodie, 2005).

The driver training industry that trains operators of large tractor trailers, emergency vehicles (e.g., firetrucks), trains, and specialized heavy equipment can use high-fidelity simulation technology such as the National Advanced Driving Simulator at the University of Iowa (www.nads-sc.uiowa.edu/projects/projects.htm). This simulator, owned by the National Highway Traffic Safety Administration, can re-create the sights and sounds of driving on highways; busy city streets; and narrow, winding country roads. Road conditions, weather conditions, and time of day or night are among the many parameters that can be simulated. In addition, during training the driver's reaction to a range of environmental distractions (e.g., blown tires, cell phones) are recorded via the simulator's video cameras and sensors (O'Neil, 2001).

More industries and organizations such as car dealerships, financial services firms, and business and consulting companies are turning to virtual interactive gaming systems as a way to train their employees. Simulated games, tailored to meet training needs, allow employees to rapidly practice skills, learn new processes, and test their knowledge before they tackle the demands of a real work setting (Brodie, 2005). Again, one must remember that simulation is not a stand-alone training solution but rather a complementary tool to real-world instruction and application.

Simulation in Occupational Therapy

Occupational therapists and occupational therapy assistants use various tools to enhance a client's ability to function in his or her natural environment and to engage more fully in community life. Simulation is one such tool or modality that is used in virtually all occupational therapy settings and is appropriate for use with people who have a variety of functional impairments that affect their participation in daily activities. Simulation can be effective as a therapy tool regardless of the client's age, gender, or ethnic or cultural background.

In occupational therapy, simulation intervention shares some of the same characteristics and benefits as simulation in other industries and professions. While simulating an activity or situation, the occupational therapist or occupational therapy assistant and the client can control the practice intensity, context, and environment of the clinical intervention. Through this modality, the practitioner can also provide feedback to the client and is able to measure the outcome of the intervention. As in other situations, simulation training by the therapy practitioner is an adjunct to real-world intervention with the client. The client's interaction with the natural setting is crucial to maximize his or her ability to engage meaningfully and practically in real-life occupations.

VIRTUAL REALITY

Virtual reality uses interactive computer-based simulations and has been used in occupational therapy for many years as a tool for evaluation and treatment of clients with physical, cognitive, and psychological impairments. Virtual reality therapy provides the clinician with a variety of meaningful, motivating, and fun activities with which to engage the client. These activities, which imitate natural situations, can be individualized, measured, graded, and adapted to facilitate the rehabilitation process (Weiss, Rand, Katz, & Kizony, 2004).

Users of virtual reality intervention can interact with displayed images and manipulate virtual objects in environments that appear to be similar to those in real life. The essence of reality in virtual interaction is being enhanced by the sense of touch (through the field of haptics) whereby a person can feel and manipulate objects in virtual environments. The *PHANToM* is one example of a haptic device (SensAble Technologies, 2009) that may have applications in occupational therapy. This computer input device allows the user to feel and handle virtual objects as if they were real. The device exerts an external force on the user's fingertips to provide information about the shape and texture of solid virtual objects. By means of this haptic interaction with the virtual environment, a user can improve motor coordination to control a virtual pencil or paintbrush and draw or paint using movements that are free and unimpeded in virtual space. As the client focuses on the virtual task, he or she may become so immersed in the virtual world that a temporary separation from the real-world environment may occur. The client's interaction with, and sense of presence in, the virtual environment may contribute certain useful information and insights that facilitate improved performance (motor and cognitive) while in the virtual world. Newly acquired skills may then be transferred to real-life situations and lead to improved functional ability in the natural environment (Weiss et al., 2004).

A new addition to the intervention tools available to occupational therapists and occupational therapy assistants is the Nintendo Wii (http://wii.com). The Wii is a virtual gaming system that has direct applications as a supplement to other occupational therapy interventions and can be used with clients of all ages to address physical, cognitive, and social interaction deficits. The Wii Remote, or Wiimote, is a wandlike motion-sensitive remote control that transmits the motion to the console using short-range wireless communication technology. The console plugs into the television, and the user interacts with Nintendo games on the television screen from up to 10 meters away. The user has a large area in which to make the appropriate body movements required to simulate playing games such as baseball, tennis, golf, and bowling (Connolly, 2008).

The Wii is also well suited to older people, who can perform real-life movements and exercises to build endurance, strength, and coordination to stay fit. They can reap such benefits while enjoying participation in virtual leisure and sport activities that impose less physical stress on their bodies. The Wii can play an important role in the rehabilitation of people with neurological (e.g., stroke) deficits and orthopedic and other musculoskeletal injuries. Using the device, clients can move in a safe environment while the therapist facilitates performance skills such as motor, praxis, sensory, visuospatial orientation, and visual perception. In addition, cognitive skills (e.g., attention, memory, decision making, judgment) and social skills (e.g., turn taking, assertiveness, fair play) may all be addressed therapeutically while the client enjoys a virtual game or sport. The improvements in functional abilities gained through the intervention can then be used to address the client's performance of real-life occupations in a natural environment.

In psychotherapy and in mental health occupational therapy, therapists use role play as an educational tool. Participants understand that they are participating in an imaginary situation, and role play provides clients with situations in which they can act out imaginary scenarios. By participating in this kind of simulation, a client may begin to understand problems, learn other ways of dealing with a situation by observing a variety of solutions, and improve his or her skills and behaviors. Role play provides the participants with simulated examples of how others act in specific situations and how they themselves may act (Corsini & Cardone, 1966). Role play also involves the repeated performance of situations in a therapeutic environment, which allows practice while encouraging exploration and spontaneity.

Mental health occupational therapy practitioners may provide interventions for clients with phobias and anxieties. Intervention using computerized simulations of the feared situation has been called *virtual reality therapy*. This kind of therapy has been used successfully by psychologists and is available to occupational therapists. For example, a client may have an irrational fear of driving. The equipment used in therapy may consist of a computer monitor with a vibrating platform, steering wheel, and brake and gas pedals; the client wears earphones and wide-range goggles. The computer is programmed with a range of road and weather conditions and with scenery that can be adjusted (Ellin, 2003). The client gets a sense of being present and immersed in a fear-inducing and anxiety-provoking driving situation. After repeated practice with the simulated driving experience (i.e., without the risks and danger of a real setting), the client may become more at ease and less fearful of driving. The goal, of course, is to get the client away from the simulation and back behind the wheel, driving safely in the real world with an increased sense of ease.

Occupational therapists plan treatment by designing activities that simulate real life. Occupational therapists and occupational therapy assistants identify activities to simulate on the basis of client evaluation data. If a client is capable of participating in the selection of activities, the practitioner should work in collaboration with him or her to select one that is appropriate. After determining which activities to simulate, the practitioner selects and creates an opportunity to engage in those activities in the occupational therapy clinic, the classroom, the home, or a community setting. While the client is engaged in the activities, the practitioner uses cues and assistance to allow the client to work through challenges that are useful and that he or she can tolerate to ensure a positive learning experience. These treatments often involve the imagination because the practitioner asks the client to imagine the circumstances and the context in which he or she will perform the occupations.

In Exercise 12.5, you were asked to use simulation to target completion of one task that is important to your client. You created the context in which your client played the role of task performer, and you provided the structure that was necessary to match the client's abilities and be sufficiently challenging; the task was also important and meaningful enough to motivate the client to work hard. The occupational therapist can control some aspects of the

---

EXERCISE 12.5: AN ADOLESCENT WHO HAS A BELOW-ELBOW AMPUTATION

You are working with a 14-year-old boy who recently underwent right below-elbow amputation as a result of a traumatic injury. The boy was previously right-hand dominant. As a result of the occupational therapy evaluation, you outline goals with input from both the child and his parents. One long-term goal is for the boy to perform activities of daily living and schoolwork using the right upper extremity (which has been fitted with a mechanical prosthesis) as an assist. Another goal is to retrain the boy to use his left upper extremity as dominant. Describe one activity that you could use to meet the goal of changing dominance. After you have described the activity, answer the following questions:

- How have you set up the treatment environment to replicate the real-life setting in which the activity will take place?
- What are the differences between your simulated environment and the real-life environment?
- How does the activity itself differ from real life in your simulation?
- How can you change the demands of the activity and the structure of the context to meet the client's changing needs as his skills improve?

CASE SCENARIO 12.4: COMMUNITY-BASED CENTER

Brenda is an occupational therapist who works in a community-based center. Her clients are primarily people who live on the street and do not work. Brenda works in a program with social workers, psychologists, and vocational rehabilitation counselors. One goal of the program is to improve the clients' work habits and skills. Her group meets for 3 months. The members start by talking about what they would like to do in the future and what steps are necessary to reach their goals. After a short period, attendance and participation in the group activities become the work of its members.

---

simulation and, therefore, he or she can design it to meet the client's needs and abilities at any given time. For example, early in the process the occupational therapist may plan the activity so that success is very likely. Later, the client can accept more of the responsibility for success. The following case scenarios illustrate this point.

Brenda's community-based program provides a clear example of an effective use of simulation in the community setting. During the group meetings, members discuss work behaviors such as grooming, timeliness, and punctuality. During some sessions, Brenda encourages group members to role-play specific situations. The group members then begin to work in the center's gift shop to further develop their work skills. Group members, who are group employees at this point, punch time clocks and meet with their supervisor on a daily basis. In addition to working in the gift shop, the members continue to meet in their discussion group. During the discussion group, they learn interviewing skills, how to write a résumé, and how to complete a job application. Group members play the roles of the interviewer and the interviewee to practice job interviews. At this point, group members can apply for specific jobs in the center's shop. For example, some people are interested in working in the stockroom, others are interested in working as cashiers, and others are interested in management.

The clients and the group leaders then work together to answer newspaper advertisements and work with job placement services. Clients go to their interviews, sometimes with a job coach or assistant, and begin their jobs with the help of their job coach. This level is the highest level of simulation; the situation is not quite real life because the job coach influences performance and success by assisting, supervising, and encouraging the client. The job coach continues to work with the client for the required amount of time and then removes himself or herself. At this point, the client is in real life in terms of working. The client may contact the group leaders at any time, and the group leaders often ask graduates of the group to return to talk to new members about the process and the result.

The ways in which occupational therapists and occupational therapy assistants use stimulation as part of their interventions are similar in all areas of practice. The process begins with a comprehensive evaluation, development of specific goals, determination of which performance components need improvement and, finally, identification of the performance skills that would benefit from a simulated situation. Of course, the client's motivation, interests, and values are key factors to consider before engaging him or her in a simulated activity. For some clients, simulations are motivating and fun. For other clients, simulations may have no apparent value, and they may perceive the simulations to be like children's play. Occupational therapists and occupational therapy assistants should thus endeavor to provide age-appropriate simulations. Practitioners should clarify or explain the value of the simulated activity in preparing the client for the real-life occupation.

As noted earlier, early recovery is when treatment appears to be least representative of real life. The simulation is rather abstract. After mastery, or partial mastery, of the individual components of an activity, the client compiles and performs the components in a protected environment. The treatment context is a safe place in which to practice each individual component and many combinations or collections of components. This context allows clients to make mistakes and learn from them, to explore alternatives, and to develop strategies for improved performance. Initially, the occupational therapist sets up the environment to protect the person from distractions and to encourage successful completion of the task.

CASE SCENARIO 12.5: BELLE

Belle, a 75-year-old woman who had a cerebrovascular accident, needs to improve her toileting skills. Initially, Belle participated in tasks and exercises focused on individual steps in the activity. The occupational therapy program included the following:

- Activities in sitting to improve balance and the ability to shift weight
- Activities in sitting that encourage weight bearing through the upper and lower extremities
- Activities requiring a forward weight shift and removing weight from the buttocks
- Fine motor activities and bimanual tasks, in preparation for lower extremity garment management
- Activities in standing to improve balance
- Activities to improve compensation for a visual field cut.

CASE SCENARIO 12.6: BELLE'S NEXT STAGE OF INTERVENTION

At the next stage of intervention, the occupational therapist uses one or more treatment sessions to bring Belle to a private bathroom where she can practice transfers to and from the commode. During these sessions, the therapist does not address other components of the activity such as lower-extremity garment management and hygiene after toileting. At some point, the client will transition these simulated activities to actual performance. Belle will toilet with assistance at first, then with supervision as she masters all of the skills required for safe toileting. Tasks that are difficult can be identified and practiced during simulations.

Other occupational therapy sessions focus only on lower-extremity garment management. For example, during part of one treatment session Belle worked on buttoning and unbuttoning buttons and zipping and unzipping zippers on a dressing board. The occupational therapist designed the activity to begin with large buttons and loose buttonholes and move on to progressively smaller buttons and tighter buttonholes. Another treatment session began with large zippers on slippery tracks and moved on to smaller zippers with more resistant tracks. Once Belle mastered the tasks on the dressing board, the next step was to lay a pair of pants smoothly in her lap. The therapist assisted by holding the clothing taut, exposing the zipper, or holding the buttonhole steady. As Belle gained the ability to perform the tasks, the therapist provided less assistance. The next step in the sequence was to have Belle practice the tasks of buttoning, unbuttoning, zipping, and unzipping on her own pants. After she mastered this step, the therapist and Belle worked on removing and replacing the lower-extremity garments in preparation for toileting.

Other interventions focused on the activities of toilet paper management and hygiene. These interventions followed the same procedure of practice and mastery. The therapist used different activities to address other areas in which Belle had difficulty. For example, the therapist used paper-and-pencil tasks, bed making, and computer games to increase her awareness of the visual field cut.

As you can see from this example, practitioners address each component of an activity individually. The client practices and masters the tasks and components of each activity and then groups them together until he or she has addressed the entire occupation (in this case, toileting) sufficiently.

When Belle is able, she completes each activity by herself. This may occur, however, only when conditions are optimal, such as when she is already in her wheelchair and wearing supportive shoes with nonslip soles. In the evenings, when Belle is fatigued, she may continue to require assistance from her husband to perform self-care activities safely. When planning treatment with Belle, her long-term goal is to toilet independently regardless of the time of day, the type of clothing she is wearing, or even the layout of the bathroom. When she is able to achieve this goal, Belle will be independent in performing this task in real life, and her occupational therapy sessions will no longer address this goal.

SIMULATIONS TO ENSURE THAT ACTIVITIES ARE PURPOSEFUL

The following are a few examples of the ways in which occupational therapists and occupational therapy assistants use simulation to ensure that occupational therapy activities are purposeful. Work-centered rehabilitation often uses simulation. Work samples such as *Valpar Work Samples* (Valpar Corporation, 1974) and work simulation and evaluation systems such as the Ergos II Work Simulator (Simwork Systems, Tucson, AZ; see Figure 12.5) replicate various job skills. Work samples and work simulations can be used to evaluate a client's functional capacity and abilities; target training of specific work skills; and provide objective, replicable data to measure the progress a client makes toward being able to work. Occupational therapists may use a work simulation system to evaluate the client's ability to perform the basic requirements of a specific job as described in the *Dictionary of Occupational Titles* (www.occupationalinfo.org/) published by the U.S. Department of Labor (personal communication, J. Martinez, February 12, 2009). Job training simulations include material handling (e.g., lifting, carrying, pushing, pulling) and postural abilities (e.g., climbing, reaching, stooping, bend-

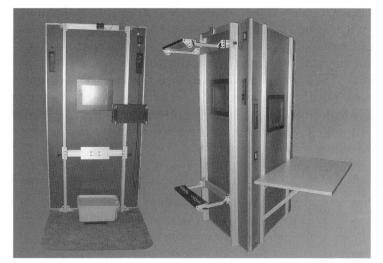

Figure 12.5. ERGOS II. Work simulation system has changed the way work capacity assessments, functional ability evaluations, and functional capacity evaluations are conducted throughout the world.

Note. Photo courtesy of Simwork Systems. Reprinted with permission.

ing). Once the simulated work training is completed, the client is reassessed to determine whether he or she has met the return-to-work goals as indicated by the U.S. Department of Labor job description. Recommendations may be made for ergonomic adjustments to the client's work space, or modification of the job requirements, to allow the client to perform the actual job.

In one Valpar activity, the user must piece together three small metal objects and place them in moving holes on a round track. The rate of movement is adjustable so that the holes move faster as the person's fine motor coordination and speed increase. The occupational therapist may adjust the time allotted for this activity to meet or challenge the user's endurance. The practitioner counts the number of sets of objects placed in the holes while the person works. The practitioner and client can track progress in several ways: by noting the client's ability as the speed quickens, by noting the length of time in which the client participates in the activity, and by noting the number of sets that the client completes in a fixed or consistent amount of time. This Valpar activity simulates the manipulation of small objects and in turn simulates repetitious assembly-line work. It is useful for several reasons, including preparing an assembly-line worker for return to work, improving a person's fine motor and bimanual coordination, increasing endurance for fine motor tasks, or even increasing tolerance for repetitive work. This tool may be appropriate for people with various disabling conditions, including traumatic hand injury, medical conditions such as diabetes that involve associated sensory impairments, visual impairments in which the purpose of occupational therapy is to improve tactile compensatory strategies, and mental illness that affects a person's concentration and attention span.

Another work-centered simulation involves adults in work rehabilitation who simulate jobs (Ellexson, 1989). In a work-hardening program, activities simulate those work skills on which the client must concentrate. Inpatients or outpatients may take contracts from other companies to complete work. For example, a cohort of adults with developmental disabilities may work in a program that has a contract to package plastic knives, forks, and spoons. This job includes counting the utensils, placing them in bags, sealing the bags, labeling the bags, and placing the bags in boxes. This activity demonstrates how simulation allows an occupational therapist to organize the environment, break tasks down into components, and offer clients purposeful activity as a treatment tool.

Occupational therapy clinics have long included specially built treatment areas so that therapists can provide treatment to clients in a setting that simulates their home. Examples include specific areas in the occupational therapy department such as a kitchen, a bathroom, or a bedroom or living area in which clients practice certain basic activities of daily living skills and instrumental activities of daily living tasks. These treatment locations are useful when the client has improved to the point at which a more realistic setting than the occupational therapy clinic or laboratory would encourage further progress. A training apartment, for example, may be useful after the client has completed wheelchair transfers in a hospital room and meal preparation in the occupational therapy kitchen area. A client's family members may join him or her in the training apartment so that they can practice caregiving skills before discharge. The training apartment offers a transition between the contrived and simulated activities in the clinic and the performance of activities in real life (in this case, at home).

Occupational therapists and occupational therapy assistants working with children and adolescents often use simulation as part of their interventions. Simulation is often the key to engaging young children in a meaningful learning activity. Children use play to explore and learn about their environment by using their imagination and to receive the sensory stimulation that they need for development. Children with disabilities may be unable to use their imagination or to participate in play sufficiently to meet these needs. The practitioner's role is, in part, to create an environment in which children can use their imaginations to develop new skills or to become secure or confident in their abilities.

Jacobs (1991) discussed the importance of introducing various activities that simulate adult roles in making the transition to becoming an adult worker. She discussed the use of exploratory play and role-playing activities even in children as young as preschool age. During these activities, children can explore the physical properties associated with various careers. Children are also able to try out different social skills and behaviors necessary for leadership and teamwork. Throughout school, these skills facilitate the development of work behaviors. Behaviors such as punctuality and preparedness are necessary early in a child's schooling, and mastering these skills prepares a child for behaviors that will be necessary later in life at work. Older children may participate in programs in which they develop a mock business and provide some service or product to others.

In the recent past, several rehabilitation departments across North America have begun to use sophisticated, visually appealing, functional simulations of various environments called *Easy Street Environments* (Habitat, Inc., 1998). These custom environments include more than 30 areas of activity such as a park, restaurant, bank, supermarket, department store, office, theater, and automobile. Easy Street Environments provide convenient, safe, low-risk, weather-free treatment spaces in which occupational therapists and occupational therapy assistants can effectively treat clients of all ages who have a wide range of disabilities. With Easy Street Environments, the practitioner and client may address discharge readiness, community reentry, client and family member training, evaluation of possible home adaptations, and assistance needed by the client in the community.

Easy Street Environments are at a level similar to that of the training apartment discussed earlier. These environments introduce the real-world and everyday occupations into the clinical setting and fill the gap between the occupational therapy clinic and real life. When a client demonstrates the ability to perform contrived and simulated activities in an occupational therapy clinic but is not yet ready for community reentry, the client may

CASE SCENARIO 12.7: RICARDO

Ricardo is a 5-year-old boy in kindergarten who has a learning disability and attention deficit hyperactivity disorder. He attends regular classes and has occupational, physical, and speech therapy three times weekly. Ricardo switches hand dominance for different activities; he throws a ball with his left hand but writes and uses scissors with his right hand. The occupational therapist observed these problems during writing activities in the class-room: impaired fine motor coordination in both hands, associated reactions in the left hand and arm, squeezing the pencil too hard, pressing too hard on the paper, and difficulty releasing the pencil when finished and repositioning it when writing.

The occupational therapist, Izzy, decides that Ricardo needs a fun way to learn to regulate pressure and to grasp and release the pencil appropriately. Izzy decides to play Blockhead™ with Ricardo. Blockhead is a game in which the players take turns balancing oddly shaped wood blocks on top of one another until one person causes the tower to topple. The person who causes the tower to topple is the "blockhead."

Ricardo does not have the attention span, motor skills, or perceptual skills to play Blockhead. Izzy adapts the game using the same rules and blocks made out of Styrofoam and paper. These materials require Ricardo to regulate his grip pressure and to use larger gross motor skills. Izzy has Ricardo play the game while assuming different positions and with both hands. Sometimes Ricardo plays while seated at a table, and other times he plays while standing. Sometimes Ricardo plays while lying in a prone position and resting on his forearms when upper-extremity weight bearing is necessary. Izzy talks with Ricardo's mother, who reports that she bought Blockhead and that he enjoys playing at home with her and with his older brother. After playing a simulated Blockhead game, Ricardo has learned the appropriate rules and developed an adequate attention span to play the real game. Izzy notes that Ricardo's writing skills have also improved.

EXERCISE 12.6: QUESTIONS ABOUT RICARDO

Think about this case scenario and answer these questions: (1) What real-life activity does this therapeutic intervention address? (2) How did the occupational therapist use simulation to imitate the real-life activity? (3) What modifications did the therapist make to the environment and the demands of the activity? (4) How do the therapist and the family members provide assistance to make the activity possible?

EXERCISE 12.7: QUESTIONS ABOUT RICARDO FROM A PRACTITIONER'S PERSPECTIVE

Take a few minutes to think about more activities that could serve the same purpose for Ricardo. If you were the occupational therapist or the occupational therapy assistant, what would you do? How would you set up the environment? How would you alter the assistance given to meet the child's changing needs? How would you help the parent and siblings to do this?

---

practice addressing environmental, community, and work-related obstacles and challenges in the Easy Street Environments. Practitioners who have used these simulated environments have claimed that their clients' confidence in performing instrumental activities of daily living increased and that the therapists can then use their time more efficiently (Habitat, Inc., 1998). The more realistic the simulation is in the controlled setting, as in Easy Street Environments, the easier or smoother the client's transition may be when performing these activities in the natural environment.

Simulation is useful in outpatient settings and can provide an even smoother transition to real life. Clients can work on a certain skill during their therapy sessions and practice the skill at home or in another real-life setting. This homework is actually an advanced form of simulation because although it is still somewhat contrived, it is useful in maximizing a person's ability to perform an activity. When clients try techniques at home, they can bring questions back to therapy, and the practitioner can devise simulated activities to use during treatment that target those specific problems. Each time a client masters a skill in the clinic, he or she can perform the skill at home or in the real-life location as a check. As the client performs activities satisfactorily at home, the goals for treatment change. The therapist can document progress and indicate whether occupational therapy should continue after satisfactory performance of the occupation in the real-life situation.

Occupational therapists and occupational therapy assistants must not make the mistake of thinking that an excellent simulation supersedes real-life training and application. Simulation, by definition, merely gives the appearance of or imitates what is real. Intense and time-consuming simulation training in occupational therapy may ease the transitioning of skills to real-life performance. Success in simulation, however, does not automatically guarantee success in real life.

ADVANCED ASSISTIVE TECHNOLOGIES AND SIMULATION

As technology advances, simulations also advance, and the distinction between simulation and real life narrows. One particular technology that illustrates this point is the brain–computer interface, or BCI. In this case, technologies are being developed that allow the operation of a computer or computer controller device via brain function. For people with physical disabilities, BCI could mean that movement would no longer be needed to operate a computer. People with conditions such as quadriplegia and locked-in syndrome resulting from diagnoses such as spinal cord injury, brain stem stroke, and amyotrophic lateral sclerosis may be able to participate in work, leisure, and their own self-care when technologies like BCI are refined and perfected (Cincotti et al., 2007). One BCI system generates computer control by translating the visual evoked potential recorded from the user's scalp over the visual cortex. Another uses electroencephalograph signals generated by the user's intent to define the output (Wolpaw, Birbaumer, McFarland, Pfurscheller, & Vaughn, 2002). BCI technologies are currently under development and are being used to generate control over computers and other robotic devices, which could lead to increased participation by people with disabilities.

As with BCI, the lines between simulation and real life are merging in other areas. For many years, simulations have been used in both the evaluation and the training of drivers with disabilities. Vehicle modifications are available so that people with disabilities can drive or ride in vehicles such as cars, vans, and trucks. Developers continue to use and adapt technologies so that people with disabilities can experience and participate in a wide variety of activities. A retired NASCAR race car, for example, has been configured with a moveable driver's seat to allow transfers into and out of the vehicle and with hand controls. Such adaptations allow drivers with disabilities to experience racecar driving—an activity that may have been considered off limits to people with disabilities. The photograph in Figure 12.6 shows the racecar with the driver's seat in position to facilitate a transfer. Figure 12.7 shows the hand controls in place.

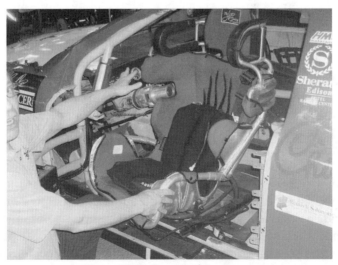

Figure 12.6. Racecar driver's seat.

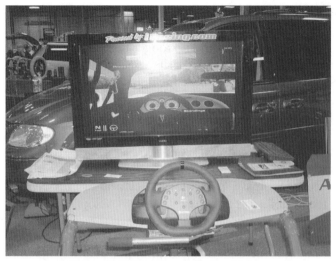

Figure 12.7. Hand controls for driving.

The company that developed this technology also developed an interface to allow the use of vehicular modified control to drive computer-based driving games such as those made for the PlayStation 2.

Real Life

The ultimate goal of occupational therapy is for the client to be successful in his or her occupations. All of the examples included in this chapter demonstrate how simulations are used to prepare clients for real-life activities and occupations, and the transition to real life is the final step in this process. In occupational therapy, the client learns problem-solving skills and other strategies that will enable him or her to generalize information to various real-life environments and situations. *Real life* is the usual environment in which any given occupation takes place and includes settings such as the home, workplace, school, places of leisure enjoyment, and private and public transportation. The occupational therapist and occupational therapy assistant can foster the transition to real life by keeping the focus on real life in treatment throughout the habilitation or rehabilitation process.

During therapy, occupational therapists and occupational therapy assistants must address the foundations of performance components and purposeful activities that are necessary to engage in real-life occupations. Addressing the psychosocial requirements of an activity is essential, including the appropriateness of the methods and equipment; feelings of embarrassment or pride associated with performance; and support of family members, friends, and others. Real-life performance includes using all of the appropriate activities to engage in an occupation. Real life includes performing activities in the conventional manner, performing activities with alternative techniques and compensatory strategies, and performing activities with assistive technology.

Indeed, when addressing activity performance in the real-world environment, occupational therapists and occupational therapy assistants often prescribe and provide adaptive equipment and assistive technology devices. Practitioners may focus on simulations with devices and ensure that the client can use them competently to complete activities in the clinic environment. Everything changes at home, and occupational therapists and occupational therapy assistants must therefore address home issues. In Phillips and Zhao's (1993) study of technology abandonment, they described patterns of clients' abandonment of the devices recommended or provided to them in a physical rehabilitation setting. Four factors were significant in abandoning technology: (1) lack of consideration of user opinion, (2) ease of device procurement, (3) poor device performance, and (4) changes in user needs or priorities. The practitioner's role is to address those factors. By ensuring that the device performs as it should, both in the protected therapeutic environment and in the real-life situation, the practitioner can help to provide the best possible solution to clients who require assistive technology. The client's home and other real-life environments should be the focus of treatment, and one should avoid assumptions such as "If it works in the hospital room, it will work the same at home."

In a related study, Bell and Hinojosa (1996) interviewed 3 participants who had spinal cord injuries regarding the effect of assistive devices on their ability to perform their daily routines. They concluded that successful use of these devices in the clinic setting did not necessarily transition to successful use of these devices at home. Rather, follow-up at home and in-home training are crucial to successfully using assistive devices or compensatory techniques in the real-life, postdischarge setting.

The occupational therapy intervention to prepare a client for real life is of course limited in scope. Predicting all of the environments in which a client may interact, for example, is impossible for the practitioner. It is essential, but not entirely possible, to plan for the unexpected. By addressing occupations in many of the more likely environments through simulation, it is possible to facilitate but not to guarantee the transition to real life. In addition, we should note that both the human and the nonhuman context in which the client performs any activity influences the realism of the simulation. For example, pretending to lift a heavy object in the proper way in an occupational therapy clinic is different from lifting an object of a similar weight on a busy factory floor. In the latter situation, the context includes noise, the space available, the presence of a supervisor and coworkers, and many distractions. These factors make real-life activity performance much more complex than simulated activity. Again, successful performance in a clinic does not necessarily guarantee success in real life.

Summary

As occupational therapists and occupational therapy assistants become more experienced, evaluating clients' long-term goals becomes easier. In turn, planning and organizing simulated activities to address their needs becomes easier. The visualization of the outcome of occupational therapy may not always be accurate because of the unpredictable nature of human beings, the unpredictability of the setting, and the other demands that influence performance. We believe that as a practitioner gains more experience and builds a repertoire of goal setting and treatment skills, his or her predictions will be more accurate or will more often be accurate. The practitioner can outline trends in performance and move from contrived to more purposeful real activities in various environments that range from clinical or simulated to real. The ultimate goal is independent activity performance in a real environment; practitioners use simulation in this effort. As in various industries, simulation in occupational therapy allows clients to test and practice techniques in a safe and controlled environment. Practitioners can address problems, gain insights, and explore solutions before attempting real-life performance. Some practitioners believe that the ultimate setting for providing occupational therapy intervention is the client's work site or the client's own home or community. In these cases, simulations are already in the real-life setting, which fosters the successful transition to optimal real-life performance.

References

Barrett, R. (2007, February). Virtual world. *Metal Bulletin Monthly, 434*, 36.

Bell, P., & Hinojosa, J. (1996). Perception of the impact of assistive devices on daily life of three individuals with quadriplegia. *Assistive Technology, 7*, 87–94.

Brodie, J. (2005). In the game. *HR Magazine, 50*, 91–94.

Bruck, L. (2008). Second Life: Test-driving real-world innovations. *Hospital and Health Networks, 82*, 50.

Cincotti, F., Mattia, D., Aloise, F., Bufalari, S., Marciani, M. G., Schalk, G., et al. (2007). Non-invasive brain-computer interface system to operate assistive devices. *Engineering in Medicine and Biology Society, 29th Annual International Conference of the IEEE, 22*(26), 2532–2535

Connolly, C. (2008). KUKA robotics open architecture allows wireless control. *Industrial Robot, 35*, 12.

Corsini, R. J., & Cardone, S. S. (1966). *Roleplaying in psychotherapy: A manual.* Chicago: Aldine.

Eastlack, J. O. (1968). New products for the seventies. In J. O. Eastlack & J. Tinker (Eds.), *New product development* (pp. 142–148). Chicago: American Marketing Association.

Ellexson, M. T. (1989). Work hardening. In S. Hertfelder & C. Gwin (Eds.), *Work in progress* (pp. 67–126). Bethesda, MD: American Occupational Therapy Association.

Ellin, A. (2003, April 17). Driving along a virtual road to recovery. *The New York Times*, p. G3.

Fiorino, L. (2009, January 2). Commentary: Need a Second Life? Have your avatar call my avatar. *The Daily Record*. Retrieved July 28, 2009, from http://findarticles.com/p/articles/mi_qn4183/is_20090102/ai_n311737281

Habitat, Inc. (1998). *Easy Street Environments product literature*. Tempe, AZ: Author.

Hansen, M. M. (2008). Versatile, immersive, creative, and dynamic virtual 3-D healthcare learning environments: A review of the literature. *Journal of Medical Internet Research, 10*(3), e26.

Howarth, N. (2009). A whole new world. *e.learning age Magazine, 12*. Retrieved July 28, 2009, from http://findarticles.com/p/articles/mi_qa5402/is_200812/ai_n31426021/

Jacobs, K. (1991). *Occupational therapy: Work-related programs and assessments*. Boston: Little, Brown.

O'Neil, J. (2001, October 10). Mistakes are measured here, not towed away. *The New York Times*, p. H12.

Phillips, B., & Zhao, H. (1993). Predictors of assistive technology abandonment. *Assistive Technology, 5*(1), 36–45.

Merriam-Webster's online dictionary. (2009). Retrieved February 28, 2009, from www.merriam-webster.com/dictionary/simulation

SensAble Technologies. (2009). *Haptic devices*. Retrieved July 28, 2009, from http://www.sensable.com/products-haptic-devices.htm

Valpar Corporation. (1974). *Valpar work samples*. (Available from Valpar Corporation, 3801 East 34th Street, Suite 105, Tucson, AZ 85713)

Visual Thinking International. (1998). *SIMUL8* [Software]. Retrieved from www.vtil.com/simul8.htmwww.VTIL.com/simul8.htm

Weiss, P. L., Rand, D., Katz, N., & Kizony, R. (2004). Video capture virtual reality as a flexible and effective rehabilitation tool. *Journal of Neuroengineering and Rehabilitation, 1*, 12.

Winarchick, C., & Caldwell, R. (1997). Physical interactive simulation: A hands-on approach to facilities improvements. *IIE Solutions, 29*, 34–36.

Wolpaw, J. R., Birbaumer, N., McFarland, D. J., Pfurtscheller, G., & Vaughn, T. M. (2002). Brain–computer interfaces for communication and control. *Clinical Neurophysiology, 113*, 767–791.

13

Leisure Occupations

Laurette Olson, PhD, OTR

Leisure is . . . freedom from the necessity of labor. (Aristotle, 1943)

*L*eisure has been described as what people do in their spare time when they are not engaged in self- or family management tasks or in work or educational activities. In leisure, people are free to participate, or not to participate, without consequence. In leisure, the goals of the activity and the direction the activity takes come from oneself. Leisure activities or occupations have no external judgment of success or failure imposed on them; only the participant can decide whether his or her level of participation is adequate for personal enjoyment. Thus, leisure affords people with great opportunity for self-determination. The research related to leisure reveals the striking potential power of leisure to support people's physical and mental health, family and community relationships, and development. Larson and Verma (1999) stated that the play and free-time activities of children and adolescents provide more opportunities for development of initiative, organization, and regulation of action than adult-defined activities such as household labor and schoolwork.

Leisure embodies a broad range of activities. Distinguishing between the kinds of leisure and the roles they play in a person's life across the lifespan is important so that professionals can work to design environments and activities that target the particular leisure needs of a population, group, or person. Across the lifespan, leisure has been broadly divided into those activities in which a person invests time, energy, and serious attention; activities that are personally interesting and engaging; and activities in which a person engages casually or passively to relax or distract oneself from the stresses of daily living (Brown, McGuire, & Voelkl, 2008; Kleiber, Larson, & Csikszentmihalyi, 1986).

Some leisure occupations require new learning that provides a challenge and intellectual stimulation. Some leisure occupations may resemble adult work, a child's school, or self-care activities. A business person may use leisure time to explore the Internet, write a novel, or refinish old furniture; a high school student may explore astronomy or create a Web site; a retired teacher may volunteer a few days a week in a nursing home; and a home-maker may design and make clothing in his or her free time. Other leisure occupations use skills that people have already acquired and may be relaxing, such as reading a novel, knitting, or gardening. These activities fit the definition of *serious leisure* because they enhance quality of life and can provide a person with a sense of achievement, an appreciation of beauty in nature or the arts, a feeling of identification with his or her community, or a sense of fulfillment of his or her potential (Campbell, Converse, & Rodgers, 1976). Kleiber et al. (1986) labeled a similar category of adolescent leisure as *transitional leisure,* in which the activities prepare an adolescent for the serious aspects of the adult world. These activities promote concentration and challenge and may include extracurricular school activities, individual hobbies such as playing a musical instrument, or developing high-level painting or dancing skills. This type of activity participation correlates with adult occupational prestige and adult civic participation (Putnam, 2000). Kleiber et al. (1986) identified another category of adolescent leisure—*relaxed leisure*—which encompasses those activities that are pleasurable but not challenging, such as listening to music, watching television, or socializing with friends at a local mall or park.

How people in Western society spend their leisure time has dramatically shifted as personal computers and other electronic media have become more sophisticated, interactive, and portable. Such electronic media not only have affected the use of leisure time but have also had a significant impact on social participation, worldviews, and everyday behavior (Figure 13.1). Children and retirees alike now maintain a wide social network through the Internet and spend hours surfing the Web—hours that used to be devoted to other activities. Computer games are common, from casino games to crosswords. Adolescents share their thoughts and experiences with close friends,

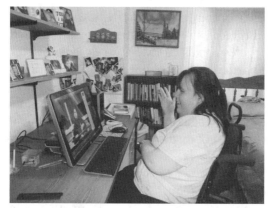

Figure 13.1. Young woman interacts with a friend through the Internet.

and more casual acquaintances, through sites like Facebook and MySpace. Online gaming engages both adolescents and adults (Griffiths, Davies, & Chappell, 2004). People from around the world now participate in virtual worlds. Six million people from around the world, for example, participate in Second Life, a collaborative virtual community that has duplicated the physical world with the exception that participants can design their virtual selves to look as they wish.

Ivory (2008) reported that 83% of children live in a home with a video game console and that the survey respondents reported spending an average of 1 hour, 8 minutes daily playing video games. Ivory also reported, in a 2007 Harris poll, that the average 8- to 12-year-old plays video games for 13 hours per week and the average 13- to 18-year-old plays for 14 hours per week. Bandura (2002) wrote about the disinhibiting effect of television. Exposure to violent television and video game content has been related to more aggressive behavior in children. MP3 players have made it possible for adults and youth alike to enjoy the relaxed leisure that music provides almost anywhere. One can listen to a self-chosen selection of music on the way to work, in the car, or during exercise. It is not uncommon for a family or a group of people to listen to their individual MP3 players as they travel together in a car or on public transportation. Music influences one's emotional state, but its power is intensified by the images that accompany it in music videos. These new trends in leisure participation, and the related research about the impact of the technologies that allowed their development, are important for professionals to consider as they help their clients compose healthy and productive leisure occupations.

Needs Met Through Leisure

People of all ages participate in leisure occupations for personal enjoyment and to fulfill a range of personal needs. Throughout life, participation in leisure occupations is a critical safeguard of people's mental health. When the external world of school, work, or everyday living does not seem to offer people affirmation and a sense of mastery, they retreat into leisure to fend off depression and engender optimism in themselves and their abilities. People can use these leisure activities as a springboard for redirecting their lives in a more satisfying and productive way. Researchers have attempted to create a taxonomy of leisure to more clearly identify the needs met through par-

---

EXERCISE 13.1: PERSONAL LEISURE ACTIVITIES

Describe your active and passive leisure activities. What activities do you do for relaxation, fun and stimulation, entertainment, and personal development? What are your major leisure occupations?

ticular activities (Tinsley & Eldredge, 1995). In this chapter, we discuss the needs commonly identified as being met through leisure.

SELF-EXPRESSION

In modern societies, social control is necessary for humans to maintain order and function every day. As members of a society, people need to fulfill certain roles and put aside their own wishes and impulses for immediate gratification. Sometimes people must contain their emotions so that work can proceed harmoniously. In modern societies, leisure provides opportunities for people to put their commitments aside and to experience freedom in activities that satisfy their interests. Moreover, participation in leisure occupations provides people with opportunities to express their desires and their true range of emotions. Such expression of emotions is also done with the approval of other people (Neulinger, 1981). For example, in a creative writing group an adolescent can write painfully honest poetry about loss and longing and receive praise from others for the beauty of and depth of emotion in his or her writing. If the adolescent had shared these feelings at his or her part-time job, coworkers might be nervous or look on the adolescent as a very troubled youth. At football games, the fans cheer and jeer loudly while simultaneously feeling an intense camaraderie. This level of emotion, expressed in daily life, would be seen as inappropriate or deviant.

BELONGING AND SOCIAL ENGAGEMENT

Throughout people's lives, the activities that help them develop, maintain, or strengthen relationships with others are most often leisure occupations. People plan and share special activities and events with family members or friends so that all participants experience pleasure and relaxation (Figure 13.2). When activities have the desired results, people associate the positive experience with those with whom they have interacted, which cements relationships. People will most likely seek out these same people when they are looking for companionship in future activities. They may also come to rely on these people when they need assistance in their daily lives and will likely be willing to help them as needed. People will more likely tolerate and resolve disagreements and frustrations with others when they occur within a relationship that has a strong history of pleasurable interactions. People most often sustain friendship throughout the lifespan through shared positive experiences that they associate with leisure.

Leisure relationships can be developed or sustained in a variety of ways. Morrison and Krugman (2001) described how the Internet allows for increased interpersonal communication and opens up opportunities to connect with new groups of people. Gibson, Willming, and Holdnak (2003) described how sharing with others the experience of being a serious football fan can provide a sense of belonging and identity across one's lifespan.

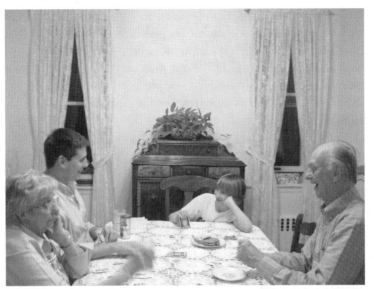

Figure 13.2. Family card games are an important time to socialize and bring families together.

Putnam (2000) explored how team sports and communal cultural activities provide opportunities for developing common ground and building positive regard and relationships among diverse community members or building relationships among different communities. Putnam stated that bowling or singing together does not require a shared ideology or social identity. He also described how civic and service activities can deepen relationships among community members.

LEISURE AS RELAXATION

Activities that help people relax are typically familiar and routine. They allow people to escape from novelty and require little physical or intellectual exertion. Leisure scholars have described this leisure as providing opportunities to rejuvenate oneself from the drudgery and stresses of everyday life (Kraus, 1994; Neulinger, 1981). Some people seek relief by withdrawing from human interactions to read the newspaper or tend to their garden in solitude. Others revive their spirits through enjoying a special meal or drinks with others to create a relaxed mood for conversation and social interaction.

LEISURE FOR COGNITIVE, EMOTIONAL, AND PHYSICAL INVIGORATION

Leisure occupations provide opportunities for people to learn more about themselves, to explore their interests, and to develop skills in the activities that bring them pleasure. In people's free time, they engage in leisure occupations that are interesting to them without concern for their usefulness to others (Neulinger, 1981). People may learn to dance, kayak, paint, or play an instrument for no other reason than the pleasure that it brings them. Developing proficiency in an activity supports people's internal sense of mastery and physical sense of control. Traveling may increase people's awareness of other cultures, expand their understanding of themselves and others, and foster an appreciation of activities from other cultures.

Engaging in leisure occupations also has the power to influence people's mood and perspective on the possibilities of everyday life. Success in a leisure activity can be an antidote to a negative experience in another part of life and can lead a person to have renewed belief in his or her capacity to be effective in all parts of life. Moreover, leisure activities and experiences can be a springboard for people to make real changes in other areas of their lives. Some people who have become depressed or feel alienated benefit from taking up a new interest (leisure activity) that challenges them physically and mentally. The value of the physical challenge that participating in a leisure activity can bring has been reported by Gulick (1998) in teenagers with spinal cord injuries who took up scuba diving and by Manuele (1998) in adults with disabilities who learned to ride horses. In these cases, people who may have felt dependent and less competent than their peers without disabilities found that in spite of their physical limitations, they could have adventures, meet the physical challenges of an active sport, and experience the physical and mental excitement of participation. Training and participation in these active leisure activities is reported to have a positive impact on the participants' mental and physical state, which extends into their everyday functioning in other occupations.

People also seek leisure for emotional stimulation. Elias and Dunning (1986) stated, "Unless an organism is intermittently flushed and stirred by some exciting experience with the help of strong feelings, overall routinization and restraint . . . are apt to engender a dryness of emotions, a feeling of monotony" (p. 73). During leisure activities, people can potentially experience the full range of human emotions that they avoid in everyday life. Many children, for example, love to frighten or be frightened on Halloween (Figure 13.3); adults pay high ticket prices to become engrossed in the pain and suffering of characters in a play. Sloan (1979) reported studies suggesting that the heartbeat and stress level of fans at sporting events can be similar to those of the athletes participating. Although tension and stress increase, these feelings are different from the tension and stress in everyday life and indeed are pleasurable. Aristotle's view that music and tragedy have a cathartic effect and move people's souls in the same way as sports relieve physical tension and energize the body is an idea that leisure theorists still assert today (Neulinger, 1981).

Leisure, as an acceptable social arena for loosening nonleisure restraints, is found in all societies and cultures. At a sporting event, a crowd may loudly express very aggressive intentions toward an opposing team that would not be acceptable in a work environment. Roughness and aggression in game

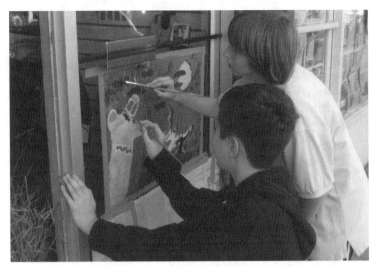

Figure 13.3. Halloween painting involves works of scary art.

play, within the confines of the rules of the game, facilitate enjoyment of watching or playing the game. Aggression guarantees the participant and the fan a high degree of competitiveness and human drama (Zillman, Sapolsky, & Bryant, 1979). Adolescents can express their sexuality more openly in social dance than they can in other environments. In some cultures, the expression of emotion is condoned more than it is in others. A difference likewise exists in the openness with which people of different ages show their tension and excitement through bodily movement. Older adults are generally more restrained than teenagers.

Spectator sports can ensure a strong emotional bond between members of a team. Spectators can feel a sense of belonging to a larger meaningful group. When the team wins, the spectators get to "bask in reflected glory" (Sloan, 1979, p. 235). Gibson et al. (2003) highlighted the sense of group identity; the title of their article "We're Gators . . . Not Just Gator Fans" captures the sense of experience that serious sport fans can have. Although fans cannot attain a direct sense of achievement as can a team player, they can experience a sense of triumph through cheering on their favorite teams. Spectator sports also facilitate social interaction between fans while watching the game or after the event. Without the common focus on sporting events, a group of people may have little to say to each other, yet a shared love of sports can be the basis for days of enjoyment and stimulating conversations for the same group of people (Figure 13.4).

Leisure occupations can provide an outlet or an adaptive way to ease the frustration of daily life. Through telling jokes, children and adults alike can share and laugh about the absurdity of life events that might otherwise produce intense anger or hurt. Adults may tell jokes about incompetent bosses or thoughtless spouses; children tell jokes about teachers and parents. Thinking about the absurdity of the antagonist removes the sting of the interaction.

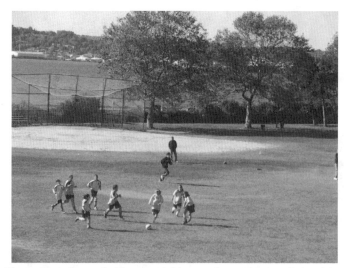

Figure 13.4. Sports facilitate social interaction and peer relationships.

For many people, pets are an important part of our leisure time. Pets fulfill the needs for companionship and love that might not be met by people's everyday human interactions. A relationship with a cat or a dog is fraught with fewer complications than relationships with other people (Figure 13.5). A pet owner can lavish attention on a pet in ways that he or she may not feel comfortable doing with other people. An animal is dependent on its owner for sustenance; the pet's life is focused on its owner. The pet is always present and provides its owner with a routine and companionship, unconditional acceptance and, potentially, affection.

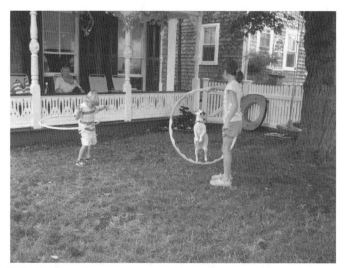

Figure 13.5. Our pets give us companionship and opportunities to learn new skills.

LEISURE AS SELF-DEVELOPMENT

Exploring new leisure activities within a structured group can lessen anxiety for learning and promote camaraderie and friendship that fosters enthusiasm for living and affirmation of the self. Developing the discipline needed to master a new activity is often easier when participating in a group of like-minded and equally skilled people. The initial work of mastering a skill or preparing for participation can seem less daunting when one experiences the camaraderie of others. When people are in the same boat, they can share small triumphs and easily give support to each other when they stumble or make mistakes. Joining in with others and working harmoniously fosters engagement and continued interest in a challenging activity. In the United States, many nonprofit clubs and for-profit companies offer structured group activities. These groups afford various options for people to discover and explore new leisure activities with others.

Independent mastery of a leisure occupation gives people pleasure. When people become overly compliant with external demands and sacrifice their individuality to the needs and desires of others, their individuality disappears and life becomes meaningless. In people's solitary time, they may learn to play a musical instrument, write, read, or participate in a range of other activities for their own individual pleasure. In an individual leisure occupation, people's activity pace is likely to be unhurried, and their imaginative and creative abilities can flourish in the presence of only the self. Through this process, people get to know themselves more deeply and gain an awareness of what moves them beyond being with people that they love. Storr (1988) discussed two opposing human drives: (1) the drive toward closeness and intimacy with other human beings and (2) the drive toward independence and self-sufficiency. Although love and friendship are important parts of what makes life worthwhile, solitude has great value. When people learn to make good use of solitude, they have the opportunity to focus on their own desires and interests, separate from the needs and desires of others.

LEISURE FOR SOCIAL CONSCIOUSNESS, ALTRUISM, AND SERVICE

People can also fulfill the need to be altruistic through leisure in ways that most work occupations do not meet. Many people use some of their leisure time to help others and in doing so feed their own spirits. Altruistic acts often result in a feeling of invigoration, effectiveness, and control for the doer.

Putnam (2000) discussed how the Internet may be part of the solution to the problem with civic engagement in society. He described it as not about technology but about bidirectional communication among people and the exchange of information. By limiting the prejudices that naturally develop among people on the basis of physical attributes, virtual communities can be more egalitarian than face-to-face communities typically are. People typically engage in virtual communities differently than they do in real-life communities. Cyberspace interactions typically develop around one interest about which group members feel passionate and typically remain focused around that issue. Face-to-face communities may begin that way but tend to grow multidimensionally as members observe and interact with other. Putnam pointed out how interactive video connections such as Skype can decrease the psychological distance and remedy the weak social cues that can be prevalent in Internet communications.

Although research on general television watching has suggested its negative influence, prosocial television programming can have prosocial effects. It can reinforce a sense of community throughout the viewing area, whether it be a city, state, or entire nation. This sense of community was observed in the positive engagement of many Americans during the 2008 presidential election and after the September 11, 2001, terrorist attacks in New York City and Washington, DC. Along with the Internet, public television programs not only inform citizens about issues but also engage people emotionally and propel them to use their leisure time for altruistic community purposes. For youth, participation in extracurricular activities, both school linked and independent, is also a means to increase civic and social involvement in later life. In their 2009 study, Wood, Larson, and Brown found that youth reported developing a perspective of themselves as responsible citizens through participating in youth programs.

Factors Affecting Leisure Participation

The focus of leisure may be different at different points in people's lives. During childhood, engaging parents or other children for fun and stimulation is a primary objective. Children need to engage others to receive sufficient nurturing, support, and stimulation for healthy development toward adulthood. Children also need physical activity for skill development and physical well-being. Leisure is often a means through which children challenge their physical skills without conscious effort and in turn develop the coordination and strength necessary for many human occupations.

Adolescents and young adults may focus on activities that are physically exciting and that offer the opportunity to meet new people. Finding a partner and establishing a satisfying adult life separate from the family of origin may be an outcome of leisure pursuits. Dating relationships that develop into marital ones in Western societies typically grow from sharing many positive leisure experiences before marriage. Participation in selected leisure activities during young adulthood may provide a career direction for later life. Adolescents and children often discover lifelong leisure or work interests through their leisure pursuits. For example, a passion for exploring the outdoors may lead to a career as a naturalist or to lifelong participation in hiking and other outdoor activities.

Throughout adulthood, leisure activities provide a means to reconnect emotionally to spouses, children, and other adults; they allow respite from work and reaffirm or establish a sense of self that may have been lost in everyday routines and responsibilities. In old age, leisure activities may be a means of making connections to others, defining a sense of identity and purpose, and bringing personal meaning to life.

PERSONAL TRAITS

Temperament, the inborn style with which we approach and respond to the environment, influences one's leisure pursuits. People's temperament affects their activity level, approach and withdrawal tendencies in new situations, adaptability to change, sensory threshold, quality and intensity of their mood states, persistence, and attention span (Chess & Thomas, 1984). When a person has a low activity level, he or she may seek out more sedentary leisure activities. When a person has a high activity level and a high sensory threshold, he or she may seek out high-intensity pursuits such as skydiving or hunting.

Likewise, people's personalities direct the activities in which they choose to participate and the extent to which they participate in them. If people are extraverted, they tend to take advantage of many social opportunities and enjoy a variety of group activities. If people are introverted, they may spend more time in solitary pursuits or those requiring the participation of only a few people.

Another personal trait that may influence people's leisure activity selection is their physical stamina and skills. Some people are physically more suited to strenuous physical activities such as skiing, swimming, or tennis. For those with less coordination, skill, or stamina, participation in these activities may feel like work.

Finally, people's cognitive skill level or interests may determine the leisure activities in which they are comfortable participating. Those with highly abstract cognitive abilities may choose to play chess, do crossword puzzles, or play word games. People with different cognitive skills may find these same activities boring, confusing, or too demanding. People with lower levels of cognitive skill may find that participation in these activities feels like work.

CULTURAL FACTORS

People's family values and culture greatly affect their leisure participation. If one's culture values productivity and usefulness within the family and the community, leisure activities may revolve around activities related to organized religion or hobbies that produce functional products. In families who believe in the centrality of the family unit, leisure pursuits may be focused on family activities. In these situations, free time and creative talents focus on enhancing family life and celebrating family events. In families who believe in self-fulfillment as a person, each member of the family is encouraged to direct his or her time and energy toward exploring individual interests, which may lead to a person's spending more time in solitary activity or in activities with like-minded people outside of the family.

Cultural beliefs and values also affect how gender or age determines leisure activities. Some cultures delineate appropriate activities by age, gender, or marital status. Some have specific rules about how and when men and women may participate in selected activities. For example, some cultural groups expect married women to spend their leisure time within the family and not in the community at large.

PERSONAL CHOICE CONSIDERATIONS

How people use time outside of leisure may affect how they view and use leisure time. Some people view their choice of activities relative to what they do in their career or vocation. Neulinger (1981) postulated that people choose leisure activities that are the direct opposite of their daily work routine. A person who works at a desk or a computer may spend his or her free time in physically strenuous outdoor sport activities (e.g., bike riding, hiking); a mother who spends most of her time tending to the needs of the family may seek out solitary activities in which she can lose herself such as jogging, painting, or dancing; a person who spends a significant amount of time in solitary work may actively seek group activities within a family or social network. Others, however, seek leisure activities that are related to their chosen career or vocation. Some examples are a person who attends conferences and socializes with members of his or her profession, a high school English teacher who chooses to read novels and attend poetry readings, or a carpenter who builds a boat in his free time.

ENVIRONMENTAL CONSIDERATIONS

People's personal access to leisure environments, materials, and equipment strongly influences how they spend their free time and what activities they explore to meet their needs. If people live in a rural environment, they are likely to have the opportunity to explore and develop skills in many outdoor activities. In a city environment, people have a greater opportunity to participate as a spectator in a range of sporting and creative arts events. Thus, the physical aspects of one's community influence leisure participation. When people have economic resources, they can buy any materials or equipment that they need to participate in an activity of interest. Thus, personal resources also hold significant influence over the leisure activities people choose to pursue.

The Internet has opened up new opportunities for leisure. People of all ages and abilities can now find online groups, games, and virtual communities even when their physical geography, physical limitations, or economic resources may limit participation in their real-life communities. A person who lives in a remote area of the Northwest can participate in a book discus-

---

EXERCISE 13.2: LEISURE PURSUITS

Think about your leisure pursuits. What factors influence your choice of these leisure activities?

---

sion with like-minded readers through discussion boards or live chats. Nintendo has allowed people to participate in a range of virtual sports. Second Life allows virtual trips to faraway places and access to virtual night clubs, university lectures, and music concerts at no cost.

Barriers to Participation in Leisure Activities

For some people, work and responsibilities seem to fill every waking hour. They may see leisure activities as frivolous. For others, leisure is threatening, frustrating, or a burden. People may be more comfortable with a consistent routine made up of required activities than with an expanse of time that they must fill with their own planned activities. To have leisure means to step outside of one's daily routine. It requires people to challenge themselves to participate in activities beyond those that are required for self- or family maintenance or work. People have the right not to participate in leisure activities and to be passive in their free time. This lack of participation, however, can be isolating and may lead to alienation and depression.

In the United States, people have many opportunities to be passive in their leisure time. Although watching television can help fill people's leisure time in a way that makes them feel momentarily better than if they had nothing to do, it can lead people away from learning to truly experience their leisure time. Putnam (2000) reported that television is the only leisure activity that seems to inhibit participation in other leisure activities. It encourages lethargy and passivity. Kubey and Csikszentmihalyi (1990) found that heavy television viewing was associated with a great deal of free time, loneliness, and emotional difficulties. This finding is consistent across cultures. People who engage in do-it-yourself projects at home are more likely to play a sport in their leisure time or to engage in public speaking. People who attend more movies are more likely to attend club meetings or dinner parties or to visit friends. Putnam (2000) also reported that people participate in television watching at the expense of nearly every social activity outside of the home. The only activities positively linked to heavy television watching are sleeping, resting, eating, housework, and listening to the radio.

When exploring alternative leisure activities, people must recognize that a significant amount of corporate profit in Western society is related to mass consumption of leisure equipment and experiences. Corporations barrage people with advertising about the "perfect" use of leisure time that may interfere with the search for personal definitions of ideal leisure. Relentless advertising attempts to convince people that they want what the ads are offering. Some people then begin to value only those leisure activities that are heavily advertised. The "right" pair of running shoes or sports equipment, belonging to the "right" gym, or going on the "right" vacations may become tied to social status, which may result in people working more hours to afford leisure versus actually enjoying leisure. People may participate in fewer leisure activities or passive activities because they believe that participation in leisure activities requires a great deal of money.

Quart (2003) addressed the powerful negative influence of youth-targeted marketing on adolescents' values and spending habits. She reported that U.S. teens have more than $155 billion in discretionary income. As a group, U.S. teens are easy prey for marketers because of their openness to the media, their insecurities, and their desire to be included in their peer group. By marketing certain products and services through teens who represent popularity, a growing segment of U.S. youth has developed strong desires for expensive, name-brand merchandise and seeks the physical perfection that mass media push on them. More teens are working extra hours to buy those products and services that are heavily advertised; their money and time are being consumed, leaving less for productive adolescent leisure pursuits.

Stereotypes can be a barrier to leisure participation, especially for school-age children, teens, and older adults. A group of children may decide that one child is strange and therefore exclude that child in playground activities or in child-initiated clubs. Adolescents identify themselves and each other with crowds who share certain observable behaviors (Brown, 1990). Typical clique identifications in a high school may include "jocks," "brains," or "druggies." Certain cliques have higher social status than others. An adolescent who is associated with an unpopular or negative clique may experience rejection and discomfort when trying to participate in leisure activities that are associated with another clique. A healthy elderly person may feel less included in some community activities that are typically associated with younger adults. She or he may need to prove competence before gaining acceptance in some leisure group activities.

Other barriers to access to leisure activities are people's personal traits and internal resources, racial background, religious practices, sexual orientation, community resources, and certain select negative habits or behaviors. Some people have personal character issues that interfere with their ability to engage in leisure activities with others. These people may lack the internal resources (i.e., coping skills) or social skills to explore interests or connect with others through personally meaningful and productive activity. Whalen, Jamner, Henker, Delfino, and Lozano (2002) found that adolescents with attention deficit hyperactivity disorder (ADHD) symptoms were more likely to spend their time in passive, entertaining leisure pursuits as opposed to hobbies and structured activities. The participants with ADHD in this study were 10 times more likely to have smoked and 4 times more likely to have consumed alcohol than adolescents without ADHD. Adolescents with ADHD may lack the skills to modulate their attention, which is important for skill development in active and productive leisure activities.

If communities do not have the resources or facilities for creative arts or organized sports, then these leisure activities are not available to people in those communities. Shann (2001), in a study of four inner-city middle schools, found that the children did not participate in after-school activities. The children reported that they primarily participated in unstructured and passive leisure activities such as watching television and hanging out with their friends. Shann advocated for greater development of after-school and weekend activities programs for inner-city children (Figure 13.6).

For elderly people, a lack of transportation to their local senior citizens' center can severely limit their ability to participate in community activities housed there. Sallis, Sirard, King, and Albright (2007) found that adults' perceptions about the availability and safety of their community environment also influenced their participation in leisure activities.

Finally, some barriers to participation are caused by a person's negative habits or behaviors such as abuse of drugs or alcohol and participation in gangs, petty crime, or violence, which may inhibit relaxation, excitement, and connecting with others. Even when substance abuse and illegal activities cease, people who have been habitually involved in these activities may lack the skills to find and participate in satisfying leisure activities. Farnworth (2000) found that her sample of adolescent offenders on probation spent 57% of their time engaged in passive leisure activities such as watching television and listening to music. They reported being bored 42% of the time.

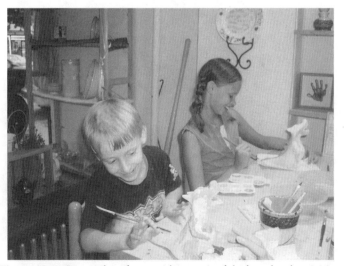

Figure 13.6. Arts and crafts provide meaningful afterschool activities.

Leisure Experiences Across the Lifespan

As people grow and mature, their leisure activities change. Leisure activities reflect a person's developmental maturation and developing interests. Leisure activities are also influenced by social and cultural factors.

INFANCY AND EARLY CHILDHOOD

Leisure for children includes solitary activities and activities with caregivers or peers. Children's first leisure experiences are play. Play is a child-initiated activity that an adult has not structured for the purpose of teaching specific skills. The child engages in the activity because he or she wants to and because it is fun (Figure 13.7). The child is free to participate independently or to negotiate sharing the activity with another. A parent might approach an infant with a busy box, and the infant may bang on it for a few minutes but then crawl away and pick up a pot to bang. The infant is in control of the activity. Thus, this same infant may look toward the parent for an indication of when he or she wants the infant to join or move away and when he or she wants the infant to play alone. An older child may build with LEGOs™ or do a puzzle because he or she finds the activity

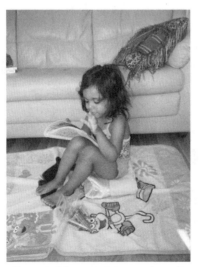

Figure 13.7. Reading as a leisure activity can be solitary and relaxing.

interesting rather than because a parent or teacher instructed the child to complete the activity.

Erikson (1963) said that children's play "is not the equivalent of adult play . . . it is not recreation. The playing adult steps sidewards into another reality, the playing child advances to new stages of mastery" (p. 222). Children's play concerns exploration and discovery in all spheres of human existence. It continuously evolves, and what was once interesting is now boring. Children develop new skills and use them in novel ways during play. Although building skills is not the purpose of play, through play, children become more competent in all areas of human functioning. They develop a capacity to cope with their environment and develop ego strength and an investment in life (Cotton, 1984).

Playfulness is an important aspect of children's play. Playfulness exists when a child is intrinsically motivated, internally controlled, and able to suspend reality (Bundy, 1997). *Intrinsic motivation* means that the child is driven to participate in particular activities because of the innate rewards experienced in the activity. The child does not participate in play activities because he or she is expecting a reward or praise. The child gets involved to have fun. *Internal control* refers to the child's having primary control over what occurs in the activity. When a child suspends reality, he or she uses objects in new ways to discover new uses for everyday things or engages in make-believe (e.g., imaginary play or games). A child frames an activity by giving cues to others as to how they should act toward him or her. A child, for example, might cue a playmate that they are now going to play house and he or she is going to be the parent. A child who wants to play superheroes and be the "bad guy" may frame the activity so that his or her peers must now fight or run away. These manipulations allow the child to experience life from the perspective of another.

Play begins in infancy when an infant learns to attend to the faces of caregivers. Caregivers smile and make soft sounds at infants and wait for infants to respond in kind. Over time, infants are ready to play peek-a-boo or to imitate facial expressions and sounds that caregivers make. Infants begin to initiate the play, and both they and caregivers receive pleasure from the interaction. This mutual interaction evolves to social play by making a different face or a sound. Through parent–child play experiences in infancy and early childhood, children develop the coping skills necessary for more complex play. The most important variable in a young child's development of coping skills is his or her mother's leisure experiences with him or her, which is the mother's enjoyment of the play (Figure 13.8; Murphy & Moriarity, 1976).

Playing and interacting with other children is an important part of the leisure experiences of a child from preschool age onward. Children share similar levels of physical activity, exuberance, and open emotional expression that make them more attractive to each other than adults are to them. Children share their interests with peers, and their enthusiasm for certain activities increases or decreases depending on the reactions of valued peers

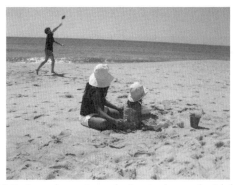

Figure 13.8. A mother enjoys playing in the sand with her child.

to those activities. Children will more likely take chances and participate in new activities when other children are participating. Through leisure play experiences, children learn the joys of friendship and camaraderie and to negotiate and compromise in the interest of maintaining peer relationships.

The supportive guidance of caregivers provides young children with confidence in their capacity to successfully participate in an activity and have fun, based on past experiences and pleasures. As children grow and enter middle childhood, some leisure activities become recreational ones; these activities have playful elements to them, but they are now structured activities that occur as part of a team game or within a club. Children who enter these activities have begun to accept rules as necessary for group activity. Without defined rules and some accepted order to activities, little pleasurable activity would occur.

Leisure for children begins to involve more complex games and group activities. Children master games of chance first, followed by games requiring strategies. In games of chance, children learn first to modulate their intense excitement related to the process of being in the lead and then to accept losses as "just a game" rather than a statement about their competence. They learn to follow the rules and to inhibit negative emotions that might lead them to quit a game prematurely or to become aggressive when a game does not end in their favor. Depending on children's temperament and innate skills, learning games may initially be challenging to both children and their caregivers. Children may be slow to learn or to acclimate to rules. Younger children often change the rules and cheat to win until losing becomes less threatening to them. Once children understand games and begin to accept rules, their animation, physical tension, and excitement in a simple game such as Old Maid can bring almost as much enjoyment to caregivers as it does to children.

McHale, Crouter, and Tucker (2001) found that in making the transition to adolescence, children who participated in structured activities such as hobbies and sports were more likely to be well-adjusted adolescents. Children who spent their free time just hanging out were more likely to exhibit

---

Exercise 13.4: Childhood

Think about a child that you know well. What activities does that child participate in that you would consider play or leisure? Why? What underlying skills does the child have that support his or her participation? What needs do you think the activities meet for the child? What effect, if any, do you think that the child's participation will have on his or her overall development?

---

less adaptive functioning, including poor school grades and more conduct problems.

Singer, Singer, D'Agostino, and DeLong (2009) reported that in the past two decades children's participation in spontaneous activities and play has diminished as a result of the popularity of television, computer games, and other technological products and because of parents' fears about children's physical safety, the shortage of quality play spaces near children's homes, and the reduction of recess time in schools. Results of this study showed that mothers reported that the most common activity for children while not in school was watching television. Many mothers reported being worried about lack of play space and the safety of their children in facing real or imagined dangers. Thus, they allowed children to stay indoors and watch television. The authors speculated that parents may be reluctant to allow their children outdoors because of fears generated from the violent content of television news and shows.

Larson and Verma (1999) reported that because leisure activities are at least partly self-chosen and involve self-control or peer-group control of action and attention, they may provide opportunities for the development of initiative, self-regulation, and social skills. However, many of the leisure activities that young people choose may involve little structure or challenge and provide little stimulus for growth. Higher rates of television viewing among children of lower socioeconomic status may be attributable to limited options for other, more rewarding leisure choices. Children often choose television to fill hours of free time. Television watching requires little active self-regulation of attention or behavior from participants; it is also related to obesity and depression. Television can be a default relaxing activity when other activities are not available, or it may displace functionally similar activities such as attending movies, listening to music, or empty time spent idling.

Adolescence

American adolescents spend up to 40% of their time in leisure pursuits (Csikszentmihalyi & Larson, 1984). Adolescents' moods are the most positive and their activity level is the highest when they are engaged in leisure activities as opposed to work or school activities (Fine, Mortimer, & Roberts, 1990). How they use their large block of leisure time is important to their psychosocial development.

Peer groups and peer culture are the central focus of adolescent leisure in the United States (Brown, 1990). Peer friendships serve as a primary source of activity, influence, and support for most adolescents. Adolescents report enjoying activities with friends more than they do with family members—feeling most understood by friends and that they can be most fully themselves in the company of friends (Savin-Williams & Berndt, 1990). Adolescents tend to see themselves and their agemates as fitting into particular groups. Group leisure opportunities for adolescents increase or decrease depending on where the particular adolescents fit within the culture of their school or community. A football player may get invited to many parties, and the president of the chess club may not. Although being a part of a high-status crowd may increase the number of group activities in which an adolescent is included, it may not enhance the adolescent's experience of leisure. Less popular teens may actively pursue individual or small-group activities for which they have a passion and may have deep and satisfying friendships.

Larson, Hansen, and Moneta (2006) studied the developmental experiences of young people as they participated in different categories of organized leisure activities including sports, performance and fine arts activities, and community-oriented and service activities. Organized sports stood out as settings that supported adolescents in developing initiative, including setting goals, applying effort, and learning time management. They also have the potential for supporting emotional regulation. Service activities were distinguished from other activities by how they connected young people to adult networks and provided positive relationship experiences. Although unstructured interactions with peers (i.e., hanging out) have the potential to provide them with rich developmental activities, young people reported higher rates of negative influences in their interactions with peers than in organized activities. Participation in music, arts, and service organizations most often engages an adolescent with a prosocial peer group and with older mentors.

Wood et al. (2009) reported that youth programs can be important contexts in which young people can develop a sense of responsibility. Although they may have limited opportunities to develop responsibility in other contexts, youth programs can provide opportunities for participants to develop responsibility in meeting task, role, and time demands as they execute meaningful tasks for their groups. Besides describing themselves as active agents in their group's success, young people reported feeling compelled by the negative consequences that nonadherence would have for their future opportunities, both within their youth group and with respect to their standing with leaders and peers in the program. Findings also highlighted the importance of young people's identifying their own goals; adult leaders should not expect that they can simply impose demands on young people and expect positive outcomes. In productive groups, these young people took ownership of demanding tasks and roles, the expectations of leaders and peers were high, and the consequences associated with the demands were meaningful and important to participants, so fulfilling demands was compelling.

Transitional leisure pursuits can be a sanctuary for adolescents. These activities most often occur in safe and familiar settings that nurture self-expression and exploration. They may involve visiting the science laboratory or the art room of a favorite teacher after school or they may involve participating in a club or extracurricular class. For example, Wilson (as cited in John-Steiner, 1985) studied the experiences of a group of high school students in art. The art room in a public high school was a retreat from the demands of the school environment. In the room, these adolescents were able to "transcend the limitations of the structure, to engage in acts which are creative or ludic or subversive and to participate in a kind of communitas" (Wilson, as quoted by John-Steiner, 1985, p. 94). *Communitas* refers to a community in which a strong feeling of equality, solidarity, and togetherness exists.

Modell and Valdez (2002) highlighted the potential of leisure participation to contribute to the successful transition of adolescents with disabilities. People with disabilities who have greater access to recreation and leisure report more satisfaction in their lives than those who have limited access.

When adolescents participate solely in relaxed leisure activities, they are more likely to be less focused and at risk for developing behavior problems that negatively affect their development. Without activities to channel their energies positively, they may be more likely to seek out adventure through drinking, drug experimentation, or early sexual activity. In contrast, adolescents who discover their particular talents, and develop habits to cultivate these talents, invest a significant amount of time in related activities and develop comfort and the ability to use solitude effectively. As a result, they have a stronger grasp on their developing self-identity, and peers are less likely to influence them negatively. These teens tend to be more open to new experiences and exhibit higher levels of concentration than do other teens. Interestingly, many of these adolescents spend more time with their parents in leisure activities. Parental engagement provides them with a sense of support and consistency, encourages their intensity and self-direction, and enhances their attentional capacities for finding and mastering challenges (Csikszentmihalyi, Rathunde, & Whalen, 1993).

EXERCISE 13.5: ADOLESCENCE

Think back to your adolescent years. Describe your participation in leisure activities at that time. What activities were you regularly involved in that might be described as relaxed leisure activities? What activities were you regularly involved in that might be described as transitional leisure activities? How did these activities influence your experiences as an adolescent and your roles as an adult?

YOUNG ADULTHOOD

As people transition from adolescence into adulthood, shifts in leisure activities occur as they continue their education and begin their first real jobs. Many young adults move out of their family homes and enter a different world from that of their childhood and adolescence. This period becomes one of defining oneself outside of the family of origin. Leisure time may lessen because of work responsibilities or may increase for college students who do not work and who may now live independently with people their own age.

When young adults decide to go to college, they pursue courses of study that expand their base of knowledge into new areas. They may develop interests in areas about which they were previously unaware and may come to find that their prior interests are less compelling. The college environment provides numerous new opportunities for leisure activities with new people to befriend. Many young adults who enter college continue to have a great deal of leisure time. Living independently on a college campus with roommates offers increased opportunities to explore and experiment. New leisure opportunities may be available at college that were not available in students' communities of origin. Young adults from a large city may find themselves in rural areas that provide opportunities for outdoor activities such as bike riding, canoeing, hiking, or skiing. Young adults from rural areas may find themselves in a major metropolitan center and discover a love for live music and theater that they have never experienced before. New friends may come from different backgrounds and expose young adults to new social opportunities. Additionally, activities that were chores during adolescence may now become valued leisure activities. For example, preparing a meal in one's own apartment for friends may be a way of expressing identity and a way of relaxing; painting and decorating a dorm room or apartment may be a work of self-expression for a young adult.

This time may also involve the loss of treasured leisure activities as a result of relocation or the responsibilities of being a college student. The transition may be accompanied by difficulty coping with the changes in tasks and activities in addition to the lack of opportunity to engage in pleasurable activities and activities in which success is guaranteed. At this time, many young adults are testing their abilities in preparation for the pursuit of a future career.

The leisure activities of young adults who enter the workforce may likewise change. They are entering a new cultural forum in which ethnicity, culture, and gender may be minimized because their presence is tied to performing a job. Pressure may exist to conform to the culture of the majority, and young adults must learn to adjust their personal values and conduct in the work environment. Leisure is a critical occupational area for workers to explore so that they may find activities that reaffirm their sense of identity, allow them to develop areas of interest and talent, reaffirm a sense of belonging to specific cultural groups, and rejuvenate the soul and spirit. Workers may continue some of the leisure activities of their school years, such as participating in local adult sport leagues; participating in music bands; and attending spectator sports, movies, or live music events. These adults may remain in the same geographical area and may socialize with the same or similar friends. The major change in their lives is that of going to work full-time, which results in a notable decrease in their amount of leisure time compared with high school. Their leisure time is now limited to the weekends or days off from work.

For all young adults, a considerable amount of leisure time may focus on establishing relationships with a significant other, and sharing leisure activities is a central part of courtship in Western culture. Through leisure activities, young people socialize in a nonthreatening, neutral environment in which they share a mutually interesting activity (such as dinner, a movie, a sporting event, or a bike ride). Such activities allow a relationship to develop in a relaxed manner. When like-minded people share leisure activities, a bond of friendship may develop. Furthermore, sharing an activity or adventure with another person provides a situation in which one learns about oneself and about the other person.

People may reflect their pleasure in the joint activity by developing a positive regard for each other and may want to learn more about the other as a person. As a meaningful relationship with a potential partner develops, young adults adjust their time commitments to fit the other person's leisure interests. Couples negotiate how much leisure time they will spend together, especially when they have different individual leisure interests and pursuits. Each person in a couple adjusts leisure expectations in the interest of the relationship: One person may give up socializing in a bar or participating in a league sport to please a partner; another person may adjust to a partner's hobby by developing an interest in that hobby to increase shared leisure time. The couple may take up a new activity together, such as ballroom dancing, to deepen their bond. Couples begin to share holidays, family traditions, and family events. They begin entertaining friends and family members together. A young wife, for example, may need to accommodate her husband by learning to participate in his traditional Italian family dinner every Sunday.

Young adults with physical disabilities may have limited opportunities for socializing and for pursuing leisure activities that interest them. People with disabilities may be limited by the availability of family members for transportation and for their company as they participate in leisure activities outside of their homes. Becoming less engaged with family members and more engaged with peers in leisure pursuits may not be possible or may be much more difficult than it is for able-bodied young adults. Although virtual communities do not replace actual human contact, the Internet has expanded leisure opportunities for people with disabilities.

In healthy young adulthood, people maintain solitary or group leisure interests that have developed during their lifetimes. Certain activities become part of one's persona, support self-esteem, and rejuvenate the participant. A person may have a longstanding love for cars that develops into an interest in restoring vintage cars. Sewing, knitting, or jewelry making may be someone's way of expressing an artistic side, although he or she may work as a store clerk. Others may join adult community sports leagues or coach children's sports teams. Many young adults who enjoyed biking as children and teenagers join biking clubs to maintain physical fitness and rejuvenate their physical bodies. More and more adults are becoming involved in virtual communities and in Internet gaming.

Drinking alcohol during social events is often part of the passage from childhood to adulthood in Western culture. The use of substances such as drugs and alcohol may stem from a search for pleasurable feelings that substances can induce (Kraus, 1994). Alcohol can lower one's inhibitions and make socialization easier. When drinking, however, dominates how people spend their leisure time, enjoyment of this activity (and other activities) diminishes.

MIDDLE ADULTHOOD

Whether adults choose to marry or remain single or to have children influences how they conceptualize and use their leisure time during middle age. Those who marry are likely to change how they use some of their leisure time to include their spouses and extended family members. Taking care of children and sharing leisure pursuits with children occupy a large amount of parents' leisure time.

Single adults continue to seek, establish, and maintain long-term relationships with significant others, but they are likely to pursue and further develop their skills in the hobbies and activities in which they have engaged across the lifespan. Single adults are likely to be settled in their careers and have adjusted to single adulthood; they have time to devote to enhancing skills in lifelong leisure activities and pursue new interests. In the process, they discover more about themselves as people and their potential to contribute to society in ways other than caring for children. In midlife, some people may become more reflective about community issues or politics and decide that they have the personal skills and resources to have a positive effect on their community. Others may turn past hobbies into part-time careers; they may write, buy and sell antiques, or design jewelry.

In some ways, single life presents a greater challenge but more opportunity for the development of a rich adult leisure life. Single or childless people confront expanses of unstructured time unencumbered by responsibilities to children or a spouse. People may perceive this unstructured time as freedom or as a burden. They can pursue interests without the restraint of the needs or disapproval of immediate family members. Without an active approach to leisure participation, a single person may experience isolation and discontent. Having solitary leisure interests can be helpful to these adults because others may not be immediately available for interaction. Finding companions for joint leisure activities is a more active process for single adults than for those with children or spouses. For some, a lack of companionship can present a serious barrier to leisure participation; for others, it is an opportunity to develop new relationships, deepen older relationships, and expand leisure opportunities through varied companions. Single adults are more likely to participate in group travel or adult leisure organizations than are people with families or spouses. Single adults may be more independent and willing to take risks to participate in activities that interest them. Single women may not experience the retreat from the exploration of their own abilities and personal interests that many married women encounter during their childbearing years.

Women's roles notably change when they become parents. Parenting changes a woman's work life or career to a greater extent than it alters a man's, even if a woman continues to work after childbirth. Although men share in child care and home maintenance activities, most mothers fill the role of primary caregiver. Women's former leisure experiences tend to decrease more notably than do their husbands.' Men may share equally in leisure activities with children, but women typically provide more instrumental child care.

Leisure activities of parents who do not work outside the home are usually home centered. Activities may include gardening, sewing, home crafts, cooking, and parent–child play. These parents intersperse these activities among house and child maintenance chores. In families in which both parents work outside the home, family leisure activities are often limited to evenings and weekends. These activities are special because the time together is short. Eating a family meal, reading a book together, and playing a game may be more important than household maintenance activities.

The leisure activities of a family undergo many transitions as children grow. As infants, children may greatly curtail parents' leisure activities as parents adjust to parenthood. Leisure may revolve around playful interaction with the infant or sharing parenting experiences with other parents or with older adults who can provide support and guidance to the new parents. Satisfying leisure needs with infants and young children requires effort on the part of the adults (Figure 13.9). In addition to home-based leisure activities, parents of young children often visit parks and other public places where other parents and children congregate. They may attend religious functions, parent–child drop-in centers, or gym activities designed to facilitate parent–child interaction and interaction with other families. These community activities provide parents with an opportunity to interact with children in the proximity of other parents, which allows adults to share their parenting joys and frustrations. During these activities, children have opportunities to meet other adults and children.

Some parents make connections to their children by sharing their own leisure passions. Parents may teach their children sports, take them to sport-

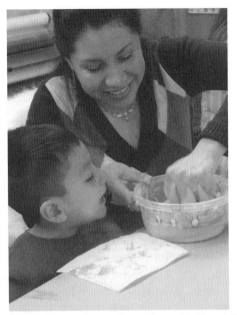

Figure 13.9. A mother and son play with Play-doh®.

ing events, and share the experience of cheering for their favorite team. If a child shows an interest in learning a sport that interests a parent, the sport may provide a means through which the parent and child can relate to one another. Positive feelings about the activity become closely associated with positive feelings toward one another, and the sport can bring the two closer together. Parents may return to the leisure activities of their youth as part of their role as parent. A parent may have loved soccer as a child and now coaches his or her child's soccer team.

Parents of children with disabilities face challenges to participation in leisure activities and challenges in facilitating family-based leisure activities. Children with disabilities make greater demands on parents' time because of added responsibilities for managing for their children academic or self-care activities that parents of typically developing children can turn over to the children themselves. Gaining access to leisure activities that are appropriate for children with disabilities is often difficult because of fewer community offerings and competition for the opportunities available.

When children reach adolescence, family-focused leisure time may occur less frequently. Although adolescents may still participate in selected family, religious, or cultural activities, they tend to begin to move beyond their immediate family for leisure pursuits. Parents may feel loss, abandonment, or a new sense of freedom as their adolescent children's leisure increasingly focuses on activities outside the family unit. Parents may experience jealousy as their teenagers' leisure activities become more exciting than their own. Activities in adolescence are very different from watching young children participate in the leisure activities of scouting or sports. This change may lead parents to question and reevaluate their own leisure activities. The leisure triumphs of an adolescent may facilitate parents' positive moods and interests in activity participation (Steinberg & Steinberg, 1994). In their study, Larson, Pearce, Sullivan, and Jarrett (2007) found that adolescents' participation in youth groups can serve as a catalyst for parents supporting adolescents' autonomy.

As children grow into adults, parental satisfaction in activities outside their role as parents provides a buffer to the experience of turmoil during the transition. In Steinberg and Steinberg's (1994) qualitative study, parents who were not engaged in satisfying activities beyond that of parenthood were vulnerable to severe distress as their children became adolescents. Steinberg and Steinberg (1994) interpreted their findings as suggesting that activities such as individual hobbies or community service provide a distraction and support parents' sense of personal competence and self-worth as they adjust to the loss of spending a great deal of time with their children.

When children move on to start their own adult lives, middle-aged adults must refocus their leisure pursuits. Although women are more likely to experience psychological turmoil during their offspring's adolescence before the children leave home, women adjust more easily to the "empty nest syndrome" than do fathers (Steinberg & Steinberg, 1994). Women are more likely to be engaged in exploring new careers, new interests, or community activities than men. Some believe that this change may occur because young women may surrender their own desires in the interest of their husbands and growing families; once their children are grown, women may seek to reclaim their sense of individuality and pursue activities that provide personal satisfaction (Labouvie-Vief, 1994; Niemela & Linto, 1994).

During later middle age, a couple may pursue new joint activities or a parent may reinvest his or her newly acquired time in individual hobbies. Work demands may have lessened, and time previously spent focusing on career building may now be available for leisure pursuits. Leisure travel may become more frequent because children place fewer demands on parents' time and finances when they become independent. Middle to older adulthood can be a time to do some of the activities that one has always wanted to do but never did. Adults also begin to see a time limit on their opportunity to participate in those activities. Some people run their first marathons at age 50, and others use late middle age to challenge themselves intellectually in ways that they wished that they had done as younger adults. Some adults reenter education to finish a high school degree, pursue a college degree for the sake of knowledge, or pursue another career that they expect may be more fulfilling than their first career. For others, late middle adulthood is an opportunity to connect with other adults in ways that were not possible when they were raising children or focusing on their careers. They may develop new or revived passions for activities such as gourmet cooking, golf, bridge, travel, or book clubs.

This time is when people may have to begin to think about their physical abilities as they become aware that minor physical injuries take longer to

---

EXERCISE 13.6: PARENT INTERVIEW

Interview a parent. Discuss the effect of children on his or her participation in leisure activities. What does a parent value in his or her leisure time? How much leisure time does he or she have per day or per week? How does he or she spend it? What leisure activities does he or she participate in alone, with children, and with other adults? Compare his or her leisure experiences with those of a single adult whom you know.

---

heal and affect function longer than in their younger years. People inevitably experience a decrease in visual acuity as they age and perhaps a change in body metabolism that may contribute to weight gain or obesity. Some people in middle adulthood may also develop high blood pressure, diabetes, or high cholesterol. These changes and dysfunctions associated with age may interfere with participation in leisure unless people make accommodations in their routines or activities.

OLDER ADULTHOOD

Besides successfully avoiding disease and disability, successful aging requires the maintenance of physical and cognitive function and engagement in social and productive activities (Hultsch, Hertzog, Small, & Dixon, 1999; Rowe & Kahn, 1997). The importance of elderly people's establishing or maintaining meaningful occupations was demonstrated in the Well-Elderly Research Study (Jackson, Carlson, Mandel, Zemke, & Clark 1998), which found that identification and engagement in meaningful occupations has an effect on the overall well-being of elderly people. Participating in leisure is the most important predictor of well-being among older adults (Zimmer, Hickey, & Searle, 1997). Carey (2009) reported that older adults who spend 3 or more hours per day in demanding mental activities such as doing crossword puzzles were more likely to maintain their cognitive function and to stave off dementia. Activities such as playing bridge that combine social connection with strong cognitive demands seem to be the most powerful in maintaining the function of elderly people. Schooler and Mulatu (2001) summarized their research findings as suggesting that more complex leisure activities increase intellectual function and less complex leisure activities decrease intellectual function.

When older adults retire from paid employment, they have a new opportunity to explore their interests, evaluate who they have been during their lifetime, and think about who they would like to be for the remainder of their lives. If they have maintained some leisure interests throughout their lives, retirement may allow them to expand on those interests and devote more time to the activities that they love. For others, retirement leads to depression or a crisis as they attempt to adjust to a new way of life. When confronted with unstructured time, these older adults may not have the initiative to pursue new leisure activities or reconnect with old ones. A grieving process may be related to loss of the previous role. The role of worker is one of the most important roles with which people identify throughout their adult lives.

Past participation in leisure activities typically determines the activities that a retiree seeks out. Optimally, people who have neglected developing leisure occupations throughout the earlier part of their lives will begin to explore leisure activities within their community and learn what they really enjoy and value beyond the daily routine of their life's work. Volunteer work in hospitals, schools, or community organizations can provide a structure that organizes daily life in similar ways as paid employment did previously and may offer the older adults an opportunity to find a new life purpose, enhance self-worth, and increase social contact with others (Morrow-Howell, Hinterlong, Rozario, & Tang, 2003; Singleton, 1996).

People's bodies and minds respond differently to the aging process. Although many elderly people may seek out more solitary and sedentary activities, many healthy elderly people are gregarious and seek out regular exercise. They may swim a few miles every week, go in-line skating, enter marathons, take tai chi or yoga classes, or go biking. Others maintain an interest and regularly participate in outdoor activities. Some older adults actually increase their involvement because they have more discretionary time. Many people retain solitary interests that have sustained their spirits throughout their lifetimes, including writing, playing an instrument, or painting. As their social obligations lessen, elderly people may become more focused on these activities.

Leisure pursuits may markedly change when adults become grandparents, especially if the grandchildren live nearby. Time spent with family members may now revolve around entertaining and engaging grandchildren. Grandchildren can bring out a relaxed ability to nurture and play that may not have been possible with one's own children. Grandparents may have increased discretionary time and the wisdom of experience to be able to enjoy the time they spend with their grandchildren more. Learning how to play virtual Wii games and activities can support older adults' engagement with their grandchildren. It can also open up older adults to new, productive ways to maintain their physical and mental fitness.

Older adults living alone report fluctuations between extremes of involvement with others and projects and periods of isolation (Siegel, 1993). An issue for these adults is how to find a balance in their time and make the time that they have left to live more valuable and meaningful for themselves. Some people may have difficulty managing this life stage; others seek and find inner creative powers that they had not recognized during earlier years of their lives.

For some mature adults, senior citizens centers become important places of social interaction. Regularly attending meetings and activities may provide the structure and support that some older adults need to deal with the loss of their jobs and former roles at retirement or with the loss of spouses and friends to death. Activities such as bingo, weekly card games, and day trips with local organizations demonstrate a shift from independent activity to activities that are more interdependent or involve dependence on others. Within the structure of these centers, older adults may find new ways to contribute to their communities, for example, they may make blankets for infants or participate in making products for nonprofit fundraising.

As older adults experience the loss of lifelong partners and close friends, they may find themselves burdened with feelings of isolation and disconnection. Although family members are often key to the physical well-being of elderly people, friends are more consistently related to well-being than are family members (Larson, Mannell, & Zuzanek, 1986). Friends provide unique companionship that transcends the mundane requirements of everyday life; they most typically share similar life experiences and view one another differently than do family members who see the older adult and themselves in their lifelong roles. Although family members are related to lifelong physical well-being, Larson et al. pointed out how friends influence one's immediate well-being, enjoyment in living, and participation in active leisure activities.

Because many of the daily activities of elderly people are voluntary rather than required work, it is easier to retreat from activity participation. Support groups with adults experiencing similar losses often help them in coming to terms with these experiences and in finding ways to reconstruct meaningful lives. In summarizing the experiences of 56 older women who participated in her qualitative study on aging, Siegel (1993) stated that

> [W]ith each death of a loved one, . . . we learn something more about more about who we are within that relationship and who we are without the presence of that person. With each loss, we also learn more about death and dying and about how to cope and survive. (p. 184)

As people near the end of their lives, they may be unable to participate in some past leisure activities because of the infirmities of old age. Some may cease participation and not seek new activities that interest them, but many older adults replace physically active pursuits with more passive ones in which they can readily participate ("Prevalence of Health-Care Providers," 2002; Zimmer et al., 1997). It is not uncommon as one gets older to need to shift from more active occupations to less active occupations, which is not to imply that people find less satisfaction in these occupations (Parker, 1996). Older adults who are likely to feel most in control of their lives will adapt their former interests to their bodies' changes in old age and will work to improve their bodies' functioning for participation in their activities through regular exercise, good nutrition, and mental activity (Baltes & Baltes, 1990; Everard, Lach, Fisher, & Baum, 2000).

Frail elderly people may become homebound and gradually lose interest in many leisure activities, including social ones. They may spend more time reflecting on the past and become dependent on adult children or community services for social interaction. In some situations, the adult may require adaptations or assistive devices (e.g., a magnifier to read a book or newspaper, adaptations to a telephone to amplify sound) to participate in leisure activities.

Considering Leisure in Prevention and Occupational Therapy Intervention

The occupation of leisure is a critical aspect of life. Developing the occupation of leisure in clients should be a primary concern for occupational therapists and occupational therapy assistants interested in prevention or working with people with disabilities. As described earlier in this chapter, when people are able to fully participate in the occupation of leisure, they are more likely to support their mental and physical health.

Leisure can be used to prevent secondary health issues that result from sedentary behavior, social isolation, or lack of cognitive stimulation. It can play a crucial role in health promotion. Leisure activities can promote self-regulation and support coregulation among family members. Panksepp (2008) highlighted the relationship between the rich physical play of children and children's learning about social dynamics, which may strengthen children's inhibitory resources for interacting sensitively with others. A study of older adults by Brown et al. (2008) supported the link between serious leisure activities and successful aging. Leisure is important across the lifespan and provides opportunities for personal growth and a sense of competency, and active social participation supports health and positive identities in the aging process. Krane and Orkis (2009) reported that people with disabilities who are physically active are more likely to be employed and more likely to report greater overall life satisfaction, to be more sociable, to have stronger support networks, and to be more positive about life prospects than people with disabilities who are not active.

As discussed earlier, leisure skill development as prevention is applicable across the lifespan, yet it may be particularly important for adolescents, people approaching retirement, and elderly people. Members of these cohorts may have more discretionary time that may potentially enrich their lives, but free time that is not productively used for activities of interest may be experienced as disorganizing or depressing. Occupational therapists and occupational therapy assistants who are cognizant of the centrality of meaningful occupation in mental health are the ideal health care providers to assist people in developing healthy leisure habits. People approaching retirement, early retirees, and elderly people may have developed activity limitations or participation restrictions caused by arthritis, diabetes, or pulmonary or cardiac dysfunction and may need to reconsider their choices of leisure activities, develop new interests, or adapt how they participate in favored activities. As noted earlier, it is not uncommon to need to shift from more active occupations to less active occupations as a person ages, which is not to imply that one finds less satisfaction in occupations (Parker, 1996).

The Well Elderly Study established occupational therapy as an effective preventive treatment for the population of well elderly people (Jackson et al., 1998). This study demonstrated that occupational therapy services focused on the power of occupation enhanced the health and functioning of the participants. The participants who were provided with education on a variety of topics relevant to the engagement in meaningful occupations and had opportunities to experience meaningful activities of their choice had the more positive gains. Overall, those receiving occupational therapy had more positive gains and fewer declines in function than those who took part in a social activity program only.

In many communities, limited exposure to the many possibilities for leisure engagement and limited support in developing skills for participation in those activities leaves many people with developmental disabilities with a narrow range of interests that may be passive and not supportive of their physical and mental health. For example, studies have suggested that adolescents and young adults with Down syndrome typically participate in passive and sedentary recreational activities such as watching television or listening to music for as much as 5 hours per day (Heyne, Schleien, & Rynders, 1997). These inactive and passive leisure pursuits are likely to be a contributing factor to the obesity and passivity often observed in people with this disorder.

Assessment

Client-centered practice has been defined as "an approach to service which embraces a philosophy of respect for, and partnership with, people receiving services" (Law, Baptiste, & Mills, 1995, p. 253). This approach focuses on the occupational problems identified by the client as it relates to his or her ability to carry out role-related occupations. This top-down, occupation-based approach supports the assessment of the occupation of leisure. The Canadian Occupational Performance Measure (Law et al., 1994) is one client-centered assessment tool used as an individualized measure to detect changes in a person's perception of his or her performance and satisfaction with occupational performance. Leisure is one of the areas of occupational performance assessed.

To have the potential for leisure satisfaction, it is important that clients be guided to recognize the importance of leisure in their lives, develop an awareness of their abilities and skills needed for leisure participation, and also have an awareness of how to identify and use leisure resources (Coyle, Lesnik-Emas, & Kinney 1994). Stebbins (2008) stated that identifying the particular kinds of serious or project-based leisure activities that would enhance the life of people with disabilities is a challenge for health professionals. They must take into consideration the physical, cognitive, and emotional limitations related to a particular disability while also introducing leisure activities that go beyond relaxation.

New assessment tools have been developed that help clinicians explore what leisure interests and activities mean to clients in addition to uncovering what activities clients are interested in and how often they participate. Meaning is central to occupation. For example, Henry (2000) developed the Pediatric Interest Profiles, paper-and-pencil surveys of play and leisure for children and adolescents ranging in age from 6 to 21. The profiles are designed simply so that children or adolescents can complete them independently or with minimal assistance from an adult in 20 to 30 minutes. A practitioner gains concrete information about a child's or adolescent's interests, actual participation, and view of his or her own participation. These data are meant to be used to facilitate a focused discussion with the child or adolescent about the meaning of their leisure interests, present participation, and desire for further development of their leisure occupations.

The Activity Leisure Profile (Mann & Talty, 1991) is specific to those who are addicted to alcohol. The Leisure Interest Profiles (Henry, 1997a, 1997b) look at the client's interests and participation in play or leisure activities for adults and seniors.

The Barth Time Construction (Barth, 1988), a time chart on which a client pastes colored strips of paper to depict the categories of activities and the amount of time devoted to particular activities over the course of a day and week before a psychiatric hospitalization, is an effective assessment tool for many clients, especially clients with substance abuse disorders. The Barth Time Construction provides clients and the occupational therapist with a graphic picture of time use over the course of a week. Clients with substance abuse disorders are frequently struck by the amount of time that they have devoted to obtaining and using alcohol or drugs and recovering from the effect of the drugs before seeking treatment. The time chart that clients create can generate a deep discussion about the lack of or minimal amount of meaningful leisure activities in these clients' lives and about their individual desires for occupational development for a healthy lifestyle.

INTERVENTION

A client-centered, occupation-based approach to the client should be at the center of occupational therapy intervention. Effective occupational therapy results from an understanding of a client's underlying abilities and needs. Depending on a client's disability, a practitioner may use a variety of frames of reference to assist the client in developing skills, or in altering the task or environment, for participation in leisure interests. Through applying the Sensory Integration and Motor Learning Frames of Reference, a practitioner may help a child develop sufficient balance and bilateral coordination for bicycle riding or in-line skating. To assist a client who has had a hand injury in developing the fine motor strength, endurance, and dexterity necessary to play a musical instrument again, a practitioner may use a biomechanical frame of reference. Adolescents with attention deficit disorder may learn how to modulate their attention and physical states to optimally participate in after-school clubs through working with a practitioner skilled in using an intervention approach that combines concepts of sensory integration with cognitive theory (e.g., Williams & Shellenberger, 1994).

Facilitating clients' development of active and social leisure participation may be hindered by the initial resistance to physical activity caused by difficulty with fine motor and gross motor skills. When a child has a learning disability or other cognitive disabilities, parents may struggle with interacting with the child in leisure activities. The child may avoid or be unable to attend to learning the typical leisure activities that parents teach and share with the child. The child may stay focused on familiar and repetitive activities or may be emotionally labile or withdrawn when confronted with leisure experiences that are pleasurable to other children. This may result in power struggles between parent and child or a more distant parent–child relationship in which the parent and child are mutually feeling sad, frustrated, and angry.

Occupational therapists and occupational therapy assistants can help parents guide their children in discovering individual and family leisure activities that are meaningful to both the parents and the child. The therapist may guide parents in learning how to provide support and assistance to their children in confronting new activities or new challenges in old activities. Parents may learn how to modify and adapt activities to foster their children's participation. Parental engagement in helping children in this way facilitates children's development of attentional and coping capacities that are necessary for future engagement in independent leisure activities. At the same time, satisfying parent–child leisure interaction has positive effects on both the parents' and the children's sense of competence and mood (Olson, 2006, 2010).

Adult clients may also avoid leisure occupations that interest them if they expect to fail because of pain, being physically unfit, being unprepared to undertake the activity, or having limited skill development. Assisting clients in adjusting their expectations for their participation and guiding them in adapting activities or locating adaptive equipment that would allow their participation and in developing the physical skills that they have for participation are important intervention strategies for occupational therapists and occupational therapy assistants to consider. Karan (2009) described how the Wii, the Nintendo virtual game system, is being used in rehabilitation centers as a means to engage clients in the physical activity necessary to regain maximal functioning. The Wii allows clients who might not be able to go bowling or to play golf to enjoy virtual versions of the sports. This can spark interest and engage clients with one another or family members while also providing needed physical exercise.

An occupational therapist or occupational therapy assistant may help a client make a connection with an organization such as the Tetra Society of North America (tetrasociety.org) or may work collaboratively with such a volunteer organization in guiding a person with a disability toward participation in leisure occupations of the person's own choosing. The Tetra Society is a volunteer organization developed by a person with tetraplegia who was active in many outdoor sports before his injury. At present, he participates in sailing and many other outdoor activities with adaptations. Tetra is dedicated to finding volunteer engineers and other professionals who work with people with disabilities to design and fabricate assistive devices to make participation possible in particular activities that are important to each person with a disability.

Guiding clients to adapt their environment so that they can readily participate in activities is a treatment strategy that occupational therapists and occupational therapy assistants regularly use with clients with all levels of disability. A parent may need to simplify game instructions so that a child with a learning disability can play with his or her family members. Reducing extraneous visual or auditory stimuli in the environment may greatly improve the ability of a person with developmental disabilities to participate in a leisure activity.

Other clients may have or may develop sufficient skill during the course of therapy but lack sufficient external resources for regular participation in activities that interest them. A therapist may then need to evaluate clients' present and required levels of resources necessary for satisfying leisure. A single adult with a physical disability may be interested in travel, or a senior citizen may be interested in finding partners for playing bridge. Helping clients find virtual communities, or actual physical community resources, or connecting them to another professional or agency that can find the appropriate external resources are important interventions.

Chronic physical or mental illness in a family may severely weaken marital and parent–child relationships, which reduces the amount and quality of emotional support that children receive from their parents or that spouses receive from each other. Joint leisure activities may be the first activities that family members sacrifice as stress increases, and playful and relaxed interaction may be minimal or nonexistent. Reexperiencing positive family leisure activities can have a major positive effect on each family member's mood and on the family's overall emotional atmosphere. Occupational therapists and occupational therapy assistants can help family members to alter their joint leisure activities in response to the effect of the illness and the change in family activities.

Adolescents with disabilities may be isolated from their mainstream peer group and may believe that they have few options for activity outside of school. Leyser and Cole (2005) found that students with disabilities were engaged in fewer activities with peers and family members than their typically developing peers. They also conversed less with their peers about leisure interests such as movies, music, television, food, or pets. Adults with brain injury may lose previous friendships and the ability to participate in some leisure pursuits as a result of reduced cognitive functioning. Loss of leisure-related occupations can have a major effect on every area of life functioning. The person may become depressed, passive, and dependent. Participating in a group that focuses on the occupation of leisure may help a person explore potential leisure interests; develop activity, social, and time management skills for leisure participation; learn how to reduce barriers to leisure participation; and develop a network of similar people who are interested in joint leisure activities. Developing a personally meaningful leisure life is likely to result in a generalized sense of well-being, independence, and personal control.

Regardless of whether depression is a primary disability or a secondary one related to a physical disability, it can have devastating effects on a person's everyday functioning. Developing leisure interests, and experiencing successful participation in them, may lessen the negative effects of difficult life situations and give the participant a new perspective on his or her life and ability to exert control over everyday activities. New interests may reduce a person's sense of alienation and make him or her more available for interaction with others. Some may need to find leisure outlets to express strong emotions that they cannot express in other everyday activities. Actively participating in sports or games or watching spectator sports, for example, may provide a socially acceptable outlet for aggressive impulses. Developing the habit of writing in a journal or composing poetry may provide a means for expressing and working through intense feelings for another person.

Adolescents with behavior disorders may have little awareness of their own individual interests, talents, and potential to develop as contributing members of society. They may be solely focused on their role within a negative peer group. Practitioners may engage such adolescents in exploring leisure activities and discovering previously unknown individual interests and talents. For example, one adolescent may find that he really enjoys the solitary experience of baking, which may give him time to relax away from peers and to think about his own life issues. Baking may lead to more prosocial individual action on the part of the teen at other times of the day. In addition, he may become aware that he has a talent for baking, may be motivated to participate in baking activities regularly, and may begin thinking about education or employment in food services or culinary arts. For an adolescent with autism spectrum disorder, transitional or serious leisure interests may be crucial for social participation and for establishing long-term personal relationships.

Throughout the intervention process, practitioners should be cognizant of clients' innate temperaments. Practitioners' expectations and style of intervention are affected by clients' temperament. People who are generally positive and easily adapt to changes in their physical status or life circumstances are likely to put a practitioner at ease and increase the practitioner's expectation of successful intervention. People who tend to have difficulty

---

EXERCISE 13.7: COMPARE LEISURE VALUES AND EXPERIENCES

Compare the leisure values and experiences of the people of all different ages that you talked to or thought about while reading and studying this chapter. What did you learn about leisure across the lifespan?

---

persevering, have typically negative states of mind and mood, or are slow to adapt to changes may be frustrating to practitioners, who may then lower their expectations of what the client and practitioner can achieve together. People who are slow to adapt to changes may also need more support at any life stage when they attempt to pursue new leisure activities.

It is critical to address clients' leisure needs, despite the pressures to address and meet their other rehabilitation needs and the high demands of the health care system. Helping clients to develop a rich and personally meaningful leisure life may facilitate their achievement of all other goals of intervention that our society values more than leisure.

Summary

Although leisure is often a second thought rather than a first and something that one may consider only after completing the required and routine activities of daily life, it can be a powerful buffer for the stresses and negative events of other occupations. Leisure can facilitate relationships and allow a person to discover a true vocation or life purpose. Through activities that help express the full emotional range in socially acceptable activities, a person is able to maintain emotional equilibrium. One can experience the benefits of leisure only by truly engaging in activities that capture one's interest and possibly even one's soul. Leisure is a challenge; it requires as much focus and energy as other human occupations. Without the active pursuit of a leisure life, free time may be a burden instead of a pleasure. It may become a time of passivity, boredom, disconnection, unhappiness, confusion, or loneliness and may thus negatively affect one's engagement and full participation in other daily occupations.

References

Aristotle. (1943). *Politics II: The treatises* (B. Jowett, Trans.). New York: Modern Library.

Baltes, P. B., & Baltes, M. M. (1990). Psychological perspectives on successful aging: The model of selective optimization with compensation. In P. B. Baltes & M. M. Baltes (Eds.), *Successful aging: Perspectives from the behavioral sciences* (pp. 1–34). London: Cambridge University Press.

Bandura, A. (2002). Social cognitive theory of mass communication. In J. Bryant & D. Zillmann (Eds.), *Media effects: Advances in theory and research* (2nd ed., pp. 121–153). Mahwah, NJ: Erlbaum.

Barth, T. (1988). Barth Time Construction. In B. Hemphill (Ed.), *Mental health assessment in occupational therapy: An integrative approach to the evaluative process* (pp. 117–129). Thorofare, NJ: Slack.

Brown, B. B. (1990). Peer groups and peer culture. In S. S. Feldman & G. R. Elliot (Eds.), *At the threshold: The developing adolescent* (pp. 171–196). Cambridge, MA: Harvard University Press.

Brown, C. A., McGuire, F. A., & Voelkl, J. (2008). The link between successful aging and serious leisure. *International Journal of Aging and Human Development, 66*(1), 73–95.

Bundy, A. C. (1997). Play and playfulness: What to look for. In L. D. Parham & L. S. Fazio (Eds.), *Play in occupational therapy for children* (pp. 52–66). St. Louis, MO: Mosby.

Campbell, A., Converse, P., & Rodgers, W. (1976). *The quality of American life: Perceptions, evaluations, and satisfactions.* New York: Russell Sage Foundation.

Carey, B. (2009, May 21). At the bridge table: Clues to a lucid old age. *The New York Times.* Retrieved from www.nytimes.com

Chess, S., & Thomas, A. (1984). *Origins and evolutions of behavior disorders: From infancy to early adult life.* New York: Brunner/Mazel.

Cotton, N. (1984). Childhood play as an analog to adult capacity to work. *Child Psychology and Human Development, 14,* 135–144.

Coyle, C. P., Lesnik-Emas, S., & Kinney, W. B. (1994). Predicting life satisfaction among adults with spinal cord injuries. *Rehabilitation Psychology, 34*(2), 95–112.

Csikszentmihalyi, M., & Larson, R. (1984). *Being adolescent.* New York: Basic Books.

Csikszentmihalyi, M., Rathunde, K., & Whalen, S. (1993). *Talented teenagers: The roots of success and failure.* New York: Cambridge University Press.

Elias, N., & Dunning, E. (1986). *Quest for excitement: Sport and leisure in the civilizing process.* New York: Blackwell.

Erikson, E. H. (1963). *Childhood and society* (2nd ed.). New York: W. W. Norton.

Everard, K. M., Lach, H. W., Fisher, E. B., & Baum, M.C. (2000). Relationship of activity and social support to the functional health of older adults. *Journals of Gerontology, Series B: Psychological Sciences and Social Sciences, 55B*(4), 208–212.

Farnworth, L. J. (2000). Time use and leisure occupations of young offenders. *American Journal of Occupational Therapy, 54*(3), 315–325.

Fine, G. A., Mortimer, J. T., & Roberts, D. F. (1990). Leisure, work, and the mass media. In S. S. Feldman & G. R. Elliot (Eds.), *At the threshold: The developing adolescent* (pp. 225–253). Cambridge, MA: Harvard University Press.

Gibson, H., Willming, C., & Holdnak, A. (2003). "We're Gators . . . not just Gator fans": Serious leisure and University of Florida football. *Journal of Leisure Research, 34*(4), 397–425.

Griffiths, M. D., Davies, M. N. O., & Chappell, D. (2004). Online computer gaming: A comparison of adolescent and adult gamers. *Journal of Adolescence, 27*(1), 87–96.

Gulick, A. (1998, July/August). Project tide. *Alert Driver,* pp. 39–43.

Henry, A. D. (1997a). *Leisure Interest Profile for Adults* (Research version 2.0). Boston: University of Massachusetts Medical Center.

Henry, A. D. (1997b). *Leisure Interest Profile for Seniors* (Research version 2.0). Boston: University of Massachusetts Medical Center.

Henry, A. D. (2000). *Pediatric Interest Profiles: Surveys of play for children and adolescents.* San Antonio, TX: Therapy Skill Builders.

Heyne, L. A., Schleien, S. J., & Rynders, J. E. (1997). Promoting quality of life through recreation participation. In S. M. Pueschel & M. Sustrova (Eds.), *Adolescents with Down syndrome: Toward a fulfilling life* (pp. 317–340). Baltimore: Paul H. Brookes.

Hultsch, D. F., Hertzog, C., Small, B. J., & Dixon, R. A. (1999). Use it or lose it: Engaged lifestyle as a buffer of cognitive decline in aging? *Psychology and Aging, 14*(2), 245–263.

Ivory, J. D. (2008). The games, they are a-changin': Technological advancements in video games and implications for effects on youth. In P. E. Jamieson & D. Romer (Eds.), *Changing portrayal of adolescents in the media since 1950* (pp. 347–376). Grand Rapids, MI: Calvin.

Jackson, J., Carlson, M., Mandel, D., Zemke, R., & Clark, F. (1998). Occupation in lifestyle redesign: The Well Elderly Study occupational therapy program. *American Journal of Occupational Therapy, 52,* 326–336.

John-Steiner, V. (1985). *Notebooks of the mind: Explorations of thinking.* New York: Harper & Row.

Karan, E. (2009, March 2). Yes, Wii can: Virtual reality in rehab. *ADVANCE for Occupational Therapy Practitioners,* pp. 29–30.

Kleiber, D. A., Larson, R., & Csikszentmihalyi, M. (1986). The experience of leisure in adolescence. *Journal of Leisure Research, 18,* 169–176.

Krane, D., & Orkis, K. (2009, February 12). *Sports and employment among Americans with disabilities.* Retrieved July 3, 2009, from www.dusa.org/pdf-files/surv/dsusa-srv09.pdf

Kraus, R. (1994). *Leisure in a changing America: Multicultural perspectives.* New York: Macmillan College.

Kubey, R. W., & Csikszentmihalyi, M. (1990). *Television and the quality of life: How viewing shapes everyday experience.* Mahwah, NJ: Erlbaum.

Labouvie-Vief, G. (1994). Women's creativity and images of gender. In B. F. Turner & L. E. Trol (Eds.), *Women growing older: Psychological perspectives* (pp. 140–165). Thousand Oaks, CA: Sage.

Larson, R., Hansen, D., & Moneta, G. (2006). Differing profiles of developmental experiences across types of organized youth activities. *Developmental Psychology, 42*(5), 849–863.

Larson, R., Mannell, R., & Zuzanek, J. (1986). Daily well-being of older adults with friends and family. *Psychology and Aging, 1*(2), 117–126.

Larson, R. W., Pearce, N., Sullivan, P. J., & Jarrett, R. L. (2007). Participation in youth programs as a catalyst for negotiation of family autonomy with connection. *Journal of Youth and Adolescence, 36*(1), 31–45.

Larson, R.W., & Verma, S. (1999). How children and adolescents spend time across the world: Work, play, and developmental opportunities. *Psychological Bulletin, 125*(6), 701–736.

Law, M., Baptiste, S., Carswell, A., McCall, M. A., Polatajko, H., & Pollock, N. (1994). *The Canadian Occupational Performance Measure* (2nd ed.). Toronto, ON: Canadian Association of Occupational Therapists.

Law, M., Baptiste, S., & Mills, J. (1995). Client-centred practice: What does it mean and does it make a difference? *Canadian Journal of Occupational Therapy, 62,* 250–257.

Leyser, Y., & Cole, K. B. (2005). Leisure preferences and leisure communication with peers of elementary students with and without disabilities: Education implications. *Education, 124*(4), 595–604.

Mann, W. C., & Talty, P. (1991). Leisure activity profile measuring use of leisure time by persons with alcoholism. *Occupational Therapy in Mental Health, 10*(4), 31–41.

Manuele, E. (1998). My rebirth. *NARHA Strides (Spirit Club News Insert), 4,* 2.

McHale, S. M., Crouter, A. C., & Tucker, C. J. (2001). Free-time activities in middle childhood: Links with adjustment in early adolescence. *Child Development, 72*(6), 1764–1778.

Modell, S. J., & Valdez, L. A. (2002). Beyond bowling: Transition planning for students with disabilities. *Teaching Exceptional Children, 34*(6), 46–53.

Morrison, M., & Krugman, D. M. (2001). A look at mass and computer-mediated technologies: Understanding the roles of television and computers in the home. *Journal of Broadcasting and Electronic Media, 45*(1), 135–161.

Morrow-Howell, N., Hinterlong, J., Rozario, P. A., & Tang, F. (2003). Effects of volunteering on the well-being of older adults. *Journals of Gerontology, Series B: Psychological and Social Sciences, 58B*(3), S137–S145.

Murphy, L. B., & Moriarity, A. E. (1976). *Vulnerability, coping, and growth: From infancy to adolescence.* New Haven, CT: Yale University Press.

Neulinger, J. (1981). *The psychology of leisure.* Springfield, IL: Charles C Thomas.

Niemela, P., & Linto, R. (1994). The significance of the 50th birthday for women's individuation. In B. F. Turner & L. E. Trol (Eds.), *Women growing older: Psychological perspectives* (pp. 117–127). Thousand Oaks, CA: Sage.

Olson, L. J. (2006). *Activity group in family-centered treatment: Psychiatric occupational therapy approaches for parents and children.* Binghamton, NY: Haworth.

Olson, L. J. (2010). Social participation frame of reference. In P. Kramer & J. Hinojosa (Eds.), *Frames of reference for pediatric occupational therapy* (3rd ed., pp. 306–348). Baltimore: Lippincott Williams & Wilkins.

Panksepp, J. (2008). Play, ADHD, and the construction of the social brain. *American Journal of Play, 1*(1), 55–79.

Parker, M. D. (1996). The relationship between time spent by older adults in leisure activities and life satisfaction. *Physical and Occupational Therapy in Geriatrics, 14*(3), 61–71.

Prevalence of health-care providers asking older adults about their physical activity levels—United States, 1998. (2002). *MMWR, 51*(19), 412–414.

Putnam, R. D. (2000). *Bowling alone.* New York: Simon & Schuster.

Quart, A. (2003). *Branded: The buying and selling of teenagers.* Cambridge, MA: Perseus.

Rowe, J. W., & Kahn, R. L. (1997). Successful aging. *Gerontologist, 37*, 433–440.

Sallis, J., Sirard, J. R., King, A. C., & Albright, C. L. (2007). Perceived environmental predictors of physical activity over 6 months in adults: Activity counseling trial. *Health Psychology, 26*(6), 701–709.

Savin-Williams, R. C., & Berndt, T. J. (1990). Friendship and peer relations. In S. S. Feldman & G. R. Elliot (Eds.), *At the threshold: The developing adolescent* (pp. 277–307). Cambridge, MA: Harvard University Press.

Schooler, C., & Mulatu, M. S. (2001). The reciprocal effects of leisure time activities and intellectual functioning in older people: A longitudinal analysis. *Psychology and Aging, 16*(3), 466–482.

Shann, M. H. (2001). Students' use of time outside of school: A case for after school programs for urban middle school youth. *Urban Review, 33*(4), 339–356.

Siegel, R. J. (1993). Between midlife and old age: Never too old to learn. In N. D. Davis, E. Cole, & E. D. Rothblum (Eds.), *Faces of women and aging* (pp. 173–185). Binghamton, NY: Harrington Park Press.

Singer, D. G., Singer, J. L., D'Agostino, H., & DeLong, R. (2009). Children's pastimes and play in sixteen nations: Is free-play declining? *American Journal of Play, 1*(3), 283–312.

Singleton, J. F. (1996). Leisure skills. In C. B. Lewis (Ed.), *Aging: The health care challenge* (3rd ed., pp. 106–125). Philadelphia: F. A. Davis.

Sloan, L. R. (1979). The function and impact of sports for fans: A review of theory and contemporary research. In J. H. Goldstein (Ed.), *Sports, games, and play: Social and psychological viewpoints* (pp. 219–262). Hillsdale, NJ: Erlbaum.

Stebbins, R. A. (2008). Right leisure: Serious, casual, or project-based? *NeuroRehabilitation, 23,* 335–341.

Steinberg, L., & Steinberg, W. (1994). *Crossing paths: How your child's adolescence can be an opportunity for your own personal growth.* New York: Simon & Schuster.

Storr, A. (1988). *Solitude: A return to the self.* New York: Ballantine Books.

Tinsley, H. E. A., & Eldredge, B. D. (1995). Psychological benefits of leisure participation: A taxonomy of leisure activities based on their need-gratifying properties. *Journal of Counseling Psychology, 42*(2), 123–132.

Whalen, C. K., Jamner, L. D., Henker, B., Delfino, R. J., & Lozano, J. M. (2002). ADHD spectrum and everyday life: Experience sampling of adolescent moods, activities, smoking, and drinking. *Child Development, 73,* 209–227.

Williams, M. S., & Shellenberger, S. (1994). *How does your engine run?* Albuquerque, NM: TherapyWorks.

Wood, D., Larson, R. W., & Brown, J. R. (2009). How adolescents come to see themselves as more responsible through participation in youth programs. *Child Development, 80*(1), 295–309.

Zillman, D., Sapolsky, B. S., & Bryant, J. (1979). The enjoyment of watching sport contests. In J. H. Goldstein (Ed.), *Sports, games, and play: Social and psychological viewpoints* (pp. 297–336). Hillsdale, NJ: Erlbaum.

Zimmer, Z., Hickey, T., & Searle, M. S. (1997). The pattern of change in leisure activity behavior among older adults with arthritis. *Gerontologist, 37*(3), 384–392.

14

Work Occupations

Anita Perr, MA, OT, ATP, FAOTA
Jane Miller, MA, OT

All work, even cotton-spinning, is noble; work is alone noble. . . .
A life of ease is not for any man, nor for any god. (Thomas
Carlyle, as cited in Beck, 1980, p. 474)

Say the word *work,* and many thoughts, both positive and negative,
come to mind. Throughout the world, people are working: Children
work during play and at school and perform chores in the home; adults
have jobs, homemaking tasks, and hobbies. Whether engaged in job seeking,
paid employment, or volunteer or retirement activities, most people work.
A job, an occupation, a vocation, a trade, employment, labor, a business, a
calling, or a pursuit—work and work-related terms are very much a part of
people's lives and vocabulary. Work implies an activity of the body, mind, or
machine or of nature itself. Usually a sustained physical or cognitive effort,
work is purposeful activity, especially when it earns one's livelihood.

Work is an area of occupation (American Occupational Therapy Association, 2008) and one aspect of occupational therapy's domain of concern.
The value of working and the type of work one chooses to do are influenced,
at least in part, by one's culture and ethnic background and by influences
from family and friends.

Briefly, work and productive activities include the purposeful activities of self-
development, social contribution, and maintaining one's livelihood. The *International Classification of Functioning, Disability and Health,* developed by the
World Health Organization (WHO; 2001), defined *work* within a broader sphere
of major life areas. This chapter includes discussion of what work is, choosing
work, doing work, clients as workers, and occupational therapists as workers.

History of Work

Throughout their history, humans have worked to gather food (albeit in current times from the neighborhood grocery store or the backyard garden),

acquire clothing and housing, defend themselves from enemies, protect territory, and raise their children. People have always engaged in these tasks and activities, frequently shared with other family or community members, out of necessity, and often for survival.

Technological advances introduced during the Industrial Revolution began to make the world of work easier in some respects and more difficult in others. The horse gave way to the automobile, and other machines performed tasks once completed by hand. Little attention was paid to the health, safety, or social conditions of the worker. Women, children, and minorities were often exploited. The plight of the factory worker, as dramatized in the writings of Charles Dickens and others, heightened the public's awareness of dangerous industrial working conditions.

Sixty percent of the U.S. working population was engaged in farming in 1850 (Morris, 1976). The agricultural production sector (farming, ranching, fishing) still employs approximately 2 million people (*Career Guide*, 2002). Air travel, the Internet, and the global market are, however, just a few of the factors influencing work today in the Information Age. Computerization and robotics have forever changed the way in which people receive, process, and use information; how they perform tasks; and how they conduct business.

Categories of Work

There are many types of work and probably just as many different ways to categorize them. Categories of work help people to narrow their choices as they decide on work interests and goals (Figure 14.1). It is important to understand that many jobs fall into multiple categories. Considerations relative to each of the categories should be accounted for when working with clients.

- Physical labor
- Cognitive work

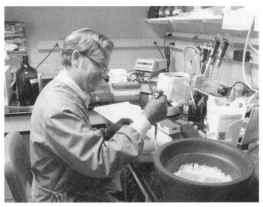

Figure 14.1. Man working in a lab.

Note. Photograph courtesy of the U.S. Geological Survey, U.S. Department of the Interior. Photo by Cathy Acker.

- Scientific work
- Artistic work
- Prestigious work
- Service
- Politics
- High- vs. low-responsibility work
- High- vs. low-paying work
- Volunteer work.

Are there other categories?

How do you categorize work? Does your approach match any in the preceding list? Are there particular settings in which different categories make more sense? When you work with different populations, do you think about work in different ways? It is important to think about all of the different ways in which people think about work—if work issues are part of your intervention, you need to be able to understand your clients' perspectives about work so that you can provide the most beneficial care.

Learning How to Work

Children are taught basic work skills and help in adult tasks as soon as they are able. In developed areas like the United States, children may often not see their parents or community engaged in remunerative work. Instead, they are permitted to spend their time at play and going to school, and their childhood games often mimic adult activities. These experiences may later affect occupational choice and work behaviors (Argyle, 1972).

Basic components of a person's work personality are established during childhood. The ability to concentrate on a task, be cooperative or competitive with peers, develop appropriate responses to authority, and understand the meanings and values associated with work and achievement will prepare the person for future work (Figure 14.2). During adolescence, teens often try out various kinds of work through home, school, and neighborhood employment. Occupational choice in modern society can include an enormous range. Several studies (Argyle, 1972; Steele & Morgan, 1991) have shown that young people are attracted to jobs that they view as congruent with their self-image or that require skills that they believe themselves to possess. By the time a person has completed formal education (e.g., high school, vocational program, college, graduate school), she or he is deemed ready to embark on a career.

The U.S. work ethic is often equated with the so-called "Protestant work ethic" (Weber, 1958). In this view, being a diligent worker indicates that one is among the elect, destined for salvation. Such ideas may permeate U.S. society, but they have probably changed over time. Work is still usually central to one's identity and establishes one's place in the community.

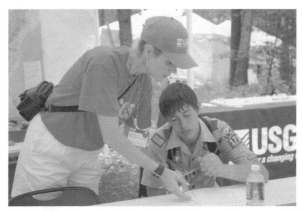

Figure 14.2. Young man learning to work in the field helps conduct a geological survey.
Note. Photograph courtesy of the U.S. Geological Survey, U.S. Department of the Interior. Photo by Tania Larso.

Trends and Forecasts in Employment

> The workplace is always in flux, always in transition, always in turmoil—It always has been, and it always will be. (Bolles, 1998, p. 11)

As a result of new technology, along with economic and political developments, the job market in various occupational fields is constantly changing. Increasing numbers of people are working at home either as wage or salaried workers or as self-employed workers. Many of these people are in white-collar occupations and use a computer for the work they accomplish at home. A 10-year projection for the U.S. workforce shows the occupations projected to have the largest growth between 2004 and 2014 to be retail salespeople, registered nurses, postsecondary teachers, consumer service representatives, janitors and cleaners, waiters and waitresses, food preparation and service workers, home health aides, nursing aides (orderlies and attendants), and general operations managers (U.S. Department of Labor, Bureau of Labor Statistics, 2005).

Unfortunately, the United States is currently in a period of high unemployment; ideas about steady growth do not seem to apply. The demographic composition of the cohort of 46- to 64-year-old workers is changing more rapidly as the baby boom generation continues to age. The projected decline in the 25- to 34-year-old group is a result of the decreased birthrates during the late 1960s and early 1970s. Service-producing industries such as health, business, social, engineering, management, and related services are expected to account for almost half of the projected growth. Health care practitioners, including technical and health care support occupations, are likely to see growth.

Occupations in the U.S. labor market are forever affected by and respond to global, societal, scientific, commercial, and legislative developments. The Balanced Budget Act of 1997, for example, has dramatically changed the employment outlook for health care providers, including occupational therapists. The health care arena has experienced mergers, downsizing, restructuring, reorganization, and consolidation. In 2002, however, the health services sector hired more workers (270,000) than any other industry (McMenamin, Krantz, & Krolik, 2003). The 2.6% growth was caused by increased demand from aging baby boomers, population growth, and technological advances.

Choosing Work

A typical college student will engage in approximately 100,000 working hours after graduating (Steele & Morgan, 1991). People's work influences their way of life—their career choices determine who their friends will be, the attitudes and values they will develop, the geographical area in which they will live, the patterns they will adopt, and how their leisure time will be spent. Work shapes and molds people's identity and gives purpose and meaning to their lives.

With all of the different possibilities for work, it can be difficult for young people to decide what type of work is best for them. For young people with disabilities, and others with disabilities who have not had job exploration opportunities, theories of career development exist that can be used to organize the process. Vocational counselors, for example, often use a selection of inventories and assessments to determine aptitudes and interests. Holland's (1997) RIASEC theory of careers is the basis for many inventories accepted today. Using a typology of personality and environments, he characterized people and their work into six groups:

1. *Realistic:* concrete and practical activity involving machines, tools, or materials
2. *Investigative:* analytical or intellectual activity aimed at problem solving or creation and use of knowledge
3. *Artistic:* creative work in the arts or unstructured and intellectual endeavors
4. *Social:* working with people in a helpful or facilitative way
5. *Enterprising:* working with people in a supervisory or persuasive way to achieve some organizational goal
6. *Conventional:* working with things, numbers, or machines in an orderly way to meet regular and predictable needs of an organization or to meet specified standards.

Holland's model provides a framework for describing what specific personal and environmental characteristics lead to satisfying and stable career decisions.

The U.S. government has a different method of classifying work. The *Guide for Occupational Exploration* produced by the U.S. Department of Labor's U.S. Employment Service (1979) groups work by the interests, abilities, and traits required for successful performance. People can identify and explore types of work that closely relate to their own skills and interests. The *Guide for Occupational Exploration* organizes data into interest areas, work groups, and subgroups. The 14 interest areas correspond to these 14 broad categories (Farr, Ludden, & Shatkin, 2001):

1. Arts, entertainment, and media (creative expression of feelings or ideas, in communicating or performing)
2. Science, math, and engineering (discovering, collecting, and analyzing information about the natural world, manipulating data, and applying technology and scientific research findings to problems in medicine, life sciences, and natural sciences)
3. Plants and animals (activities involving plants and animals, usually in an outdoor setting)
4. Law, law enforcement, and public safety (use of authority to protect people and property)
5. Mechanics, installers, and repairers (applying mechanical and electrical or electronic principles to practical situations; using machines, hand tools, or techniques)
6. Construction, mining, and drilling (assembling components of structures and using mechanical devices to drill or excavate)
7. Transportation (moving people or materials)
8. Industrial production (repetitive, concrete, organized activities in a factory setting)
9. Business detail (organized, clearly defined activities requiring accuracy and attention to detail, primarily in office settings)
10. Sales and marketing (bringing others to a point of view through personal persuasion, using sales and promotion techniques)
11. Recreation, travel, and other personal services (catering to the wishes of others, usually on a one-to-one basis)
12. Education and social services (teaching people or improving their spiritual, social, physical, or vocational needs)
13. General management and support (making organizations run smoothly)
14. Medical and health services (helping people be healthy).

Occupational therapists are listed in the medical therapy work group (14.06.01) under the broader medical and health services area (14).

EXERCISE 14.1: SELECTING A PROFESSION

Think about how you decided to enter the profession of occupational therapy. How did you discover this area of work? Did you have a role model or personal experience in this area of work? Where did you go to obtain more information? If you could, how would you have done things differently?

EXERCISE 14.2: EXAMINING VOCATIONAL INTERESTS

Read *What Color is Your Parachute* by Richard Bolles (1998). It provides excellent tips and suggestions for analyzing your vocational interests and strengths and for obtaining employment. Be sure to visit Bolles's Web site at www.jobhuntersbible.com. The site is designed to supplement his text.

Another comprehensive source for finding information about all different types of jobs is the *Occupational Outlook Handbook* (U.S. Department of Labor, Bureau of Labor Statistics, 2002). Revised every 2 years, the volume describes approximately 250 occupations and their associated job tasks and working conditions, the education and training needed, and anticipated job prospects and earnings. The Internet version is available at www.bls.gov/ oco. First published more than 60 years ago, the *Dictionary of Occupational Title Codes* (DOT; U.S. Department of Labor, U.S. Employment Service, 1991) has been replaced by (and incorporated into) an updated, Internet-based comprehensive database of worker attributes and job characteristics named the Occupational Information Network, or O*NET (U.S. Department of Labor, Employment and Training Administration, 2003; see Figure 14.3). The eight-digit O*NET code identifies each unique occupation within the related occupational group and according to worker functions. Now also

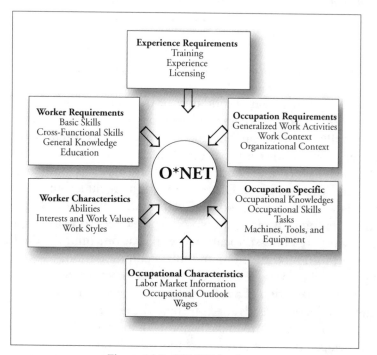

Figure 14.3. O*NET database.

available in a Spanish version, the O*NET is continually updated with occupational information and labor market research. The direct link to the O*NET database is http://online.onetcenter.org/.

Case Scenario 14.1: Defining Occupational Therapy—How Is an Occupational Therapist Described in the Occupational Outlook Handbook?

Occupational therapists (O*NET 29-1122.00, DOT 076.121-010) work in one of the fastest growing occupations. Employment in occupational therapy is projected to increase faster than average as a result of a rapidly aging population and increased demand for therapeutic services (Farr, 2003). Both the print and Web-based versions elaborate on both the pros and the cons of particular occupations. For example, the job of occupational therapy can be tiring because therapists are on their feet much of the time, and those therapists employed in home health may spend hours driving to and from appointments. Occupational therapists also face job-related hazards such as back strain from lifting clients and equipment. Required qualifications include patience, strong interpersonal skills to inspire trust and respect, ingenuity, and imagination in adapting activities and environments. Occupational therapists are increasingly taking on supervisory roles, and more than one-third work part-time. Explore the O*NET description of occupational therapy yourself, and use the Skills Search option to see whether your skills and abilities match the profession.

Role of Occupational Therapy in Work and Work Activities

Historically, work has been a modality of treatment rather than the goal of treatment. "Occupational therapy took root in a rich soil of work activities for the mentally ill. In the early 1920s, the first occupational therapists documented steps for a uniform program of curative activity" (Marshall, 1985, p. 297). Today, work and work activities are used as both the treatment approach and the end goal. These applications include but are not limited to work-related games for children; welfare-to-work, work-hardening, and work-conditioning programs; transition from school to work; supported employment; work readiness; vocational exploration; injury reduction; stress management; tool modification; and job accommodation.

Occupational therapists are uniquely qualified to synthesize information for the design and implementation of a safe work environment; they are able to establish appropriate productivity levels for homebound, sheltered, modified, or competitive work, and they are able to implement tool or job site evaluation and modification. The therapist develops and guides job-specific programs of graded activity for the worker; performs job task analysis and work station and tool modification;

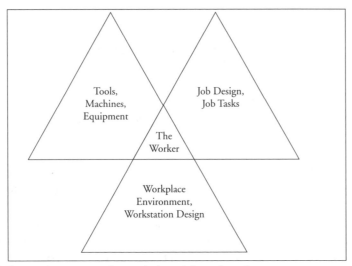

Figure 14.4. Interactions among the workplace, job, and worker.

Note. From "Ergonomics and the Occupational Therapist," by E. R. Smith. In S. Hertfelder and C. Gwin (Eds.), *Work in Progress: Occupational Therapy in Work Programs*, p. 129. Copyright © 1989, by the American Occupational Therapy Association. Reprinted with permission.

and identifies and remediates behaviors inappropriate to the work environment. The benefits to the worker, employer, and the work environment include increased productivity, decreases in worker's compensation claims and lost workdays, prevention or reduction of injury, and psychosocial benefits to the client.

Occupational therapists may collaborate with professionals who specialize in ergonomics. *Ergonomics,* the science of work, is the matching of human abilities and capabilities and job requirements within the context of the physical and social work environment. Also known as *human factors* or *human engineering,* ergonomics interacts closely with other applied and life sciences such as engineering, medicine, and psychology to preserve health, prevent injury, and maximize work efficiency. The role of ergonomics in rehabilitation is in the redesigning of the external environment to accommodate the worker with disabilities or injuries, thereby enabling each person to contribute fully and independently (Smith, 1989; see Figure 14.4). In disability prevention, ergonomists examine human factors relevant to the job, human capabilities, and the man–machine interaction or interface under given environmental conditions. *Ergonomic design* is the application of this knowledge to tool, machine, system, job, and environmental design for safe, comfortable, and effective human use. Ergonomists are often engineers (e.g., safety and mechanical) and therapists (e.g., physical and occupational) who have undergone specific educational experiences.

Examining the Workplace and the Worker

Job analysis and worker evaluation is a multiphase process: job description (which includes an objective record of the job and its components, similar to those in the DOT or O*NET), task or job analysis (which includes evaluation of selected tasks or activities in terms of human demands such as vision, hearing, cognitive processes, and muscle recruitment), and identification of worker capabilities. These phases do not always proceed in a neat or orderly sequence.

Activity analysis is at the core of conducting a job analysis evaluation. The process of job analysis examines the physical demands; cognitive factors; specific tasks, tools, and machines used; the environment; and the work's psychological and physical hazards. These techniques may be used to conduct a job evaluation: interviews with employer and employee(s), questionnaires, observation and photographic documentation (still photos and videocamera recording), anthropometric data collection, and functional and specific work assessments. Potentially hazardous or inadequate work habits, equipment, and environmental factors are noted. After analysis of the data, recommendations are offered to (1) reduce risk of work-related injury; (2) provide workers with guidelines for safe, efficient task completion; and (3) suggest possible workstation modifications.

A functional capacity evaluation is used to determine a person's level of physical ability to perform basic work tasks. This protocol may be submitted in litigation, preemployment screens, and return-to-work and work capacity evaluations. Tasks such as lifting, pulling, pushing, and climbing are measured, and numerous standardized and nonstandardized assessments are available for this purpose.

CASE SCENARIO 14.2: TYPICAL OFFICE WORKER

According to the U.S. Department of Labor's U.S. Employment Service (1991) and Bureau of Labor Statistics (2002), the job title of *administrative secretary* (O*NET 43-6011.00, DOT 169.167-014) involves the physical demands of sedentary work (maximum lift of 10 pounds) and the abilities to talk, hear, reach, handle, finger, and feel. A limited amount of walking, standing, and carrying of light objects is required. The worker must be able to extend the arms in any direction, seize, hold, grasp, turn, pick, pinch, and perceive size, shape, temperature, or texture of objects. Working conditions are inside (75% or more, with protection from weather conditions but not necessarily from temperature changes).

This job title involves overseeing and carrying out office operations, . . . and applying clerical skills . . . including planning own or others' work programs, using reasoning, using hands and fingers in typing, . . . and recording data, obtaining and safeguarding confidential information . . . recognizing and proofing copy to correct errors in spelling, grammar, and punctuation, speaking distinctly . . . and making decisions involving . . . policy (U.S. Employment Service; Bureau of Labor Statistics, 2002).

The administrative secretary, a 52-year-old woman with a 2-year employment history with Happy Socks Unlimited, was interviewed regarding her job tasks, responsibilities, and work-related health concerns. She has a below-average sick time usage (i.e., fewer than half of the allotted 12 days per year). Absences are usually because of seasonal allergies and sinus headaches. During periods of high keyboarding activity, she reports stiffness in the neck, pain accompanying neck rotation to the right, radiating pain down both arms, and nocturnal numbness and tingling in both hands.

The administrative secretary oversees the general functioning of the office and supervises full- and part-time clerical personnel. The specific job duties and tasks can be categorized as follows:

- Cognitive tasks
  - Gathers and develops information
  - Stores and retrieves information
  - Reads
  - Proofreads and edits
  - Calculates and analyzes data
  - Orders supplies
  - Inspects supplies and compares invoices
  - Plans and schedules
  - Makes decisions.
- Social tasks
  - Answers and uses the telephone and routes calls
  - Confers and meets with people
  - Works with other people.
- Physical tasks
  - Stores and retrieves documents and files
  - Writes with pen, pencil, or marker
  - Handles mail
  - Collates and sorts
  - Photocopies documents
  - Types documents from handwritten drafts or typed matter
  - Maintains calendar
  - Maintains or conducts minor repairs of equipment (e.g., fixes paper jams in photocopier, loads paper, changes printer toner)
  - Uses equipment (e.g., pencil, computer, photocopier, printer, telephone).

(continued)

Case Scenario 14.2: (cont.)

The physical demands, consistent with the O*NET/DOT description, include

- Standing
- Walking
- Sitting (75% of the time, sedentary work)
- Lifting and carrying (light objects less than 10 lb.)
- Reaching and grasping
- Handling and fingering
- Stair or step climbing (infrequently)
- Balancing, stooping, and kneeling (infrequently)
- Communicating (talking)
- Hearing
- Vision (near, mid-range, far; visual accommodation; color vision).

Anthropometric measurements were taken with a tape measure using the guidelines and standards listed in Grandjean (1988). These external body dimensions (e.g., standing height, forward reach, arm span, foot to popliteal length) were compared with group norms. A goniometer was used to measure range of motion. Hand strength, specifically grasp and pinch, were measured using a dynamometer and pinch gauge. A full upper-extremity evaluation was completed, and overall coordination, sensation, and functional abilities were assessed. The evaluation confirmed that the worker was within normal limits in all areas (for people of similar age and gender).

Work sampling was then conducted. The secretary was seated at her desk in an upright posture, and the computer, monitor, and printer were switched on. The task of keyboarding a brief memorandum from a two-page, handwritten draft was analyzed in detail. The steps included

1. Taking the draft out of the "to-do" box on the desk or receiving draft from the originator or courier;
2. Putting the draft on the copy stand;
3. Selecting the word-processing icon (software loads);
4. Creating a document file;
5. Inputting via typing on keyboard and mouse clicking;
6. Proofreading, editing, and spell-checking the document;
7. Clicking on the print icon;
8. Possibly needing to walk to the printer location, retrieve the paper from the storage bin, and load paper;
9. Walking to the printer location and retrieving the document;
10. Completing final proofreading; and
11. Putting the finished memorandum in the "out" box.

Time studies were conducted to determine the approximate hourly keystroke rate. Using a keyboarding assessment, three trials were completed.

The documents produced were well formatted; error free; and edited for content, style, spelling, and grammar. The secretary's preferred rate allowed for simultaneous conversation with others and did not appear to result in any physical complaints. If the workload warranted, she was able to perform two to three times faster than this rate; however, upper-extremity problems usually resulted from prolonged exertion.

The work site is housed in a newly renovated facility. The space includes company offices, secretarial areas, reception, and storage. A fully equipped lounge with kitchen area (e.g., sink, refrigerator, microwave oven, coffee–hot water system, table, and chairs) is available for mealtime and snacks. Accessible restrooms are located in the building.

Secretarial workstations contain standard office desks, lateral filing cabinets, shelving, an adjustable desk chair, and guest chairs. All enclosed offices are soundproof within an acceptable level. Except for the hallways, kitchen, restrooms, and storage areas, all floors are carpeted. The heating, ventilation, and air conditioning (HVAC) system is reportedly a source of irritation: It is noisy and drafty at certain locations and does not regulate the temperature well throughout the office. The secretary usually sits 24 inches (61 centimeters) from her monitor and maintains a viewing angle of 18°. Seat height, back angle, elbow angle, keyboard, and screen height are also within acceptable ranges.

Findings and recommendations: Overall, the flexibility inherent in the secretary's job allows her to pace her work. Although the work site is not perfect (e.g., HVAC system) and job demands are more stressful at times, it is usually manageable. Her capabilities and task–work requirements are normally balanced. These suggestions were made to further enhance performance, reduce work-related injury, and increase worker comfort:

- Modify the workstation by adding task lighting, a keyboard wrist rest, an angled adjustable footrest (and clearing the area under the desk to allow for more leg room), and a chair mat; changing shelf spacing and improving the arrangement of work materials; and changing the desk, if possible, to a reduced length, rounded D-shaped work surface.
- Reduce repetitive components, as much as possible, by incorporating varied job tasks, increasing freedom of motion in the workstation area (by ridding the area of nonessential storage material), taking frequent "microbreaks" (stretch and exercise periods), and use auto-suggestive techniques to relax body during activity.
- Encourage the worker to avoid excessive extension, flexion, and deviation of the wrist and constrained postures.
- Encourage the worker to vary and alternate tasks to reduce the sedentary work.

(continued)

CASE SCENARIO *14.2: (cont.)*

- Maintain comfortable environmental temperature and relative humidity; minimize static electricity and drafts.

Epidemiological Approach

An epidemiological study of a work-related disease is subject to inherent difficulties related to providing evidence of causality (WHO, 1989). Causative factors often have a complex etiology and are influenced by confounding variables such as lifestyle, work habits, and individual capabilities (Figure 14.5). A disorder requiring a long exposure time or repeated injuries such as repetitive strain injury (RSI) are more difficult to identify with a specific work activity and onset. The Person–Environment Fit Model, based on McGarth's work (Van Harrison, 1978), depicts the tenuous balance (often an imbalance) between job demands and the person's ability to satisfy those demands (see Table 14.1). The National Institute for Occupational Safety and Health, the federal agency that provides recommendations to prevent work-related illness and injury, agrees that exposure to stressful working conditions can have a direct influence on worker safety and health. Psychological and physiological strain results when demands and

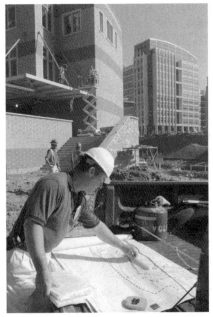

Figure 14.5. Context of work influences performance and the person's ability to deal with it.
Note. Photograph courtesy of the Public Health Image Library, Centers for Disease Control and Prevention. Photo by Greg Knobloch.

Table 14.1. Job Conditions That May Lead to Stress

Conditions	Characteristics	Examples
Design of tasks	Heavy workload; infrequent rest breaks; long work hours and shift work; hectic and routine tasks that have little inherent meaning, do not use workers' skills, and provide little sense of control	David works to the point of exhaustion. Theresa is tied to the computer, allowing little room for flexibility, self-initiative, or rest.
Management style	Lack of participation by workers in decision making, poor communication in the organization, lack of family-friendly policies	Theresa needs to get her boss's approval for everything, and the company is insensitive to her family needs.
Interpersonal relationships	Poor social environment and lack of support or help from coworkers and supervisors	Theresa's physical isolation reduces her opportunities to interact with other workers or receive help from them.
Work roles	Conflicting or uncertain job expectations, too much responsibility, too many "hats to wear"	Theresa is often caught in a difficult situation in which she tries to simultaneously satisfy the customer's needs and the company's expectations.
Career concerns	Job insecurity and lack of opportunity for growth, advancement, or promotion; rapid changes for which workers are unprepared	Since the reorganization at David's plant, everyone is worried about their future with the company and what will happen next.
Environmental conditions	Unpleasant or dangerous physical conditions such as crowding, noise, air pollution, or ergonomic problems	David is exposed to constant noise at work

Note. From "Stress at work" by U.S. Department of Health and Human Services, National Institute for Occupational Safety and Health, 1999, Publication No. 99-101.

abilities are ill matched (U.S. Department of Health and Human Services, National Institute for Occupational Safety and Health, 1999; Van Harrison, 1978; see Figures 14.6 and 14.7).

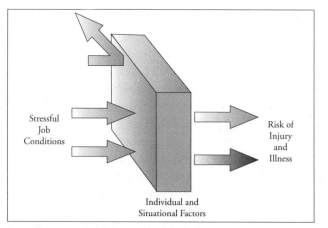

Figure 14.6. National Institute for Occupational Safety and Health model of job stress.
Note. From *Stress at Work*, by the National Institute of Occupational Safety and Health, U.S. Department of Health and Human Services (Pub. No. 99-101), 1999, p. 8.

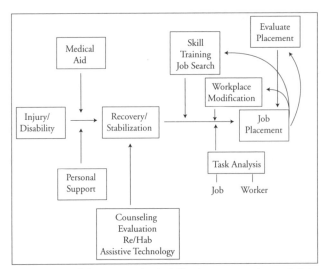

Figure 14.7. Habilitation and rehabilitation process in work injury.

CASE SCENARIO 14.3: WORK-RELATED INJURIES

Workers in food-processing, health services, manufacturing, and craft industries have long suffered work-related injuries secondary to repetitive, manual exertion. The rise of the computer in the workplace has introduced another source of work-related concerns. The work of a computer keyboard user may involve rapid, repetitive movements of the upper extremities and static loading (i.e., wrists and shoulders held in same position for extended periods). *RSI,* also known as *cumulative trauma disorder, occupational overuse syndrome,* or *repetitive motion disorder,* is a generic label given to a variety of painful and debilitating soft-tissue conditions believed to be caused by repetitive movements of the hands or arms. Activities such as stooping; sedentary work; constrained postures; and biophysiological factors such as physical size, strength, fitness, range of motion, and work endurance are thought to contribute to RSI. Psychological stressors from the job structure (e.g., scheduling, machine pacing), job content (e.g., time pressures and overload, underload, lack of control), and organization (e.g., role ambiguity, competition) can further compound the situation with anxiety, dissatisfaction, psychogenic illness, and absenteeism. A variety of conditions, many ill defined, make up RSI. Tenosynovitis, shoulder pain, neck tension, tendonitis, and carpal tunnel injury are but a few of the many musculotendinous conditions included in this disorder. People often list many complaints such as tenderness, pain, swelling, cramping, and tingling sensations.

Health in the Workplace

In the United States, more than 39 million people are hospitalized or receive emergency services for accidental injuries. More than 3 million people sustain disabling injuries on the job (Fitzgerald, 2002). Escalating costs from loss of productivity, absenteeism, retraining, and medical and disability insurance have pushed the concern for a healthy worker and a healthy work environment into the spotlight. The switch from a traditional approach of treating illnesses to a health maintenance or preventive medical approach is taking hold. The role of the employees' health services has become more comprehensive in many settings. In addition to providing medical care, industrial safety, and compliance with state and federal regulations, the employer may provide the following:

- Preplacement examinations (baseline medical profiles protect both the company and the worker);
- Periodic health and medical surveillance exams (preventive, early detection screens; Figure 14.8);
- Return-to-work and disability management (prevent accidents, reinjury, or spread of illness; proper care and rehabilitation to minimize duration of injury); and

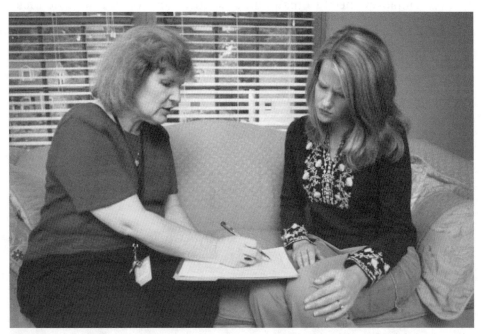

Figure 14.8. Employees' health services provide periodic health and medical exams.

Note. Photograph courtesy of U.S. Department of Agriculture, National Resources Conservation Service.

- Wellness and fitness programs (promote fitness; e.g., smoking cessation, general nutrition, weight reduction, and stress reduction).

Lower health care costs and absenteeism accompany prevention, which can be achieved through environmental protection in the workplace, safety education of workers and managers, the application of appropriate and safe work practices, and the application of basic ergonomic principles (Figure 14.9; WHO, 1989).

Work injury management and prevention is a multidisciplinary effort (Isernhagen, 1995). Medical, legal, vocational, and insurance professionals and employers and employees must communicate and cooperate to safeguard the worker and prevent job-related injuries. Work evaluation consists of evaluation of the injured worker (or potential worker), the type and method of work performed, and the employee's unique capabilities and interests. Each professional contributes to the worker's success at the work site: the rehabilitation team of occupational therapists, physical therapists, the vocational counselor, the physician, and the psychologist. Depending on the situation, occupational health and safety engineers, industrial psychologists, ergonomists, kinesiologists, personnel and human resources staff, attorneys, insurance adjustors, and workers' compensation judges may also be involved in the return-to-work process. It is therefore vital that the resulting documentation be readable, devoid of jargon or highly technical wording, and understandable to a wide audience. To ensure competitiveness in the world market, employers need to maintain a healthy workforce. Providing ongoing safety training and timely rehabilitation of sick and injured workers are sound practices.

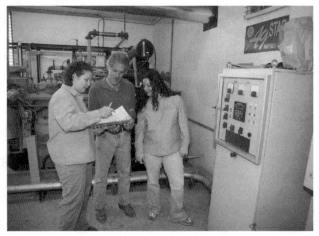

Figure 14.9. Scientists working in the lab to ensure safe working conditions.

Note. Photograph courtesey of U.S. Department of Agriculture, National Resources Conservation Service. Photo by Jeff Vangua.

CASE SCENARIO 14.4: THE TIRE FACTORY WORKER

An injured factory worker experienced a lumbosacral sprain, right knee sprain, and reported ringing in the ears. On inspection, it was noted that the factory had continuous, high-volume background noise and a slight (but noticeable) floor vibration.

Job description: The job involved identifying and marking defective tires being transported through the area by an overhead carrier, which was accomplished partly by sight and partly by touch while walking slowly behind the moving tire. Workers also removed surplus rubber left by the molding process with a sharp knife. Rejected tires were removed from the overhead carrier and placed in wheeled carts for reprocessing. The job required standing and walking throughout the work shift. Lifting a tire, weighing approximately 30 to 45 pounds, was required once every 4 to 5 minutes.

Conclusions: The lifting requirements were in excess of the worker's capabilities and likely to exacerbate his back condition. Prolonged standing and walking combined with floor vibration were likely to worsen both the knee and the back. Because of a high noise level, communication with coworkers was difficult and caused stress. It was recommended that the worker be considered for alternate employment. This job and work site environment has numerous conditions affecting other workers such as constrained work postures, uneven work rate, and vibration. A thorough ergonomic evaluation was recommended.

Compliance With State and Federal Regulations

The Occupational Safety and Health Act of 1970 established the Occupational Safety and Health Administration (OSHA) under the U.S. Department of Labor to "disseminate and enforce safety and health standards to protect employees at work" (Career Information Center, 1990, p. 55). Places of employment should be free from recognized hazards. A work site with 11 or more employees is mandated to maintain records of work-related injuries and illness and to provide medical surveillance and protective equipment. Specifically, the employer must identify chemical, physical, biological, and ergonomic hazards in the workplace. Medical monitoring for exposure to toxic elements such as asbestos, noise, and lead must be offered along with protective equipment: safety shoes, helmets, safety glasses, respirators, and hearing protectors.

Hazard communication, or right-to-know compliance, enacted by OSHA in 1983 further requires that all employers notify workers if they are exposed to or in contact with hazardous materials. All hazardous chemicals must be identified and labeled. Material safety data sheets must be obtained from the manufacturer or supplier. These technical bulletins describe a chemical and its characteristics, health and safety hazards, and precautions. Employees must receive training in the safe handling of the chemical.

OLDER WORKERS

Increasing life expectancy, low birth rate (which has reduced the number of younger replacement workers available), and an aging labor force are changing the age composition of the workplace. The Age Discrimination in Employment Amendments of 1986 abolished the mandatory retirement age. These amendments safeguard the older worker (older than age 40) from age-based distinctions in hiring, salary, promotions, and training. Cost projections of retirement for the individual worker and society are staggering. Legislative actions and policies are being proposed and implemented to extend one's working career. Some programs include

- Expansion of work opportunities and alternative work schedules via job redesign, phased retirement, job sharing, and part-time jobs;
- Legislation to outlaw age discrimination in employment;
- Retraining and second (third, etc.) career opportunities;
- Subsidized employment; and
- Pension reform for raising age of eligibility.

Physical changes inevitably occur with age. Because work capabilities vary, every older worker should be evaluated individually. Functional capacity and the ability to perform tasks or physiological activities may decline with age. However, productivity may not decline with age. Decision-making abilities are enhanced by life experiences, although reaction time slows with age. The older worker tends to be less apt to engage in risk-taking behavior (resulting in lower accident rates). Intellectual functioning does not appear to be altered with age but rather by perception, attention, health status, and motivation.

WORKERS WITH DISABILITIES

Work site accessibility involves a person's ability to overcome barriers to arrive at his or her workstation. A common simplified assumption is to equate accessibility issues only with wheelchair use. Many issues may restrict access, such as reduced endurance for walking, visual impairment, amputation, incontinence, hearing loss, difficulties with interpersonal communication, and worker–peer attitudes. Successful job placement is dependent on surmounting all barriers along relevant access routes (see Figure 14.10).

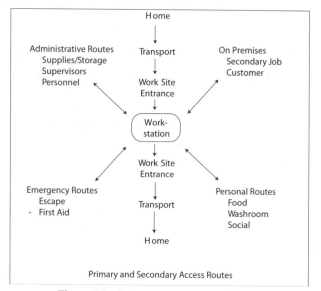

Figure 14.10. Access routes to work site.

Workstations designed to enhance user capabilities contribute to user comfort, motivation, and productivity. Poor design can result in fatigue, discomfort, and stress. Matching the worker with the job and the site often involves making changes to current conditions. Work site analysis involves identifying jobs and workstations that contain, cause, or pose risk factors for hazards. This analysis includes identification of symptoms, especially musculoskeletal, and associated risk factors such as awkward posture, repetitiveness, sustained exertions, extreme temperatures, and vibration.

Job modification via changing job assignments, tools, or the work environment to eliminate risk factors can prevent injuries and eliminate hazards. Specific strategies include alterations in method or strength required to complete the task; location and position of equipment or tools; speed or frequency; and ambient factors such as light, noise, and air quality. Common workstation changes include those in layout, seating, and handling of materials that promote neutral postures and adjustability. Training and education of employees and management staff in principles of ergonomics and safety is an effective means of preventing injury and facilitating a safe working environment.

Addressing work integration is not limited to a person's physical ability to perform the job but also to his or her ability to meet its cognitive and social demands. The work site assessment should therefore also include these factors. It may be important to identify the amount and type of supervision provided or available. It might also be important to know the physical layout of the workplace so that the social implications may be understood.

CASE SCENARIO 14.5: CLIENT WITH A CLOSED-HEAD INJURY

You are working with a client who sustained a closed-head injury 8 months ago. He has regained most of his physical, cognitive, and social abilities through inpatient and outpatient rehabilitation. He is still easily distracted, and when he becomes overwhelmed, his cognitive skills deteriorate. In your outpatient clinic, you work together to refine the skills needed for his work in a publishing company where he will be inserting advertisements into a newsletter. The ads have to be placed in the correct section of the newsletter. When you perform the work site assessment, you realize that all of the employees work in an open space to foster communication and a sense of camaraderie. You quickly realize that your client may become overwhelmed. What are some solutions to this situation? How would you make suggestions that might benefit your client?

Technology at Work

With increased use of computers and automation equipment in many industries, assistive technology can be applied to increase ease of use. Some of these tools may be as simple as a glare protection screen on a computer monitor to minimize visual fatigue, a large monitor to increase character size in proportion to monitor dimensions, and voice recognition software to eliminate the need for keyboard data entry. Once thought to be costly or impossible dreams, today's computer systems (hardware and software) incorporate many energy-efficient and accessible features. The use of robotic aids for people with disabilities has many benefits: cost-effectiveness (lessening dependence on attendant care), improved reliability (always available), and increased environmental control and quality of life. Robotic aids, such as a robotic arm, can be used in a workstation. A worker with no or limited arm function can control the robotic arm via switches (e.g., puff-and-sip, chin control, eye gaze).

Making Changes in the Workplace

Accommodation refers to the application of ergonomic principles to maximize the capabilities of all users and thus provide an optimal interface. The Job Accommodation Network (n.d.; www.jan.wvu.edu/) is a federally funded operation that assists employers in accommodating workers with disabilities. The network also provides information about the employability of people with disabilities.

The Americans With Disabilities Act (ADA), signed into law on July 26, 1990, is perhaps the most far-reaching piece of legislation of its time. The ADA's protection applies primarily but not exclusively to people with disabilities (i.e., those with a current or prior history of a physical or mental impairment that substantially limits one or more major life activities). Intended to make society more accessible, the law has five specific parts: (1) employment (must provide reasonable accommodations such as modifying equipment or restructuring jobs), (2) public services, (3) public accommodations, (4) tele-communications, and (5) a miscellaneous category prohibiting retaliation against those with disabilities. The employment title of the ADA requires that people with disabilities be considered in all aspects of work, including hiring and maintaining jobs, as would any other employee. The ADA states that a person should be considered in terms of his or her abilities to perform the job with or without reasonable accommodations.

During the hiring process, employers cannot ask about a potential employee's disabilities. Instead, employers must talk about the job in terms of its require-ments, usually identified as the job's essential functions. The determining factors for deciding what is an essential function include things such as the amount of training required to do the task, the number of other people able to perform the task, and how relevant that task is to the overall operation of the work site.

The potential employee is responsible for asking for the accommodations he or she needs. It is the employer's responsibility to determine what is reason-able. The decision is usually based on the cost relative to the company's overall assets and the impact the accommodations would have on other workers and the overall flow of work. Ideally, the communication between the worker and the employer is open, and disagreements are settled by compromise. If this is not the case, mediation or legal intervention may be necessary.

The occupational therapist is well qualified to target many areas of em-ployment. For instance, occupational therapists' expertise in task analysis and synthesis allows them to work with an employer to develop specific job descriptions that include the essential and secondary functions. In another capacity, occupational therapists may work with clients in preparation for specific jobs in a therapeutic or clinical setting.

Summary

The performance area of work is a significant aspect of occupational therapy's scope of practice. Work activities include an infinite number of purposeful ac-tivities, which occupational therapists and occupational therapy assistants use as part of interventions. For many clients, the ultimate goal of occupational ther-apy intervention is to allow them to return to work or to engage in vocations

References

Age Discrimination in Employment Amendments of 1986, Pub. L. 99592, 100 Stat. 3342.

American Occupational Therapy Association. (2008). Occupational therapy practice framework: Domain and process (2nd ed.). *American Journal of Occupational Therapy, 62,* 625–683.

Americans With Disabilities Act of 1990, Pub. L. 101–336, 42 U.S.C. § 12101.

Argyle, M. (1972). *The social psychology of work*. New York: Taplinger.

Balanced Budget Act of 1997, Pub. L. 98–473, 111 Stat. 251.

Beck, E. M. (Ed.). (1980). *Bartlett's familiar quotations* (15th ed.). Boston: Little, Brown.

Bolles, R. N. (1998). *What color is your parachute? A practical manual for job hunters and career-changers*. Berkeley, CA: Ten Speed Press.

Career guide to America's top industries: Essential data on job opportunities in 42 industries (5th ed.). (2002). Indianapolis, IN: JIST Works.

Career Information Center. (1990). *Employment trends and master index* (4th ed.). Mission Hills, CA: Glencoe.

Farr, J. M. (2003). *America's fastest growing jobs: Detailed information on the 141 fastest growing jobs in our economy* (7th ed.). Indianapolis, IN: JIST Works.

Farr, J. M., Ludden, L. L., & Shatkin, L. (2001). *Guide for occupational exploration* (3rd ed.). Indianapolis, IN: JIST Works.

Fitzgerald, P. (2002). The forensic chiropractic examiner: Duties and professional opportunities—Part 1. *Dynamic Chiropractic, 20*(13).

Grandjean, E. (1988). *Fitting the task to the man: An ergonomic approach*. London: Taylor & Francis.

Holland, J. L. (1997). *Making vocational choices: A theory of vocational personalities and work environments* (3rd ed.). Odessa, FL: Psychological Assessment Resources.

Isernhagen, S. J. (Ed.) (1995). *The comprehensive guide to work injury management*. Gaithersburg, MD: Aspen.

Job Accommodation Network. (n.d.). Retrieved April 3, 2008, from www.jan.wvu.edu/

Marshall, E. (1985). Looking back. *American Journal of Occupational Therapy, 39*, 297–300.

McMenamin, T., Krantz, R., & Krolik, T. J. (2003, February). U.S. labor market in 2002: Continued weakness. *Monthly Labor Review*, 3–25. Retrieved from www.bls.gov/opub/mlr/2003/02/art1full.pdf

Morris, R. B. (Ed.). (1976). *United States Department of Labor bicentennial history of the American worker*. Washington, DC: U.S. Government Printing Office.

Occupational Safety and Health Act of 1970, Pub. L. 91-596, 84 Stat. 1590 (29 U.S.C. 651 *et seq.*).

Smith, E. R. (1989). Ergonomics and the occupational therapist. In S. Hertfelder & C. Gwin (Eds.), *Work in progress: Occupational therapy in work programs* (pp. 127–155). Bethesda, MD: American Occupational Therapy Association.

Steele, J. E., & Morgan, M. S. (1991). *Career planning and development for college students and recent graduates*. Lincolnwood, IL: VGM Career Horizons.

U.S. Department of Health and Human Services, National Institute for Occupational Safety and Health (1999). *Stress at work* (Pub. No. 99-101). Cincinnati, OH: Publications Dissemination, Education, and Information Division.

U.S. Department of Labor, Bureau of Labor Statistics. (2002). *Occupational outlook handbook, 2002-2003 edition, Bulletin 2540*. Washington, DC: U.S. Government Printing Office. Retrieved November 25, 2003, from www.bls.gov/oco/

U.S. Department of Labor, Bureau of Labor Statistics. (2005, December 22). *Occupations with the largest job growth, 2004–14, The Editor's Desk*. Retrieved June 1, 2009, from www.bls.gov/opub/ted/2005/dec/wk3/art04.htm

U.S. Department of Labor, Employment and Training Administration. (2003). *O*NET—Beyond information—Intelligence*. Retrieved November 25, 2003, from www.doleta.gov/programs/onet

U.S. Department of Labor, U.S. Employment Service. (1979). *Guide for occupational exploration*. Washington, DC: U.S. Government Printing Office.

U.S. Department of Labor, U.S. Employment Service. (1991). *Dictionary of occupational titles* (4th ed., rev.). Lanham, MD: Bernan Press.

Van Harrison, R. (1978). Person–environment fit and job stress. In C. L. Cooper & R. Payne (Eds.), *Stress at work* (pp. 175–205). Chichester, England: Wiley.

Weber, M. (1958). *The protestant ethic and the spirit of capitalism*. New York: Scribner's.

World Health Organization. (1989). Epidemiology of work-related diseases and accidents. In *Tenth report of the Joint ILO/WHO Committee on Occupational Health* (Technical Report Series 777). Geneva: Author.

World Health Organization. (2001). *International classification of functioning, disability and health*. Geneva: Author.

15

⬦

Self-Care Occupations

Anita Perr, MA, OT, ATP, FAOTA

In this chapter, I focus on the things people do to take care of themselves. As a group, these things are called by many names: *activities of daily living (ADLs), daily living skills, basic activities of daily living, instrumental activities of daily living (IADLs), self-care skills or activities* and, recently, *occupations of daily living.* This chapter provides a framework with which one can organize evaluations of a person's self-care and design appropriate interventions for a person who has difficulty with self-care. Finally, you are asked to examine your own thoughts about ADLs related to the specific activities and your occupations.

A focus on daily life activities is part of the history of occupational therapy. Early in this history, the focus was on the importance of habits and habit training. Eleanor Clarke Slagle developed programs of habit training for people with social and psychiatric conditions. Her focus included self-care and other routine activities.

A focus on ADLs goes into and out of vogue in occupational therapy. Often, it is difficult for occupational therapists and occupational therapy assistants who feel the need to defend their profession to focus on such commonplace activities. These commonplace activities, however, make up a large part of everyone's lives. The importance of ADLs is identified in both the *Occupational Therapy Practice Framework: Doman and Process* (2nd ed.; AOTA, 2008) and the World Health Organization's (WHO's; 2001) *International Classification of Functioning, Disability and Health* (*ICF*). I use both of these paradigms in this chapter to organize the discussion of ADLs.

The focus on a person's ability to engage in self-care activities is a great service of occupational therapy. Self-care activities are fundamental to human existence and affect people's ability to function. By addressing ADLs with clients, occupational therapists influence the daily lives of those they serve.

People's specific routines vary by gender, ethnicity, age, and many other factors. These differences, or preferences, should be addressed in treatment. As the field of occupational therapy further explores the terms *occupation, activity*, and *task*, it makes sense to think about ADLs in these terms as well. At the most basic level, one can look at the category of self-care as the occupation. If occupation can be thought of as a collection of activities, then, one can think of the various components of self-care as activities. In this paradigm, the activities are things such as combing hair, sexual expression, brushing teeth, toileting, and eating. The way each person puts the activities of self-care together becomes the occupation and is grounded in personal meanings.

Two people, Grace and Jon, serve as case examples throughout this chapter. Grace and Jon lead very different lives and have different habits, preferences, values, and needs. Their occupational profiles illustrate the various aspects of ADLs that occupational therapists and occupational therapy assistants can address. The case scenarios are divided into parts and placed throughout the chapter. Each part is associated with the specific discussion. Only certain aspects of Grace's and Jon's lives are shared in this chapter. Each of their therapists would have learned this information during evaluations and ongoing intervention. Additionally, because the relationship between the client and the occupational therapist may be long term, it may change over time, and the client may share different bits of information at different stages of the relationship.

CASE SCENARIO 15.1, PART 1: GRACE

Grace is a 45-year-old woman who underwent surgery to repair a brain aneurysm. During the surgery, the aneurysm bled, resulting in a hemorrhagic stroke. The result is that she is hemiparetic on the right side. She has flaccid paralysis of the right upper extremity. Grace is right-hand dominant. Although the right lower extremity has some areas of abnormal tone and weakness, Grace is able to ambulate for about 10 ft on level surfaces without using an ambulation aid, such as a cane. She also has mild memory impairment and mildly limited executive cognitive functions.

CASE SCENARIO 15.2, PART 1: JON

Jon is a 16-year-old boy who broke his right arm while skateboarding. He has compound fractures of the humerus (midshaft) and of the ulna and radius. An external fixator is in place at the humerus. Internal fixators, plates, and screws are in place in the forearm. Jon is right-hand dominant.

CASE SCENARIO 15.1, PART 2: IMPORTANT ADL FOR GRACE

When meeting Grace, her occupational therapist was struck by her precise dressing and grooming. By Grace's report, it is important that she "look well put-together." Prior to her stroke, she wore her hair in long braids, which she braided herself. She jogged 1 to 3 miles at least three times a week. She showered each morning before leaving for work. An important occupation was cooking, during which she attended to nutritional advice and enjoyed the challenges of preparing dinner for others. Grace did not drive but used buses and subways daily, usually for more than just her trip to and from work.

CASE SCENARIO 15.2, PART 2: IMPORTANT ADL FOR JON

Jon is a social teenager who spends a great deal of time getting ready to go out with friends. He works at looking well groomed and dressing in the same way as do his friends and their role models, mainly hip-hop artists. Jon reports that he has great difficulty putting gel in his hair and getting it to look the way he wants to since breaking his arm. Jon showers at school after his gym class three times weekly. During his evaluation, Jon revealed that he is uncomfortable dressing and undressing after gym class. He works out about four times a week, primarily lifting weights and working to improve his physique, but he calls himself scrawny. He does not want his classmates to see that he is skinny. He thinks he looks like a little kid and does not understand why he is not bulking up like most of the other teens he is friendly with. Jon has no interest in cooking or preparing meals. His mother prepares meals at home for the whole family. Jon buys lunch in his school cafeteria.

Contextual Factors

Everything takes place within a context. Changing the context changes the activity. Context includes *external factors,* those that are outside the person, that influence function. When disability is discussed, the impact of the contextual factors may be magnified. Contextual factors need to be identified during the evaluation and included during the intervention. Some contextual factors are facilitators and help the person perform the task. Think about a person with limited hand function. Imagine that this person uses a dresser with large knobs for drawer pulls. Because the drawers have large knobs, the person can open them. The design of the dresser facilitates function.

Some contextual factors, however, are barriers and limit or prevent performance. Imagine the same person with a dresser whose drawers have narrow grooves carved them in to act as handles. Here, the person is unable to open the drawers and therefore needs help. As one can see, contextual factors affect people's abilities. By understanding the contextual factors, the therapist is better able to prioritize treatment and determine what is important for each individual client. The context includes both environmental and personal factors.

ENVIRONMENTAL FACTORS

Environmental factors can be further subdivided into physical, social, and attitudinal environments. During the intervention, the therapist uses environmental facilitators to improve participation in ADLs and addresses the environmental barriers to alleviate or lessen their impact. The closet shown in Figure 15.1 was previously an environmental barrier. Initially, only one rod hung in the closet, the higher one. The man in the photo could not reach into the closet from his wheelchair to get his clothes. He installed the second rod and moved the clothing that he wears the most frequently to that rod. Now it is easy to get to the clothing he

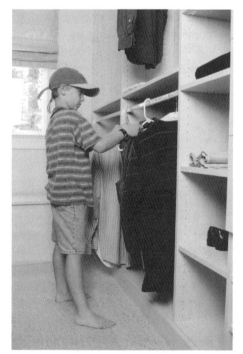

Figure 15.1. Clothes closet with a second rod is no longer an environmental barrier. The second rod is now an environmental facilitator.

Note. Photo courtesy of the Public Health Image Library, Centers for Disease Control and Prevention, Center for Universal Design.

usually wears. If he needs to retrieve an item from the upper rod, he uses a reacher.

CASE SCENARIO 15.1, PART 3: PHYSICAL ENVIRONMENT FOR GRACE

Grace lives in a studio apartment in a large East Coast city. The apartment is on the second floor, up a flight of 18 steps. The building has no elevator. Grace sleeps on a waterbed that is against the wall at the head and left side. She has a small closet in which she keeps the current season's clothing and outerwear. She also has a small dresser for undergarments. Grace's bathroom is very small. The only storage space she has in the bathroom is a small medicine cabinet over the sink. She has a clawfoot bathtub with a shower extension attached to the tub spout.

CASE SCENARIO 15.2, PART 3: PHYSICAL ENVIRONMENT FOR JON

Jon lives in the suburbs, about 2 hr from the city in which Grace lives. He lives in a two-story, four-bedroom house in which all of the bedrooms are on the second floor. Jon shares a bedroom with his 14-year-old brother. He sleeps on the bottom bunk. Jon keeps his clothes folded in dresser drawers or hung on hooks or hangers in a closet, but he reports that his room is usually messy, and he usually finds the clothes he wears on the floor or on a chair. The bathroom that Jon most frequently uses for his morning routine is shared by four children. It has a stall shower. As previously stated, Jon usually showers at school and says this is because if he showers at home there may not be enough hot water for his siblings.

CASE SCENARIO 15.1, PART 4: SOCIAL ENVIRONMENT FOR GRACE

Grace is engaged to be married about 6 months from the time of her surgery. She has no immediate or extended family nearby with the exception of her fiancé, Tony. Grace has four or five close friends with whom she spoke and spent time about five times a week prior to her stroke. Since then, they have visited regularly in the hospital and it is expected that they will remain supportive and be available to help Grace. She is very pleasant, although somewhat quiet. She has many acquaintances at work, in her gym, and at church. Grace does not have pets. Before this incident, Grace had never had any medical problems. She sees her physician annually.

CASE SCENARIO 15.2, PART 4: SOCIAL ENVIRONMENT FOR JON

Jon lives with his mother, father, and three brothers. His extended family lives in nearby states and in Taiwan. The family in the area gets together regularly. He has cousins with whom he is very friendly. Jon has a group of about 15 close friends from school. The catchment area for the school is large, and none of these boys live near Jon. Jon has one neighborhood friend: the boy next door who is about 2 years younger. His school friends do not know about his neighborhood friend because Jon is afraid his friends will tease him for being friends with a younger boy.

CASE SCENARIO 15.1, PART 5: ATTITUDINAL ENVIRONMENT FOR GRACE

Grace values her social and economic independence. Although she is very much in love with Tony, they both plan to continue to spend time with their own friends pursuing their own interests in addition to building new friendships and developing new pursuits together. She belongs to a church in her neighborhood, attends services regularly, and participates in other church activities. She met Tony during a fund-raising activity that the church sponsored. Graces enjoys yoga and meditation and is learning about Eastern religions. She celebrates her African heritage, celebrates Kwanzaa, and plans to "jump the broom" at her wedding.

CASE SCENARIO 15.2, PART 5: ATTITUDINAL ENVIRONMENT FOR JON

Jon's family is generally conservative in their political views. Jon views his family as too traditional and boring. He says that they are sometimes worried about him because he "tends to be more wild." His family is Catholic, but they do not regularly attend church or actively practice religion. Jon and his friends tend to use curse words when they are with each other, but Jon does not curse when near family members. Jon's family values education, and he is expected to go to college after graduating from high school.

EXERCISE 15.1: THINK ABOUT ENVIRONMENTAL FACTORS

In these profiles, what are the physical, social, and attitudinal facilitators and barriers to participation in ADLs for Grace and Jon? Think about your own life. What are the environmental facilitators and barriers? How do you use the facilitators? How do you deal with the barriers?

PERSONAL FACTORS

Personal factors also are contextual and include age, gender, social status, life experiences, and so on. It is easy to see that the ADLs of a 3-year-old differ from those of a teenager, which differ from those of an adult, which further differ from those of an older adult. The young child may be focusing on dressing himself or herself, wearing clothing with elastic waists and shoes with hook-and-loop closures. Most teens have mastered grooming and dressing and focus on conforming to some model. Teens may also be more focused on other activities like learning to drive or managing their own bank account. Gender-specific and sexual activities are also important activities and occupations for teenagers. Sex, an often-ignored daily life activity or occupation, is extremely important for adolescents and young and mature adults. Adults may focus on housekeeping. Older adults may have different responsibilities. If they live in a retirement community, they may not have the responsibility for lawn and garden care and may have time to focus on other responsibilities and interests.

CASE SCENARIO 15.1, PART 6: PERSONAL FACTORS FOR GRACE

At 45, Grace cannot believe that she is middle aged, does not like to think about it, and does not want to think about getting older. She is African-American and grew up in a small southern town. She has lived on her own since high school. She earned an undergraduate degree and a master of business administration degree from a prestigious New England university. Her fiancé, Tony, is Brazilian and not yet a U.S. citizen. The couple have been involved for 3 years. Grace says that their love life is healthy, that they have sex regularly, and that they are both very caring and compassionate. She says that she likes to experiment a little more than he does. Grace currently works for a small business importing gift items from Africa. She loves to travel.

CASE SCENARIO 15.2, PART 6: PERSONAL FACTORS FOR JON

Jon is a 16-year-old Asian-American. He attends high school, where his grade-point average is 2.42. He and his male friends often skip school. He has lived his entire life in the same home. He has slept over at friends' houses but not for more than 1 night consecutively. Jon does not have a girlfriend and is extremely hesitant to talk about close personal relationships. Jon says that he is not sexually active.

Functioning and Disability

All people participate in activities and occupations. The assortment and variety of activities and occupations varies from person to person. As previously established, contextual factors influence people's ability to participate. Other factors influence participation as well. The structural make-up of a person's body provides him or her with a capacity to do something. When an impairment of body structures exists, a person's body functions may be hindered. When body functions are hindered, participation is limited. Using *ICF* (WHO, 2001) terminology, these difficulties are referred to as *participation restrictions* and *activity limitations*. Body functions and body structures can be compared with the component level of the third edition of the *Uniform Terminology for Occupational Therapy* (AOTA, 1994).

CASE SCENARIO 15.1, PART 7: BODY STRUCTURE FACTORS FOR GRACE

Grace suffered a left parietal lobe infarct during the surgery to clip an aneurysm. She presents with muscle imbalance in the trunk and extremely low tone in the right arm. She has spotty decreased strength in her right leg.

CASE SCENARIO 15.2, PART 7: BODY STRUCTURE FACTORS FOR JON

Jon suffered multiple fractures in his right arm and has an external fixator in place for 5 to 7 weeks. He also uses a sling and bolster to support his arm when standing. Jon's arm should also be raised and supported when he is seated, but he says that he is usually not able to do this. Open wounds exist at the pin sites where the external fixator protrudes from his arm.

CASE SCENARIO 15.1, PART 8: BODY FUNCTION FACTORS FOR GRACE

Since the neurologic insult, Grace has become quieter and now perceives herself as shy. She also complains that she does not know how people will react or whether she will be able to follow the nuances of conversations. She is somewhat downhearted about her condition and her impending wedding. Her motivation fluctuates from day to day. She tends to be sleepy most of the time and cannot tell whether it is from the new medication because she "just feels crummy." She has mild short-term and long-term memory impairment and mild impairment of high-level cognitive functions. Sensory functions are intact. Grace has a mild balance impairment in standing and mild to moderate impairment in endurance.

CASE SCENARIO 15.2, PART 8: BODY FUNCTION FACTORS FOR JON

Jon's mental and sensory functions are intact and age appropriate.

Evaluation and Intervention

To help a client become more independent in ADLs, it is important to complete a thorough evaluation. A comprehensive evaluation identifies the areas of limited participation and how disability limits participation. The most reliable information is learned by performing the activity in its usual environment, but this is frequently impossible to do. Therapists who work in home-based practice have the advantage of using the client's own environment and materials during the evaluation and the intervention. In most situations, however, the evaluation and intervention do not take place in the usual environment. An alternative is to have the person perform the activity using the real tools, such as his or her own clothing or toothbrush, in a simulated setting like a hospital room or an area of an occupational therapy clinic. Care should be taken to bring as much of the usual environment into the evaluation and intervention context, including taking into account the client's values and beliefs and his or her roles and responsibilities. The evaluation should capture all of this.

Some facilities use their own ADL evaluations; some use tools that are commercially available. The evaluation the therapist uses should allow him or her to collect information about self-care, mobility, IADLs, caring for others, and other personal self-management tasks (see Box 15.1). The evaluation should include a reliable and valid rating scale. Some rating scales use words to describe performance, such as *independent, moderate assistance,* and *dependent.* The ICF uses the qualifiers *no problem, mild problem, moderate problem, severe problem,* and *complete problem* (WHO, 2001). Other ADL evaluations use a numeric scale, such as one ranging from 1 to 7, that delineates levels of independence. The preference for the type of rating scale is up to the evaluator as

Box 15.1. Evaluation Categories

Self-Care Activities	**Mobility**	**IADLs**
Sexual expression	Transfers	Housekeeping
Toileting	Mobility	Money
Bathing	Indoors	management
Grooming and	Home	Caring for others
hygiene	Community	Other
Dressing	Transportation	
Other	Other	

Note. IADLs = instrumental activities of daily living.

EXERCISE 15.2: EVALUATION

Before moving on to intervention, think about Grace and Jon and perform an imaginary evaluation on them. What areas of ADLs are going to be limited? What are the causes for the limitations? Are they body structures? Body functions? Contextual factors?

---

long as the measure is identified and the descriptions make sense for the people who are evaluated and for the environment in which they are evaluated.

The evaluation should also have the capacity to include information that is not actually performed. At times, therapists must rely on reports from the client, the client's family, and others involved in the client's care. This information should be labeled *by report* or similarly to differentiate it from information gained through observation.

Intervention

Occupational therapists and occupational therapy assistants provide intervention to increase a client's ability to participate in activities, in this case, ADLs. Areas of disability should be addressed during intervention. Interventions are developed to remedy impairments in body structures and body functions, to maximize facilitating contextual factors, and to eliminate or lessen barriers. The evaluation will help to identify the problem areas. Once the evaluation is completed, the next step is to identify the priorities because it may be impossible to address everything. Setting priorities helps the therapist and client focus on the most critical areas to target first. Client preferences should strongly influence the priorities for intervention; safety is even more important than client preference. Although safety is often the client's highest priority, there are instances in which the client does not identify problems in judgment and safety awareness. The prevalence of falls in older people, for instance, may be caused in part by an inability to recognize potential hazards. A client may say to a practitioner that the first thing he or she wants to work on is ironing clothes. The practitioner, however, recognizes that because of the impairments to body structures, such as those present after a spinal cord injury, the client cannot reach or use the emergency call bell in the hospital room. Everyone should be able to call for help if he or she needs it, which means that the first ADL task addressed for most hospitalized patients is using the call system to call a nurse. Frank discussions between the client and the therapist may help both parties to identify goals based on the same priorities.

EXERCISE 15.3: ADL PRIORITIES FOR GRACE AND JON

What are the ADL priorities for Grace and Jon? Are there safety concerns? First, list as many problems as you can. Then put the list in order of priority. Why did you set them as priorities? Thinking about that rationale really helps therapists to develop comprehensive treatment programs.

One ADL task that needs to be addressed with Jon is cleaning the pin sites on his arm. If these sites are not kept clean, infections can develop, slowing his recovery and perhaps leading to further disability. Jon may or may not be mature enough to realize the threat of infection, but one of the first things the therapist should do is discuss this with Jon and his parents. The first ADL priority for Jon may be washing and drying his right arm, caring for the sling and bolster, and addressing issues of positioning in sitting and standing. Did you think of that?

CASE SCENARIO 15.1, PART 9: GRACE'S PRIORITIES

Grace is having a difficult time dealing with the changes that she is undergoing. The stress of her upcoming wedding and the possibility that she may still have residual disabilities at that time sometimes overwhelms her. Through conversation, Grace and the occupational therapist decide that addressing her depression must start immediately and must pervade every other treatment activity. Other priorities are learning to swing her arm when walking and holding objects in both hands. Again, in planning for her wedding, Grace focuses on wanting to be able to carry her bouquet. In addition, she wants to dress, bathe, and groom herself so that she does not have to rely on others to help her. Improving her ability to complete ADLs independently is especially important to her because she knows how particular she is in her self-care and thinks that others are bothered by her idiosyncrasies.

CASE SCENARIO 15.2, PART 9: JON'S PRIORITIES

Jon identified as a priority being able to put gel in his hair. The therapist talked with Jon and explained the importance of wound care in healing. Jon agreed to make wound care a top priority. The therapist also talked to Jon about toileting. Jon was embarrassed and admitted that he did not use the bathroom at school because it was so difficult. After discussing it with the therapist, Jon agreed that working on toileting was a higher priority than hair care. When you did the exercise, did you identify toileting as a priority?

What are the limitations that affect Jon's ability to use a bathroom independently? What about Grace's ability to manage toileting by herself? Jon and Grace may both need to work on one-handed techniques and dominance retraining to manage lower-extremity garments and to clean themselves after toileting. Jon's therapist asked about the pants he likes to wear, and Jon decided to put away his button-fly jeans until his arm heals. He chose to use alternative clothing rather than use an alternative technique to button the buttons or a button aid or other adaptive device to help with the task. Jon also said that he was going to switch to boxer shorts because briefs are too difficult for him to manage with one hand. If the therapist had not addressed toileting, Jon may not have developed compensatory strategies for this activity. Grace preferred not to change the type of clothing she likes to wear. Instead of wearing sweat pants with an elastic waist, she learned to use a button aid and zipper pull to fasten her pants after toileting.

Activities are rarely addressed individually. Most activities occur in combinations. Although the focus for both Grace and Jon was toileting, dressing had to be addressed as well. This illustrates a common occurrence in occupational therapy practice settings: Single treatment sessions frequently address multiple problem areas and multiple goals.

WHERE TO START

In many instances, it makes the most sense to start intervention at the level of body structure and body function. By improving the status of the structure, performance of ADLs is improved. If this is the case, it is important for the therapist to discuss the relation of the body structure to the performance of ADL. Clients may then be better able to articulate the relationship between individual intervention activities and the goals and activities with which they are associated. This generalization of learning helps the client participate in activities more fully.

Therapists make the choice of which approach to treatment to use on the basis of the client, the limitation, the environment, and all the other factors influencing participation. With ADLs, the intervention is usually based on some combination of improving function and compensating for disability that cannot be changed. The compensation usually comes in two forms: (1) changing the strategy used to complete the activity or (2) adding adaptive equipment or technology. In Figure 15.2, notice that the client is using a universal cuff to hold the toothbrush. Because of paralysis after a spinal cord injury, he is unable to hold his toothbrush in the usual way. Although he tried alternate handling methods during treatment, he and his therapist determined that using the universal cuff was the easiest and most effective way for him to hold his toothbrush. The client uses adaptive equipment to compensate for his inability to hold the toothbrush from weakness caused by paralysis.

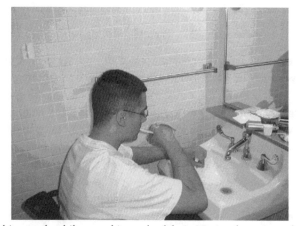

Figure 15.2. Brushing teeth while seated in a wheelchair. Notice the universal cuff on the young man's right hand into which the toothbrush is placed. Additionally, lever faucets make it easier to set water force and temperature.

USE THE INFORMATION GAINED DURING THE EVALUATION

Body structure information tells the occupational therapist about diagnosis. The anatomical structure, including the presence and extent of impairment, sets the stage for occupational therapy intervention. It is easy to see that a person with missing body parts may have difficulty performing ADLs or will perform ADLs using an alternative technique. The same is true for impairment of any body structure. During the evaluation, the extent of the impairment is identified, and the expected recovery is determined. Goals are set according to the expected recovery and the expected ability of the person to compensate for any residual impairment.

Related to body structures are body functions. How is the person able to function within the confines of the extent of impairment in any of the body structures? Occupational therapists and occupational therapy assistants focus their intervention at this level. Practitioners use purposeful activities to heal body structures and improve body functions.

Both Grace and Jon will use alternative techniques to complete their ADLs. Part of the intervention for both clients may include training in upper-extremity range-of-motion exercises. To have the potential for the highest level of independence, both Jon and Grace need to maintain the structural integrity of their arms to allow them to use their arms as fully as possible when they are able.

As stated earlier, the evaluation also provides information about the contextual factors affecting a client's participation in ADLs. How so? Think about how the physical environment could influence participation. The person pictured in Figure 15.3 has been paralyzed for many years and has always dressed himself independently. Recently, however, he started using an alternating pressure mattress to decrease the pressure over his bony promi-

---

CASE SCENARIO 15.1, PART 10: GRACE'S INTERVENTION

Because Grace had a hemorrhagic stroke during surgery, there is no way to know how much of the blood will be reabsorbed or how much residual damage there will be. The expected recovery of the neurologic system is not known. Brain function may come back as the blood is reabsorbed and the swelling resolves. Associated areas of the brain may take over for the damaged areas. The therapist may have difficulty knowing how much recovery will occur in Grace's flaccid right arm and in her cognitive functioning. Grace's overall program is designed to allow medical recovery of body structures to occur. Occupational therapy intervention will include purposeful activities to attempt to improve Grace's ability to use her right arm. She will learn alternative techniques, such as using her left arm to put her right arm in a position to act as a stabilizer when, for example, stabilizing her toothbrush while applying toothpaste with her left hand. Treatment also focuses on performing ADLs and other standing activities to improve Grace's balance and motor control.

CASE SCENARIO 15.2, PART 10: JON'S INTERVENTION

Jon has a mostly temporary disability. In all likelihood, the bones will heal. He should recover fully, although a chance exists that he will have limited mobility in his forearm, affecting his ability to supinate and pronate. Jon also is at risk for developing infection at the wound sites.

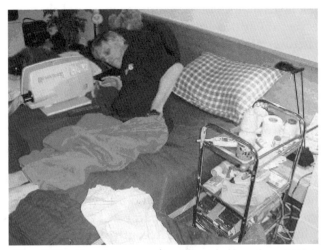

Figure 15.3. Dressing on an alternating pressure air mattress.

nences after flap surgery for a Stage III pressure ulcer. The softness and dynamic qualities of the alternating pressure mattress have made it nearly impossible for him to position himself stably and move to dress himself. The solution was to fully inflate the mattress and stop the alternating airflow while he dresses his lower extremities and performs transfers. The motor for the alternating pressure mattress is next to him on his bed, and he can manage the switch independently.

In Figure 15.4, a young man uses an alternative technique to hold a pen. He weaves the pen in between his fingers and uses tenodesis to hold the pen tightly. This technique allows him to write with enough force to see the ink. He prefers this method to using an adaptive device because he can use any pen or pencil available and does not have to remember to carry another piece of equipment with him.

CASE SCENARIO 15.1, PART II: GRACE'S SUMMARY

Grace is now on a rehabilitation unit in an acute care hospital and is likely to stay for about 3 weeks before she goes home. This environment is not similar to her home because Grace lives in a small apartment.

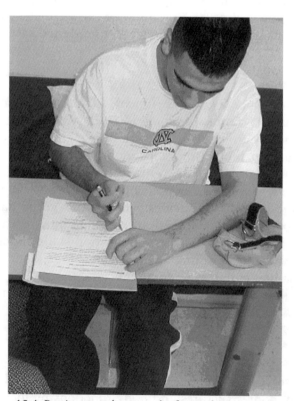

Figure 15.4. Pen is woven between the fingers for stronger control.

CASE SCENARIO 15.2, PART II: JON'S SUMMARY

Jon is treated in an outpatient occupational therapy setting. This environment is also not similar to his home because Jon lives in a large single-family house.

How will you develop your interventions to be meaningful for Grace and Jon? How can you simulate their home environments in an inpatient or outpatient clinic? Therapists process these concepts to develop interventions that will be the most useful. There are many other factors to think about. Age and gender influence the types of activities the practitioner brings into treatment. They may also influence the client's priorities. Even though Grace is a female adult and Jon is a male adolescent, both have stated that hair care is high on their list of priorities.

Other personal factors will also influence the focus of treatment and the purposeful activities used during intervention. It would be important, for example, to know that a client is a vegetarian so that cooking activities will include ingredients that the client will eat. It is just as important to know whether the person has dietary restrictions related to religion or, for that matter, because of personal taste and preferences. Tying personal factors to body functions and structures, a practitioner can see that a client wears dentures or has dysphagia and would prefer soft food that is easy to manage.

GROUP VS. INDIVIDUAL TREATMENT

Many facilities encourage group treatment. ADLs can be addressed very effectively in groups. A common example is the existence of self-feeding groups in many facilities. A group of clients with dysphagia may eat together, with a speech–language pathologist, occupational therapist or occupational therapy assistant, or nursing assistant available for cuing and assistance. Routine participation in a grooming group may be effective in helping a client with mental illness resume these activities. This routine group daily life activity uses Slagle's concept of rebuilding routines and allows each participant to develop and refine interpersonal communication skills and appropriate social behaviors. Whether working on interpersonal interactions and relationships, domestic life, mobility, or communication, a cooking activity can be developed to allow each member to work on his or her individual goals.

Summary

Good ADL intervention gets the most bang for the buck. The practitioner can treat many body structures and body functions by focusing on the activities of daily life. Identify the factors that influence the person's ability to participate in ADLs. Make the most of the factors that facilitate participation, and figure out ways to lessen the impact of those that are barriers. The end result should be the highest level of independence or the highest degree of participation in the ADL that you address.

References

American Occupational Therapy Association. (1994). Uniform terminology for occupational therapy (3rd ed.). *American Journal of Occupational Therapy, 48,* 1047–1054.

American Occupational Therapy Association. (2008). Occupational therapy practice framework: Domain and process (2nd ed.). *American Journal of Occupational Therapy, 62,* 625–683.

World Health Organization. (2001). *International classification of functioning, disability and health, short version.* Geneva: Author.

16

Care and Caregiving: Implications for Occupational Therapy

Kristine Haertl, PhD, OTR/L

Humans are social beings who give and receive care throughout the course of life, sharing in daily activities while working to create meaning and satisfaction. From the arrival of a newborn to the passing on of a valued elderly grandparent, we rely on one another to survive and thrive in the world. Consider a mother raising a toddler, a health practitioner looking after a dying patient, a sister babysitting for a developmentally disabled brother, and spouses caring for one another. All these examples encompass acts of care and caregiving. In this chapter, I present an overview of care and caregiving and examine the role of the occupational therapist in working with clients and families to assess and develop caregiving skills.

Care and Caregiving

The terms *care* and *caregiving* are often referred to in relation to one person taking care of another, as in a mother caring for a child or a daughter looking after an elderly parent. Although such cases are typical of caregiving relationships, *care* and *caregiving* are much broader terms, encompassing the care of humans and of plants and animals and in some contexts including the care of self. Interestingly, definitions for the term *care* often include descriptions such as "concern for" or "anxiety about" others. *Merriam Webster's Online Dictionary* (2009) defines care as "suffering of mind," "a disquieted state of mixed uncertainty, apprehension and responsibility," and "painstaking or watchful attention." Yet characterizations such as "regard coming from desire or esteem" are also used in relation to care. Additional descriptions of *care* include words and phrases such as "concern about," "protection," and "affection for" (*Collins Essential English Dictionary*, 2009). Thus, definitions of *care* are often dependent on the context in which the term is used.

453

Leininger (1988b) differentiated between general care and professional care. She defined *care* and *caring* as "those assistive, supportive, or facilitative acts toward or for another individual or group with evident or anticipated needs to ameliorate or improve a human condition or lifeway" (p. 9). *Professional caring* was defined as "those cognitive and culturally learned action behaviors, techniques, processes or patterns that enable (or help) an individual, family, or community to improve or maintain a favorably healthy condition or lifeway" (p. 9). Key commonalities in the definitions of *care* and *caring* generally transcend the feelings associated with the terms and generally focus on the actions required for caregiving.

Caregiving, with the root word *care*, refers to the process of providing care for another. Generally, the concept of *caregiver* refers to the person who provides the primary care and support to a person (Awad & Voruganti, 2008), yet definitions vary on the basis of culture, context, and formal vs. informal caregiving. Typically, one person is the caregiver and the other the care receiver, yet in many instances the role of caregiver may change. For example, a mother and father care for a child, but later in life the roles may change as the child takes care of an aging parent. Caregiving may also occur temporarily during instances of brief illness or disability, such as when a teenager requires extra care for a broken bone sustained in a ski accident or a sibling requires extra care during a bout of the flu.

A review of the literature reveals conceptualizations of caregiving that include both formal paid caregiving and informal unpaid caregiving; a nurse, home health aide, or occupational therapist may provide formal paid care, whereas a person may take care of a relative or friend in an informal and unpaid context. Drentea (2007) defined *caregiving* as "the act of providing unpaid assistance and support to family members or acquaintances who have physical, psychological, or developmental needs." She identified three forms of care: (1) instrumental, (2) emotional, and (3) informational. *Instrumental caring* includes facilitation of tasks that need to be done such as cooking or providing transportation for a loved one. *Emotional caring* involves providing support, emotional assistance, counseling, and emotional companionship. Finally, *informational caring*, a key type found in health care, may include education, adaptation of the environment, or training in compensatory techniques.

Although care and caregiving are related concepts, they are not identical. The term *care* is often used primarily to denote emotional feelings, affection for, and concern for the well-being of another. *Caregiving*, however, encompasses the actions and occupations required to meet the daily needs of another. According to Sachs and Labovitz (2004), *caregiving* may embody aspects of caring, yet one may care for another without providing the actual daily caregiving, as in the instance of an elderly relative living at a long-term-care (LTC) facility. Similarly, a person may take on a formal caregiving role in a health care setting, yet not have the same affection for the client as would a family member or friend. It is, however, advantageous if the care-

---

EXERCISE 16.1: CAREGIVER AND CARE RECEIVER ROLES

Identify the primary roles and occupational activities you have taken on as caregiver and care receiver in your life. Answer these questions: How have these roles changed over the course of time? Consider your daily schedule and occupational demands. Do the roles of caregiver and care receiver have a prominent place, or do other occupational roles such as being a student require most of your time? Do you have competing responsibilities and caregiving roles that create role conflict? How can you work to balance your roles? How will your experiences as a caregiver and care receiver affect you as an occupational therapist?

---

giver maintains an unconditional positive regard and has sincere concern for the well-being of the person being cared for.

CAREGIVING AND HUMAN OCCUPATION

Who are caregivers, and what are their roles and functions? Although context greatly influences the nature of caregiving, across Western cultures there are many similarities. Statistics cited by the National Family Caregivers Association (n.d.) indicate that more than 50 million Americans care for a disabled, ill, or aging family member in any given year. Of caregivers, 30% are seniors themselves (U.S. Department of Health and Human Services, 2001), and unpaid family members will likely continue to be the largest provider of LTC services (U.S. Department of Health and Human Services, Assistant Secretary for Planning and Evaluation, et al., 2003). Although most caregivers are female (Levine, 2001; Zukewich, 2003), people of all ages, genders, and sociocultural backgrounds may be called on to take on caregiving roles. Although the term *caregiving* is often used in relation to providing assistance for elderly people or a person with a disability or temporary illness, caregiving also includes taking care of infants, children, and even plants and animals.

The process of caregiving is relational and involves both those giving care and those receiving care (Figures 16.1 and 16.2). Bumagin and Hirn (2001) identified primary care recipients as including young children, teenagers, people with temporary or permanent disabilities, and elderly people. Although there may be a primary relationship between caregiver and care receiver (such as a mother taking care of an infant), caregiving may also involve complex coordination of relationships such as a special needs child receiving services from multiple academic and health services agencies. Within these situations, the role of primary caregiver may often change, and communication between caregivers is crucial to provide comprehensive client-centered care.

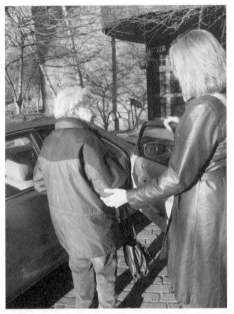

Figure 16.1. Caregiving roles may shift over time. In this setting, a well elderly 92-year-old woman is assisted by her daughter for transportation needs.

Case Scenario 16.1: John

John is a 7-year-old child with moderate mental retardation, cerebral palsy, fetal alcohol syndrome, and oppositional defiant disorder. His biological mother was a drug user and abandoned him at birth, and his father's identity is unknown. John has lived in various foster care homes throughout his life. Because of recent assaultive behaviors, he was placed in a crisis home and is currently receiving services through the home, school, and county.

Who are the caregivers in this situation? Are they formal or informal caregivers? What can be done to facilitate the coordination of care in this instance?

In the example of John, the nature of caregiving is formal and complex. John has lived in several foster homes and receives care for his basic physical, cognitive, emotional, and academic needs. The role of primary caregiver in a parental relationship is easily defined, whereas in John's situation it is far more complex because the staff at the crisis home, the case manager, and the special education professionals all have unique roles in John's care.

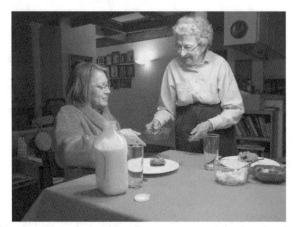

Figure 16.2. Within the same relationship, the woman cared for her daughter during a recent illness.

The occupational tasks of caregiving and care receiving may be categorized on the basis of the relationship and the informal vs. formal nature of the care provided. Lackey and Gates (2001) classified caregiving for a family member with illness into four broad categories: (1) provision of personal care, (2) provision of medical care, (3) provision of household care, and (4) spending time (emotional care) with the person. *Personal care* includes tasks such as assistance with bathing, grooming, dressing, and feeding. *Medical care* includes the daily activities that assist a person in meeting medical needs such as wound care or medication administration. *Household care* includes assistance with daily tasks such as cooking and cleaning, and *emotional care* provides support by spending time with, talking to, or praying with the care receiver. As previously discussed, Drentea's (2007) categorizations differ in broadening the scope to include instrumental, emotional, and informational tasks. Perhaps one of the most comprehensive conceptualizations of caregiving is that of Janelle Sellick (2005), who identified six domains of wellness that are crucial to both the caregiver and the care receiver. Sellick asserted the importance of maintaining wellness within the caregiver–care receiver relationship in these six domains: (1) physical (e.g., physical needs, fitness, nutrition, lifestyle, health and medical), (2) emotional (e.g., feelings expression, control of stress, problem solving, self-efficacy), (3) social (e.g., relational; respect for self and others; interaction with the environment; people, pets, community; social cause), (4) spiritual (e.g., purpose in life, morals and ethics, self-determination, love, hope, faith), (5) intellectual (e.g., lifelong learning, cognition, exploration), and (6) vocational (e.g., skill development, work, volunteerism, personal interests). Consideration of each of these domains of well-being for both the caregiver and the care receiver is crucial to enhancing quality of life and the caregiver–care receiver relationship.

EXERCISE 16.2: PRIMARY CAREGIVING

Consider your own life course. Who have been your primary caregivers in each of the preceding domains? Notice how in some situations there may be role differences (e.g., in the intellectual domain, a teacher may have played a key role but was not considered a formal caregiver). Which domains have relied more heavily on other people, and which have required self-care and self-determination? As an occupational therapist, how would you ensure that each of the domains is addressed for your clients?

GENDER AND CULTURAL INFLUENCES

The roles and functions of caregiving and the development of caregiving skills are heavily influenced by gender and culture. From people's early years, they learn about themselves and their environment by using their caregivers as role models. These models are usually their parents (Figure 16.3). The nature of the caregiving relationship may be positive, marked by mutual affection, or it may be strained, as in the instance of a child growing up with an abusive or alcoholic parent.

Yet, regardless of the circumstances, parents are generally the socializing agents for gender roles within society (Leaper, 2002). Parents often treat children differently on the basis of gender, for example, through the way they dress their children or the toys they give to them. The blending of gender roles has occurred over time, as evidenced, for example, in the increase in numbers of female doctors and lawyers and of men taking on significant roles in parenting and child care. Yet Western culture still maintains distinct

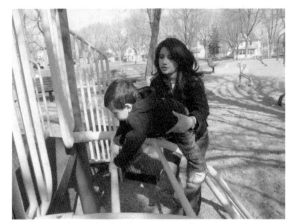

Figure 16.3. Parents are critical in role development and in supporting mastery in occupational performance.

differences between genders, as exemplified in the toy aisles of department stores or in television advertisements aimed at audiences of a particular gender. Girls are still often taught to care for and nurture dolls and boys are given trucks, cars, and action figures. Such socialization may lend itself to differing roles for the caregivers: Fathers have been shown to engage in more physical play with their children; mothers, in more imaginary play (Lindsay & Mize, 2001). Men have also been shown to use more technological approaches in socializing their children, whereas women use creative and pretend forms of play (Abrahamy, Finkelson, Lydon, & Murray, 2003). As people age and take on responsibility for older children, spouses, or parents, gender differences are perpetuated in relation to tasks, responsibilities, and psychological responses to caregiving (Coutinho, Hersch, & Davidson, 2006; Dahlberg, Demack, & Bambra, 2007; Etters, Goodall, & Harrison, 2008). Some of these caregiving roles may be planned, such as when a couple decides to have children or chooses to assist in caring for a grandchild. Some, however, are unplanned, as in the case of a spouse's traumatic injury or when an aging parent suddenly requires care.

Although the phenomenon of caring is universal, it is uniquely expressed across cultures and time. *Culture* may be described as the human values, beliefs, and activities existing within a particular setting or group. Although often referred to in relationship to ethnic background, the term is far more comprehensive and may include socioeconomic status, geographical locale, gender, sexual orientation, ability status, age, and even a particular professional cohort.

Social behaviors of caring reflect expectations of relationships through the cultural milieu in which the caregiving takes place (Figure 16.4). According to Bevis (1988), key cultural factors that influence the nature of caregiving include the values influenced by culture; the cost of services; the exclusiveness of the relationship (e.g., in a spousal relationship); the maturation of the caregiver and care receiver; personal life decisions and freedom; the stress level of the caregiver and care receiver; and the time available for providing care. Despite the subgroupings of culture, much of

---

EXERCISE 16.3: CAREGIVERS IN LIFE

Consider two caregivers in your own life as you grew up. What were the gender and cultural differences you experienced? Compare and contrast your experience of caregiving with that of someone from a different cultural background (e.g., ethnic, rural–urban, socioeconomic). What are the similarities and differences between your experience and theirs? Why is this important knowledge for an occupational therapist?

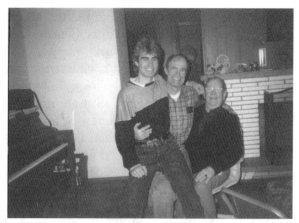

Figure 16.4. Although caregiving is often taken on by women, men also take on caregiving roles. Wayne (middle) often took care of his son, who had brain injury and epilepsy, and his 90-year-old aging father.

the literature on similarities and differences in caregiving practices is based on findings for ethnic groups.

In the United States, elderly people from ethnic minorities are more likely to be taken care of by an extended family network than is true of their European-American counterparts (Yarry, Stevens, & McCallum, 2007), and Latinos and African-Americans are less likely to be taken care of exclusively by a spouse (Sorensen & Pinquart, 2005; see Figure 16.5). Similarly, Mexican-Americans tend to want to live closer to extended kin than do

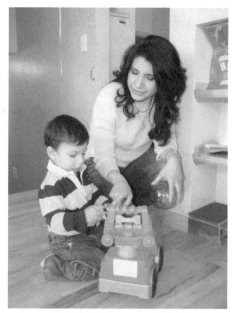

Figure 16.5. Although gender and culture influence caregiving, there are concepts universal to all cultures, including the important influence of parents as caregivers.

European-Americans (Burr & Mutchler, 1999). Yet integration into U.S. society and socioeconomic factors may also affect the extent to which financial and personal responsibility is met in extended family caregiving (Sarkisian, Gerena, & Gerstel, 2007). Similar findings in Asian culture have indicated high percentages of people taking care of extended family and aging relatives (AARP, 2001). Despite these differences, common variables exist across cultures, including learning caregiving roles from parents and kin during the developmental years; personal and cultural beliefs about the responsibility for taking care of one's own, referred to as *family* or *kin;* and the development of a unique cross-cultural custom of caregiving incorporating personal and familial beliefs, attitudes, and behaviors (Ayalong, 2004).

Models of Caregiving

Although a comprehensive presentation of caregiving models transcends the scope of this chapter, a general understanding is important for occupational therapists. Just as the second edition of the *Occupational Therapy Practice Framework: Domain and Process (Framework–II;* American Occupational Therapy Association [AOTA], 2008) addresses clients at the level of people, organizations, and populations, caregiving theories apply to all levels of service delivery. Conceptually, caregiving models vary in their focus from a global perspective on the systems and structures that support and govern caregiving to a more individualized emphasis on practitioner care and the relationship between caregivers and care receivers. Authors have described micro and macro factors that affect caregiving at all levels (e.g., Leininger, 1988a; Mak, 2005).

The Multi-Level Structural Caring Model as proposed by Leininger (1988a) is a hierarchical model used to conceptualize the scope, nature, and structures of caring. This model's highest level is a worldwide multicultural societal focus of caring. Leininger asserted that study within this level can generate information regarding broad views and theoretical underpinnings of care. At the mid-level, specific cultures and systems are emphasized, providing information about the systemic aspects of culture that influence care, such as legal, political, health care, and economic systems. At the lowest level are the individual or group foci, conceptualizing caring structures and functions within family or small interpersonal groups.

By contrast to large groupings, authors have also identified multilevel factors that influence caregiving on an interpersonal level. Mak (2005) identified macro factors affecting individual caregivers, including sociocultural factors (e.g., ethnicity, age, gender, income), interpersonal factors such as marital factors and kinship ties, structural factors such as managed care and health care systems, and clinical factors including the health of the caregiver and care receiver. Micro influences on caregiving include the individual experiences, day-to-day encounters, and occupational patterns within the caregiving relationship. A caregiving relationship may have strengths in certain factors, such as a close caring relationship, yet be negatively affected by lack of resources, exacerbation of illness, role strain, or limited health care coverage. To provide holistic client-centered services, health practitioners must plan evaluation and interventions taking all levels of caregiving into consideration.

Parenting

Research on parenting and subsequent theories and models are often focused on the relationship between parent and child on the basis of attachment theory (Bowlby, 1982), styles of parenting (Baumrind, 1967, 1971, 1996), and parental processes (Belsky, 1984). A comprehensive description of attachment styles may be found in the psychology literature. For the purposes of this chapter, I discuss the works of Diana Baumrind (1967, 1971, 1996) and Jay Belsky (1984; Belsky, Fearon, & Bell, 2007; Belsky, Vandell, et al., 2007).

BAUMRIND'S PARENTING STYLES

In her seminal work, Diana Baumrind (1967, 1971) found that parents differ in their expressions of maturity, communication, discipline, and warmth. On the basis of these dimensions, she identified distinct parenting styles, including permissive style, authoritative style, and authoritarian style. The *permissive* style of parenting governs children in an accepting, affirmative, and nonpunitive manner. In this style, parents generally make few demands of the child and maximize child input, yet do not seek to model antisocial behaviors, behavior that results in disobedience at times, or low tolerance for challenge. Over time, children with permissive parents may lack self-control and may struggle with the firm demands later placed on them in school. An *authoritative* style of parenting emphasizes autonomy and self-will; values the child's gifts, talents, and individuality; and yet sets clear expectations for standards. This type of parenting is said to lead to well-adjusted children with the ability to regulate emotion and positive social skills. In this style of parenting, parents value the child's individuality yet continue to maintain their parental authority and their role in setting limits. An *authoritarian* style of parenting seeks to shape the child's behaviors through discipline, firm expectations, and a set code of conduct. This type of parent is often strict and may use external forces and rules such as those derived from religion, specific philosophies, or an external set of beliefs to help guide parenting. Authoritarian styles may be equated with more control and less flexibility and may lead to anxious and withdrawn demeanors and poor frustration tolerance.

A final style of parenting includes *noninvolvement,* which may result in low responsiveness, low involvement, and low demands. In extreme cases, children may be neglected or left without the necessary care. Over decades of research, Baumrind (1967, 1971, 1996) concluded that the authoritative parenting style, which seeks to use warmth and guidance through listening and shaping the child's behaviors, is most effective and results in happier, better-adjusted children than the other parenting styles.

Although contextual cultural variations occur in parenting styles, Sorkhabi's (2005) work concluded that Baumrind's (1967, 1971) four parenting styles are applicable to both individualistic and collectivist cultures. She asserted, however, that the manifestations of parenting styles may not result in similar outcomes in collectivist cultures and that more research is needed to confirm this assertion. Baumrind's seminal work on parenting styles continues to be upheld and used in a variety of studies to investigate the effects of parenting practices (Brenner & Fox, 1999; Buri, 1991; Woolfsen & Grant, 2006).

BELSKY'S PROCESS MODEL

Research has revealed a link between the quality of parenting and subsequent child development (Belsky et al., 2007). Whereas Baumrind (1967, 1971) emphasized parenting styles, Jay Belsky (1984) developed a process model that sought to explain the determinants or factors that influence parenting and their subsequent effects on child development. Belsky's model asserts that "parents' developmental histories, marital relations, social networks, and jobs influence individual personality and general psychological well-being of parents and, thereby, parental functioning and, in turn child development" (p. 84).

Belsky identified three domains or determinants influencing the parental process: (1) personal and psychological resources of the parents, (2) characteristics of the child, and (3) contextual sources of stress and support. Parental personality and psychological well-being were found to be the most powerful determinants in supporting parental function and child development. This model assumes that parenting is influenced by forces both internal and external to the parent and child, along with the contextual factors in which the parenting takes place. Major contextual influences on stress and support were identified as the marital relationship, social networks, and work.

Conclusions of the model assert that parenting is determined by a multitude of factors, the determinant factors do not equally influence the parenting process, and personality and developmental history indirectly shape the parenting process through the broader context. Subsequent to Belsky's original research and model, Belsky, Vandell, et al. (2007) have found that although parenting is most influential in determining child development, the quality of early child care experiences external to the home also affects development, performance, and behavior. Through an understanding of the determinants of parenting and caregiving, therapists work to teach skills designed to enhance the relationship between caregiver and care receiver (Figure 16.6).

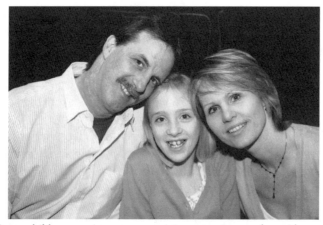

Figure 16.6. Some children require extra caregiving attention, such as Alyssa, who has spina bifida.

Stress, Coping, and Caregiver Burden

With respect to care of an elderly person or an ill person, models differ in their approach from the parenting models discussed earlier. Many of the models of caring for those with an illness or disability focus on the stress and coping demands of the caregiving situation. Yet some researchers have argued that models of caregiving that focus only on stress and burden are inadequate given the complexity of caregiving situations (Gubrium, 1995; Upton & Reed, 2006). The term *caregiver burden* refers to the emotional, financial, and physical strains resulting from a caregiving situation. Such stress is increased when additional external demands are factored in. Many contextual variables influence caregiver stress and burden, yet researchers have particularly emphasized the importance of the subjective perceptions of family members and caregivers in determining levels of caregiver burden (Bumagin & Hirn, 2001; Poulshock & Deimling, 1984). Given similar illnesses and family situations, differences occur in perceived stress. This variability is based on familial relationships, external supports, and attitudes toward the caregiving situation. Some families and individuals are more resilient in relation to the stressors resulting from caring for an elderly, sick, or disabled person, and others struggle to meet their daily obligations along with caregiving demands.

Positive coping strategies and social support have been shown to mediate the stress caused by caregiver burden (Ergh, Rapport, Coleman, & Hanks, 2002; Pakenham, 2001; Wells, Dywan, & Dumas, 2005). A sense of coherence or a perceived ability to respond to stress by using effective coping strategies is important in maintaining caregiver health and decreasing burden (Chumbler, Grimm, Cody, & Beck, 2003; Gallagher, Wagenfeld, Baro, & Haepers, 1994). Perceived self-efficacy and ability to handle caregiver situations also influence caregiver burden (Riley, 2007). Within occupational therapy, emphasis is placed on skill building and creating a client–environment fit (Dooley & Hinojosa, 2004) to maximize occupational performance and reduce stress. Everyday occupation and co-occupational involvement between caregivers and care receivers has been found to create meaning and help mitigate disruption and stress in caregiving situations (Abelenda & Helfrich, 2003; Hasselkus & Murray, 2007). For practitioners working with caregivers, emphasis is placed on providing family supports to reduce stress and maximize quality of life for both caregivers and care receivers.

Clinicians are also instrumental in the facilitation of care transition (moving from one setting to another). In addition to the stress of caring for a person at home, family members may eventually have to cope with guilt and ambivalence should a child with a disability have to be placed in a group home or an elderly spouse or family member in a nursing home. Kellet (1999) identified five themes common to family caregivers after nursing home placement: (1) a perceived loss of control; (2) a feeling of disempowerment; (3) a perceived sense of failure; (4) feelings of simultaneous sadness, guilt, and relief; and (5) the feeling of being forced to make a negative choice. Such feelings of ambivalence and loss may also be experienced when having to place a disabled child in a group home. It is important for practitioners to support the family through such transitions and to include the family in decisions regarding the extent and nature of their involvement after placement. Families and caregivers can be supported in maintaining contact and staying involved with their family member's care in several ways.

In recent years, additional emphasis has been placed on encouraging research and models of care that provide support for family caregivers and emphasize the preservation of meaning and quality of life for both caregiver and care receiver (e.g., Sellick, 2005; Vellone, Piras, Talucci, & Cohen, 2008). Hospice models designed for people at the end of life focus on dignity, comfort, and quality of life throughout the dying process. Although hospice care was initially designed for end-of-life issues, many of its goals are applicable to all caregiving situations. Lattanzi-Licht (2001) identified these goals for hospice care: The dying person and the family should be the focus,

---

EXERCISE 16.4: LONG-TERM-CARE FACILITY

Have you ever had a friend or family member placed in a LTC facility or group home? What was the impact on the family and on the person placed in the home? As an occupational therapist, what strategies can you use to facilitate family involvement after placement? How can the family still maintain meaningful occupational and social engagement with the person placed in the home? How will you, as the occupational therapist, support the family in working through these transitions?

with an emphasis on "quality of life . . . self-worth, individuality, autonomy, and security" (p. 21). Hospice care commonly addresses these goals. Overall, hospice stresses provision of support for the dying person and for that person's family members. Additionally, hospice aims to enhance dignity and approaches that fit the people involved, with comfort, pain management, and a holistic approach being paramount. This type of support continues for the family after their loved one's death, with grieving, recognition of the loss, and a period of mourning being part of the process.

Four key values identified by Lattanzi-Licht (2001) within the hospice model are (1) the worth of the person, (2) the importance of choice and self-determination, (3) provision for whole-person care, and (4) provision for family-centered care. During the transition into hospice, daily patterns and activities may shift, yet the preservation of self-worth, dignity, and meaning is imperative. In studying people in hospice, Jacques and Hasselkus (2004) found that throughout the dying process, occupational engagement takes on new meaning even in ordinary and familiar everyday activities. Provision for daily routines that support meaningful occupational engagement and co-occupation between caregivers and care receivers throughout all phases of care appears to mediate stress brought on by daily requirements of caregiving and the transition to hospice or other caregiving facilities. Practitioners serving all client populations may benefit from consideration of the goals and values of the hospice model in supporting quality of life throughout all phases of habilitation, rehabilitation, and caregiving.

Role of Occupational Therapy in Caregiving

As the demographic profiles of many industrialized nations shift toward increasing numbers of elderly people, the occupational therapy profession must work to meet the needs of increasing numbers of families who are informal caregivers for those with illness and disability. Although many health professions adhere to models of caregiving, occupational therapy holds a unique viewpoint in its emphasis on the use of occupation-based evaluation and intervention. A comprehensive review of the need for occupational therapy services in caregiving families revealed key themes, including

- The importance of emphasizing meaning and motivation in the caregiving relationship;
- The emphasis on caregiver–care receiver occupations and the use of meaningful occupation in therapy;
- The acknowledgment of gender roles that often influence occupational engagement;
- The importance of developing positive caregiving–care receiving routines and habits;
- The management and development of environmental structures and modifications to support meaningful occupation and improve outcomes; and

- The use of Person–Environment–Occupation models to facilitate positive adaptation (Coutinho et al., 2006).

The *Framework–II* cites an overarching assertion of occupational therapy's domain in "supporting health and participation in life through engagement in occupation" (AOTA, 2008, p. 626). Within the realm of caregiving, therapists work with families to ensure that caregiving skills are supported to maximize client participation, meaning, and engagement in occupations. The primary client may include the caregiver (such as a client with mental health concerns who is learning parenting skills), the care receiver (in the instance of a client with dementia whose family must be educated in the client's caregiving needs), or an entire system (as in facilitating positive environments for seniors). When considering environmental and caregiver supports to maximize occupational engagement, Haertl (2004) emphasized the importance of including the family and the extended care network (additional people involved with a client's care and daily activities) throughout the evaluation and intervention process. Key questions identified by Haertl included, for family,

- What is the role of the family in the client's life?
- Are there conflicts within the family, and what is the client's view of the family?
- To what extent is and should the family be involved in the therapy process?
- Will the client return to live with the family (or spouse)? If not, where will the client live?
- Is there agreement regarding the course of intervention between the family, health professionals, and other care providers? and
- What are the family's strengths, resources, and needs? How can the strengths be most effectively used, and how can the needs be most successfully met?

and, for the extended care network,

- Who are the important people in the client's life, and how will they be involved in the therapy process?
- Are the caregivers adequately trained, prepared, and willing to follow through with the intervention plan? What training needs exist?
- What extended care network resources are available, and how can they best be used? and
- What are the strengths and needs of the extended care network?

Support for the family and caregivers is designed to bolster resources and enhance existing strengths (Humphry & Case-Smith, 2005). Such support may include the use of direct models of intervention, education, and adaptation or home modification. Evaluation and intervention methods may be delivered at the client, family, or systems level.

Evaluation

Although care of others and care of pets are listed in the *Framework–II* as instrumental activities of daily living (IADLs) within occupational therapy's domain of practice (AOTA, 2008), limited options are available pertaining to direct occupational therapy–standardized assessment tools for parenting and caregiving. Most of the formalized instruments designed for the assessment of activities of daily living (ADLs) and IADLs focus on self-care skills rather than care of others. Sachs and Labovitz (2004) identified the use of interviews, ethnography, and the Canadian Occupational Performance Measure (COPM; Law et al., 1994) as client-based tools that may be used to identify caregiver needs and priorities. In recent years, the COPM has been updated and may be used with both clients and families to identify priorities, goals, and client–caregiver perceptions of change over time (Law et al., 2005). Therapists may also use formal and informal occupation-based self-reports, interviews, and observations to assess the caregiver relationship and to identify strengths and needs related to priorities for therapy.

Outside the field of occupational therapy, several interdisciplinary tools exist related to parenting and caregiving. The Parent–Child Relationship Inventory (Gerard, 1994) is an instrument designed to look at the parenting relationship in content areas of support, satisfaction with parenting involvement, communication, limit setting, and role orientation. The Parenting Stress Index (Abidin, 1995) is a self-report instrument often used in high-risk families to identify parents' stress levels. The inventory is designed for parents of children with physical and emotional problems, for families at risk of failing to promote normal development, and for parents at risk for dysfunctional parenting. Measurements are rated on a Likert-type 5-point scale, ranging from *strongly agree* to *strongly disagree*, in relation to child characteristics, parent personality, and contextual variables.

The Keys to Interactive Parenting Scale (Comfort & Gordon, 2005) is an observational tool designed to measure parent behaviors with children 2 months old through preschool age. A videotaped observation is conducted in a familiar environment, and parents are rated on 12 behaviors in areas such as sensitivity, involvement in child activities, reasonable expectations, and responsiveness to the child. The Alabama Parenting Questionnaire (Frick, 1991) includes both child and parent versions to assess five dimensions of parenting, including (1) positive involvement with children, (2) supervision and monitoring, (3) use of positive discipline, (4) consistency with discipline, and (5) use of corporal punishment. Although it has been used fairly extensively in research (e.g., Elgar, Waschbusch, Dadds, & Sigvaldason, 2007; Hawes & Dadds, 2006;

Locke & Prinz, 2002), it has practical application in both clinical and research settings.

Evaluation of caregivers for elderly people and for people with disabilities often includes a survey of the strengths and needs in the caregiving situation and a review of the caregiving environment. Instruments fall into both general and illness-specific categories. Several tools, including the Carers' Checklist (Hodgson, Higginson, & Jefferys, 1998), Caregiving Activity Survey (Davis et al., 1997), and Caregiver Burden Inventory (Novak & Guest, 1989), are specifically designed to assess caregiving situations for elderly people and people with cognitive disorders and dementia.

The Carers' Checklist is designed for people with dementia and their caregivers; it assesses the caregiving situation, the symptoms of dementia, the burden of care, the strengths and needs of the caregiving situation, and the impact of services. This tool may be used to facilitate intervention planning and monitor change over time. The Caregiving Activity Survey monitors use of time within the daily occupations of the caregiving relationship, including communication, transportation, dressing, eating, appearance and grooming, and supervision. An updated version (McCarron, Gill, Lawlor, & Beagly, 2002) includes bathing, toileting, housekeeping, and nursing activities.

The Caregiver Burden Inventory (Novak & Guest, 1989) reviews five dimensions of burden: (1) time-dependent, (2) developmental, (3) physical, (4) social, and (5) emotional. Additional general tools such as the Appraisal of Caregiving Scale (Oberst, 1991; Oberst, Gass, & Ward, 1989), the Caregiver Burden Scale (Elmstahl, Malmberg & Annerstedt, 1996), the Caregiving Self-Efficacy (Zeiss, Gallagher-Thompson, Lovett, Rose, & McKibbin, 1999), and the modified version of the Caregiving Appraisal Scale (Hughes & Caliandro, 1996) may be used to assess perceived burden, self-efficacy, and personal satisfaction in a variety of caregiving situations.

In addition to surveys and interviews, it is advantageous if the caregiver evaluation process involves observation and a review of the environment. The occupational therapist identifies strengths and barriers in the environment in which the daily routine typically occurs. Consideration should be given to occupational engagement in the environment and to adaptations that may be needed to enhance occupational performance. Formal tools such as the Home Observation for Measure of the Environment (Caldwell & Bradley, 1984) and the Environmental Rating Scales (Harms, Clifford, & Cryer, 1998; Harms, Cryer, & Clifford, 2003, 2007; Harms, Jacobs, & White, 1996) are useful in pediatric populations to assess environmental factors that support healthy development. For adults and seniors, the Home Assessment Profile (Chandler, Duncan, Weiner, & Studenski, 2001), a newer version of the Functional Environment Assessment (Chandler, Prescott, Duncan, & Studenski, 1991), and the Safe at Home (Anemaet & Moffa-Trotter, 1997, 1999) tools may be used to consider environmental needs in the home and to identify resources needed for the client and caregiver to maximize occupational performance and opportunities for meaningful engagement in daily

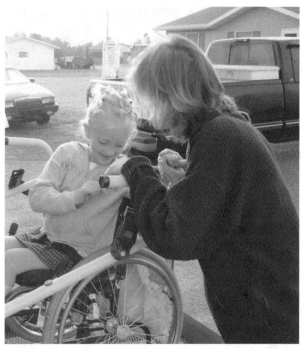

Figure 16.7. Evaluation of parenting for children with special needs should include the child, family, and extended-care network.

activities. These tools provide a review of the home environment in which caregiving takes place and identify the extent to which assistance is needed and barriers to performance exist and also give suggestions for resources and equipment. Formal assessment tools (discussed earlier) in conjunction with informal observations are used to develop an occupational profile and priorities for intervention (see Figure 16.7).

As the evaluation process is completed, the occupational profile results in a greater understanding of the client's past and current occupational performance, patterns of daily living, strengths, and needs (AOTA, 2008). The development of an occupational profile in a caregiving relationship should include client and contextual factors pertaining to the caregiver, the care receivers, and the systems that influence the provision of care. The resulting analysis of occupational performance should identify key priorities and outcomes for intervention.

Intervention

Therapeutic approaches to caregiving should be client centered and occupation based. Within the context of the caregiving relationship, the client may include the caregiver and care receiver along with additional family members and service practitioners (e.g., a personal care attendant) involved in the care. The *Framework–II* emphasizes the importance of guiding the intervention plan through the client's goals, values, interests and occupational needs; health and well-being; performance skills and patterns; context, activity demands, and client factors; and the best available evidence (AOTA, 2008). Within the therapist–client relationship, the emphasis is placed on maximizing quality of life for the caregiver and care receiver while fostering occupational performance and participation throughout the lifespan.

GENERAL RECOMMENDATIONS FOR INTERVENTION

Working with caregivers and families in a client-centered model may be a challenge because of the potential for disagreement regarding priorities for therapy. Family members and primary caregivers have been shown to question health professionals' decisions regarding care (Bowers, 1988; Hasselkus, 1988). Communication and discussion of priorities is critical before the onset of intervention. To move beyond the therapist's priorities and work toward a collaborative relationship, the therapist may have to suspend personal ideals and beliefs to fully discover the occupational patterns, values, and beliefs of the client and family (Gitlin, Corcoran, & Leinmiller-Eckhardt, 1995). Partnerships in therapy should engage "parents, families and other paid/formal and unpaid/informal caregivers to develop strategies that support occupational engagement and participation, health, and well-being, as well as support caregivers as they cope with the complex demands inherent in the caregiving role" (Gray, Horowitz, O'Sullivan, Behr, & Abreu, 2007, p. CE-1).

Within the occupational requirements of caregiving, Hasselkus (1988) outlined three broad goals identified by caregivers: (1) getting things done, (2) promoting the care receiver's health and well-being, and (3) maintaining the caregiver's health and well-being. To achieve these goals, the therapist uses intervention strategies that include education, skill training, adaptation, and modification. Determining the specific requirements for intervention involves understanding the dynamic interaction of the caregiver and care receiver while taking into account the contextual factors of the environment, occupational routines and requirements, and priorities. Schumacher, Stewart, Archbol, Dodd, and Dibble (2000) and Schumacher, Beidler, Beeber, and Gambino (2006) identified nine core skills important in the caregiving process:

1. *Monitoring*—Ensuring that everything is going well;
2. *Interpreting*—Making sense of observations;
3. *Making decisions*—Considering options for the best course of action;
4. *Taking action*—Carrying out daily caregiver tasks and requirements;
5. *Providing hands-on care*—Ensuring safety and comfort while providing care;
6. *Making adjustments*—Considering the best strategies;
7. *Accessing resources*;

8. *Working together* with the ill person and considering the personhood of both the caregiver and the care receiver; and
9. *Negotiating* the health care system.

For the occupational therapist, application of these core skills includes working through these processes while maximizing quality of life and enhancing opportunities for meaningful engagement in daily activities. Initial stages involve identification of the client's current state, the contextual influences of the setting in which the caregiving takes place, assessment of the care receiver–caregiver relationship, and identification of the role of the therapist throughout the evaluation and intervention process.

Sachs and Labovitz (2004) adapted four stages as outlined by Gitlin et al. (1995) in planning for caregiver intervention. The first stage involves identification of the primary caregiver and the current strategies and practices used in the caregiving relationship. The second stage involves coming to an understanding of the caregiver's perspective, daily routines, values, and beliefs. In the third stage, the therapist self-questions the knowledge gained and considers the congruency of the therapist's and caregiver's priorities and values. The final stage involves designation of the intervention. In this process, it is important to identify to what extent the caregiver and care receiver agree on priorities. For instance, a wife may be the primary caregiver for a husband newly diagnosed with Alzheimer's disease. As his illness progresses, she may believe that it is unsafe for him to drive, yet he may identify his return to driving as a priority. The therapist's communication skills in therapeutic interactions are crucial in working to find common agreement on priorities for intervention.

EXERCISE 16.5: GEORGE WITH ALZHEIMER'S DISEASE:
CAREGIVER AND CARE RECEIVER

Consider this situation: You have been working with George, a 61-year-old real estate agent diagnosed during the past year with Alzheimer's disease. Over time, George's wife has had to take on some of the higher-level daily occupations such as managing finances and paying the bills. George has continued to place high importance on his work of selling homes. His position requires him to drive clients around town, yet his wife claims he frequently gets lost and at times disobeys traffic laws. She has expressed sincere concern about the safety of his driving.

As George's wife gradually takes on a caregiving role, how would you support the two of them in this process? How would you address the disagreement about driving? What strengths and barriers do you see in this situation? What would be your role as a therapist?

An important area of consideration in this scenario is clarification of the therapist's role in working with the caregiver. Often, the therapist's primary therapeutic relationship is with the care receiver or person in need. Thus, patient privacy and the needs of the family and all those involved in the client's care must be balanced. In addition, a newly formed caregiver situation will likely require a period of transition for both the caregiver and the care receiver. The therapist serves the patient by using appropriate strategies to address the identified needs while simultaneously working with the family to implement occupational adaptations and environmental modifications that will maximize occupational performance and enhance the caregiver–care receiver relationship. In this scenario, questions particularly related to a person's competency to continue with work, transportation alternatives, available resources, and plans for the future must be answered.

In George's case, for a therapist to apply the key questions presented earlier in the chapter, the therapist would need to consider George's relationship with his wife, the context in which he will be discharged, and current and future prognosis. A comprehensive evaluation of George's current cognitive status and ability to complete activities of daily living is of importance, as is an evaluation of his discharge environment. The use of the COPM (Law et al., 1994) may prove valuable to attain input from George and his wife related to priorities, current routines and habits, and areas of meaningful engagement.

For those in the middle to late stages of Alzheimer's disease, driving is often contraindicated, although the client may continue to remember how to turn on and steer the car, navigating signs, responding to safety situations, and negotiating unfamiliar environments require higher level cognitive skills. If George continues to have some level of knowledge related to his vocation, a meeting with his employer and consideration of alternatives may be suggested. For those clients who must adapt to transition out of work, the addition of meaningful activities in the daily routine promotes quality of life. Additional questions related to the family's resources and needs should be addressed, along with the health and well-being of George's wife, and her ability to meet George's daily needs, as well as her own, in the caregiving role. Education for the family in relation to Alzheimer's disease, prognosis, and caregiving should be addressed along with any home modifications or any daily programs (e.g., adult day care) or in-home services that are advised. Preservation of meaning and family education also is important, as is close work with the multidisciplinary team.

Therapist roles and interactions within the caregiving relationship shift over time. In earlier stages, therapists serve to educate the care receiver and caregiver and facilitate adaptation to roles and responsibilities in the caregiving relationship. Perkinson, La Vesser, Morgan, and Perlmutter (2004) outlined the roles and responsibilities of the therapist and family through application of Aneshensel, Pearlin, Mullan, Zarit, and Whitlatch's (1995) three stages of caregiving: (1) role acquisition stage, (2) role enactment stage, and (3) role disengagement stage. Within each stage, the therapist and family interact in a unique manner on the basis of the situation's contextual needs.

Within the initial stage of *role acquisition*, given the challenge of a newly acquired illness, the family has to adjust to new roles, functions, and routines. During this stage of caregiving, the therapist serves as an educator regarding the illness, helps the family to identify resources, and anticipates future needs. In the *role enactment* stage, the family may need additional training related to direct care skills and advice about resources available to them. Particularly in cases of progressive illness or disease, this stage may also involve discussion of future environmental or housing needs. During this phase, the occupational therapist may be called on to expand skills training in use of special devices, home modification, and consideration for community placement. For those with a terminal illness, or perhaps children with disabilities who reach adulthood, the final stage of *role disengagement* involves major transition (Figure 16.8). Although the original model was patterned around elders and coping with death, there are also emotional stresses if a grown child is placed in a residential facility or moves away from home. During this stage, caregivers often have to work through grief, loss, and bereavement. The therapist's role is to facilitate support for the family members in coping with loss and transition. Families may require assistance to find support groups, to identify new roles should the loved one move into a community facility or group home, and to deal with grief in times of death and loss. Throughout each of these stages, the therapist works with the family to promote skills and routines that preserve time for meaningful activity and promote quality of life for all people in the caring relationship.

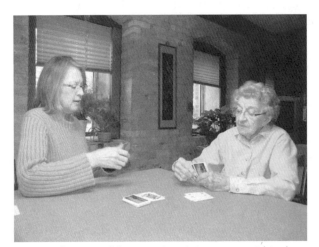

Figure 16.8. Preservation of meaningful occupations is important within the caregiving relationship.

Caregiving for Those With Illness and Special Needs

Much of the literature on caregiving is aimed at those caring for people with illness or disability, yet often it is the caregiver who has the special needs or conditions. Parents with disabilities and populations unaccustomed to providing caregiving (e.g., children) may require training and support to fulfill caregiving roles. Questions surrounding a person's competence to provide parenting or take on a caregiving role may arise, particularly in instances of cognitive or psychological impairment such as major mental illness or a severe traumatic brain injury. Similarly, caregivers may themselves develop challenges, such as an elderly woman caring for her spouse who later has a stroke or a parent who becomes physically disabled after an illness or severe injury. Although the number of people with major cognitive issues in caregiving roles has increased, services to these populations have not increased correspondingly (Kirkpatrick, 2008). A family systems approach to working with all people involved in the caregiving situation takes into account caregivers' and care receivers' needs. Programs such as those evolving from the U.K.'s Combined Skills Model emphasize the rights of people with special needs to serve in caregiving roles, yet focus on providing services to the entire family unit (Young & Hawkins, 2006).

The Social Care Institute for Excellence (2007) identified general principles of good practice for services to parents with special needs, and these principles are furthermore applicable to all caregiving situations:

- Needs arising from people who have special needs or consideration are addressed before making judgments about capacity for caregiving;
- The rights of the caregivers and the responsibilities of service organizations should be clear and transparent;
- There should be positive working relationships among service organizations, service disciplines, and the people receiving services; and
- There should be a prevention–intervention continuum.

For therapists, consideration of daily occupational patterns in caregiving situations, current skills and resources, and barriers to performance facilitates a foundation for the therapeutic relationship. The therapist generally works with an interdisciplinary team to develop strategies to ensure that caregivers' and care receivers' needs are met.

The roles and functions of the occupational therapist working with caregivers who have special needs may include evaluation of skill and competence and intervention for the purposes of training, modification, and procurement of resources. People with alteration of caregiving roles caused by a traumatic event have differing needs from those with chronic conditions (Fasoli, 2008). Techniques to prevent the decline of caregiving roles, such as in the case of an elder with decreasing physical function, may include the implementation of daily physical tasks or group activities designed to bolster physical, cognitive, and social capacities (Jackson, Carlson, Mandel, Zemke, & Clark, 1998). Services for children or teens assisting in the caregiving of a parent or sibling should include not only skills training but also consideration of their disrupted roles as students, friends, and leisure participants (Lackey & Gates, 2001). People with mental illness have often found providing care and maintaining a parenting role to be a motivating factor in agreeing to services because maintaining such roles provides a connection to the community and a way to acknowledge themselves as "normal" (Bassett & Lloyd, 2005; Gewurtz, Krupa, Eastabrook, & Horgan, 2004).

Finally, people with major physical and motor impairments often need adaptive strategies and home modification to facilitate caregiving. The use of ergonomic techniques to facilitate lifting and carrying, energy conservation techniques to minimize fatigue, and environmental modification such as adaptive cribs and changing tables help preserve the parent–child bond and facilitate maximal occupational performance in the parenting role (Fasoli, 2008). In instances in which the client is deemed unable to fully carry out caregiving roles, the therapist, multidisciplinary team, client, and family work together to identify available supports. The addition of in-home care and supportive services may be advantageous. When possible, efforts should be made to facilitate the bond between the caregiver and care receiver amid the presence of external supports.

Summary

This chapter provides an overview of the definitions of *care* and *caregiver,* a description of gender and cultural influences on caregiving, a review of current models, and a discussion of the roles and functions of the occupational therapist. Occupational therapy serves a unique and vital role in providing services to caregivers and care receivers. Through the use of client-centered occupation-based evaluation and intervention, therapists work to enhance meaning and quality of life for the caregiver and the care receiver. Service provision includes the micro (individual–family) approach and the macro (systems) approach. Unique to the profession, occupational therapy evaluates and plans intervention through assessment of the client–environment fit; daily caregiving occupational patterns; strength and barriers to health, well-being, and daily occupational performance; and development of strategies to enhance quality of life for both caregiver and care receiver.

References

AARP. (2001). *In the middle: A report of multi-cultural boomers coping with family and aging issues* [Prepared for AARP by Belden Russonello & Stewart and Research/Strategy/Management]. Washington, DC: Author.

Abelenda, J., & Helfrich, C. (2003). Family resilience and mental illness: The role of occupational therapy. *Occupational Therapy in Mental Health, 19*(1), 25–39.

Abidin, R. R. (1995). *Parenting Stress Index* (3rd ed.). Lutz, FL: Psychological Assessment Resources.

Abrahamy, M., Finkelson, E. B., Lydon, C., & Murray, K. (2003). Caregivers' socialization of gender roles in a children's museum. *Perspectives in Psychology, Spring,* 19–25.

American Occupational Therapy Association. (2008). Occupational therapy practice framework: Domain and process (2nd ed.). *American Journal of Occupational Therapy, 62,* 625–683.

Anemaet, W. K., & Moffa-Trotter, M. E. (1997). *The user friendly home care handbook.* McLean, VA: LEARN.

Anemaet, W. K., & Moffa-Trotter, M. E. (1999). Promoting safety and function through home assessments. *Topics in Geriatric Rehabilitation, 15,* 26–55.

Aneshensel, C. S., Pearlin, L. I., Mullan, J. T., Zarit, S. H., & Whitlatch, C. J. (1995). *Profiles in caregiving: The unexpected career.* San Diego, CA: Academic Press.

Awad, A. G., & Voruganti, L. N. (2008). The burden of schizophrenia on caregivers: A review. *Pharmacoeconomics, 26,* 149–162.

Ayalong, L. (2004). Cultural variants of caregiving or the culture of caregiving. *Journal of Cultural Diversity, 11,* 131–138.

Bassett, H., & Lloyd, C. (2005). At-risk families with mental illness: Partnerships in practice. *New Zealand Journal of Occupational Therapy, 52,* 31–37.

Baumrind, D. (1967). Childcare practices anteceding three patterns of preschool behavior. *Genetic Psychology Monographs, 75,* 43–88.

Baumrind, D. (1971). Current patterns of parental authority. *Developmental Psychology Monograph, 4,* 1–103.

Baumrind, D. (1996). The discipline controversy revisited. *Family Relations, 45,* 405–414.

Belsky, J. (1984). The determinants of parenting: A process model. *Child Development, 55,* 83–96.

Belsky, J., Fearon, R. M., & Bell, B. (2007). Parenting, attention, and externalizing problems: Testing mediation longitudinally, repeatedly and reciprocally. *Journal of Child Psychology and Psychiatry, 48,* 1233–1242.

Belsky, J., Vandell, D. L., Burchinal, M., Clarke-Stewart, K. A., McCartney, K., & Owen, M. T. (2007). Are there long term effects of early child care? *Child Development, 78,* 681–701.

Bevis, E. O. (1988). Caring: A life force. In M. Leininger (Ed.), *Caring: An essential human need. Proceedings of the three National Caring Conferences* (pp. 49–59). Detroit, MI: Wayne State University Press.

Bowers, B. J. (1988). Family perceptions of nursing home care: A grounded theory study of family work in a nursing home. *Gerontologist, 28,* 361–368.

Bowlby, J. (1982). *Attachment and loss. Volume 1: Attachment* (2nd ed.). New York: Basic Books

Brenner, V., & Fox, R. A. (1999). An empirically derived classification of parenting practices. *Journal of Genetic Psychology, 160,* 343–356.

Bumagin, V. E., & Hirn, K. F. (2001). *Caregiving: A guide for those who give care and those who receive it.* New York: Springer.

Buri, J. R. (1991). Parental Authority Questionnaire. *Journal of Personality Assessment, 57,* 110–119.

Burr, J. A., & Mutchler, J. E. (1999). Race and ethnic variations in norms of filial responsibility among older adults. *Journal of Marriage and the Family, 61,* 674–687.

Caldwell, B., & Bradley, R. H. (1984). *Home Observation for Measure of the Environment* (rev. ed.). Little Rock: University of Arkansas.

Chandler, J. M., Duncan, P. W., Weiner, D. K., & Studenski, S. A. (2001). Special Feature—The Home Assessment Profile—A reliable and valid assessment tool. *Topics in Geriatric Rehabilitation, 16,* 77–88.

Chandler, J. M., Prescott, B., Duncan, P. W., & Studenski, S. (1991). Reliability of a new instrument: The Functional Environment Assessment. *Physical Therapy, 71,* 574.

Chumbler, N. R., Grimm, J. W., Cody, M., & Beck, C. (2003). Gender, kinship, and caregiver burden: The case of community-dwelling memory impaired seniors. *International Journal of Geriatric Psychiatry, 18,* 722–732.

Collins Essential English Dictionary. (2009). Retrieved May 1, 2009, from www.thefreedictionary.com/care

Comfort, M., & Gordon, P. (2005). *Keys to Interactive Parenting Scale.* Cheyney, PA: Comfort Consultants.

Coutinho, F., Hersch, G., & Davidson, H. (2006). The impact of informal caregiving in occupational therapy. *Physical and Occupational Therapy in Geriatrics, 25,* 47–61.

Dahlberg, L., Demack, S., & Bambra, C. (2007). Age and gender of informal carers: A population-based study in the UK. *Health and Social Care in the Community, 15,* 439–445.

Davis, K. L., Marin, D. B., Kane, R., Patrick, D., Peskind, E. R., Raskind, M. A., & Puder, K. L. (1997). The Caregiver Activity Survey (CAS): Development and validation of a new measure for caregivers of persons with Alzheimer's disease. *International Journal of Geriatric Psychiatry, 12,* 978–988.

Dooley, N. R., & Hinojosa, J. (2004). Improving quality of life for persons with Alzheimer's disease and their family caregivers: Brief occupational therapy intervention. *American Journal of Occupational Therapy, 58,* 561–569.

Drentea, P. (2007). Caregiving. In G. Ritzer (Ed.), *Blackwell encyclopedia of sociology* (Blackwell Reference Online). Retrieved January 15, 2009, from www.blackwellreference.com/public/tocnode?id=g9781405124331_chunk_g97814051243319_ss1-7

Elgar, F. J., Waschbusch, D. A., Dadds, M. R., & Sigvaldason, N. (2007). Development and validation of a short form of the Alabama Parenting Questionnaire. *Journal of Child and Family Studies, 16,* 243–259.

Elmstahl, S., Malmberg, B., & Annerstedt, L. (1996). Caregiver's burden of patients 3 years after stroke assessed by a novel caregiver burden scale. *Archives of Physical Medicine and Rehabilitation, 77,* 177–182.

Ergh, T. C., Rapport, L. J., Coleman, R. D., & Hanks, R. A. (2002). Predictors of caregiver and family functioning following traumatic brain injury: Social support moderates caregiver stress. *Journal of Head Trauma Rehabilitation, 17,* 155–174.

Etters, L., Goodall, D., & Harrison, B. E. (2008). Caregiver burden among dementia patient caregivers: A review of the literature. *Journal of the American Academy of Nurse Practitioners, 20,* 423–428.

Fasoli, S. E. (2008). Restoring competence for homemaker and parent roles. In M. V. Radomski & C. A. Trombly (Eds.), *Occupational therapy for physical dysfunction* (6th ed., pp. 854–874). Baltimore: Lippincott Williams & Wilkins.

Frick, P. J. (1991). *Alabama Parenting Questionnaire.* Birmingham, AL: Author.

Gallagher, T. J., Wagenfeld, M. O., Baro, F., & Haepers, K. (1994). Sense of coherence: Coping and caregiver role overload. *Social Science and Medicine, 39,* 1615–1622.

Gerard, A. B. (1994). *Parent–Child Relationship Inventory (PCRI).* Los Angeles: Western Psychological Services.

Gewurtz, R., Krupa, T., Eastabrook, S., & Horgan, S. (2004). Prevalence and characteristics among people served by assertive community treatment. *Psychiatric Rehabilitation Journal, 28*, 63–65.

Gitlin, L. G., Corcoran, M., & Leinmiller-Eckhardt, S. (1995). Understanding the family perspective: An ethnographic framework for providing occupational therapy in the home. *American Journal of Occupational Therapy, 49*, 802–809.

Gray, K., Horowitz, B. P., O'Sullivan, A., Behr, S. K., & Abreu, B. C. (2007). Occupational therapy's role in the occupation of caregiving. *OT Practice, 12*(15), CE1–CE8.

Gubrium, J. F. (1995). Taking stock. *Qualitative Health Research, 5*, 267–269.

Haertl, K. H. (2004). Adaptive strategies for adults with developmental disabilities. In C. H. Christiansen & K. M. Matuska (Eds.), *Ways of living: Adaptive strategies for special needs* (3rd ed., pp. 149–183). Bethesda, MD: AOTA Press.

Harms, T., Clifford, R., & Cryer, D. (1998). *Early Childhood Environment Rating Scale–Revised (ECERS–R)*. New York: Teachers College Press.

Harms, T., Cryer, D., & Clifford, R. (2003). *Infant Toddler Environment Rating Scale–Revised (ITERS–R)*. New York: Teachers College Press.

Harms, T., Cryer, D., & Clifford, R. (2007). *Family Childcare Environment Rating Scale (FCERS–R)*. New York: Teachers College Press.

Harms, T., Jacobs, E. V., & White, D. R. (1996). *School Age Care Environment Rating Scale*. New York: Teachers College Press.

Hasselkus, B. R. (1988). Meaning in family caregiving: Perspectives on caregiver/professional relationships. *Gerontologist, 28*, 686–691.

Hasselkus, B. R., & Murray, B. J. (2007). Everyday occupation, well-being, and identity: The experience of caregivers in families with dementia. *American Journal of Occupational Therapy, 61*, 9–20.

Hawes, D. J., & Dadds, M. R. (2006). Assessing parenting practices through parent report and direct observation during parent-training. *Journal of Child and Family Studies, 15*, 555–568.

Hodgson, C., Higginson, I., & Jeffreys, P. (1998). *Carers' checklist: An outcome measure for people with dementia and their carers*. London: Mental Health Foundation.

Hughes, C. B., & Caliandro, G. (1996). Effects of social support, stress, and level of illness on caregiving of children with AIDS. *Journal of Pediatric Nursing, 11*, 347–358.

Humphry, R., & Case-Smith, J. (2005). Working with families. In J. Case-Smith (Ed.), *Occupational therapy for children* (5th ed., 117–153). St. Louis, MO: Mosby.

Jackson, J., Carlson, M., Mandel, D., Zemke, R., & Clark, F. (1998). Occupational lifestyle redesign: The well-elderly study occupational therapy program. *American Journal of Occupational Therapy, 52*, 326–336.

Jacques, N. D., & Hasselkus, B. R. (2004). The nature of occupation surrounding dying and death. *OTJR: Occupation, Participation and Health, 24*, 44–53.

Kellet, U. M. (1999). Transition in care: Family carer's experience of nursing home placement. *Journal of Advanced Nursing, 29*, 1474–1481.

Kirkpatrick, K. (2008). Working with parents with a learning disability. *Learning Disability Today, 8*, 8–11.

Lackey, N. R., & Gates, M. F. (2001). Adults' recollections of their experiences as young caregivers of family members with chronic mental illness. *Journal of Advanced Nursing, 34*, 320–328.

Lattanzi-Licht, M. (2001). Hospice as a model for caregiving. In K. J. Doka & J. D. Davidson (Eds.), *Caregiving and loss: Family needs, professional responses* (pp. 19–31). Washington, DC: Hospice Foundation of America.

Law, M., Baptiste, S., Carswell, A., McColl, M. A., Polatajko, H., & Pollock, N. (1994). *Canadian Occupational Performance Measure* (2nd ed.). Toronto: CAOT Publications.

Law, M., Baptiste, S., Carswell, A., McColl, M. A., Polatajko, H., & Pollock, N. (2005). *Canadian Occupational Performance Measure* (4th ed.). Ottawa, Ontario: CAOT Publications.

Leaper, C. (2002). Parenting girls and boys. In M. H. Bornstein (Ed.), *Handbook of parenting. Volume 1: Children and parenting* (2nd ed., pp. 189–225). Mahwah, NJ: Erlbaum.

Leininger, M. (1988a). Cross-cultural hypothetical functions of caring and nursing care. In M. Leininger (Ed.), *Caring—An essential human need: Proceedings of the three National Caring Conferences* (pp. 95–102). Detroit, MI: Wayne State University Press.

Leininger, M. (1988b). The phenomenon of caring: Importance, research questions, and theoretical considerations. In M. Leininger (Ed.), *Caring—An essential human need: Proceedings of the three National Caring Conferences* (pp. 3–16). Detroit, MI: Wayne State University Press.

Levine, C. (2001). Introduction: Nature of caregiving. In K. J. Doka & J. D. Davidson (Eds.), *Caregiving and loss: Family needs, professional responses* (pp. 5–18). Washington, DC: Hospice Foundation of America.

Lindsay, E. W., & Mize, J. (2001). Contextual differences in parent–child play: Implications for children's gender role development. *Sex Roles, 44,* 155–176.

Locke, L. M., & Prinz, R. J. (2002). Measurement of parental discipline and nurturance. *Clinical Psychology Review, 22,* 895–929.

Mak, W. W. (2005). Integrative model of caregiving: How macro and micro factors affect caregivers of adults with severe and persistent mental illness. *American Journal of Orthopsychiatry, 75,* 40–53.

McCarron, M., Gill, M., Lawlor, B., & Beagly, C. (2002). A pilot study of the reliability and validity of the Caregiver Activity Survey–Intellectual Disability (CAS–ID). *Journal of Intellectual Disability Research, 46,* 605–612.

Merriam Webster's online dictionary. (2009). Retrieved May 2, 2009, from www.merriam-webster.com/dictionary/care

National Family Caregiving Association. (n.d.). *Caregiving statistics.* Retrieved January 17, 2009, from www.thefamilycaregiver.org/who_are_family_caregivers/care_giving_statstics.cfm

Novak, M., & Guest, C. (1989). Application of a multi-dimensional caregiver burden inventory. *Gerontologist, 29,* 798–803.

Oberst, M. T. (1991). *Appraisal of Caregiving Scale: Manual.* Detroit, MI: Wayne State University.

Oberst, M. T., Gass, K. A., & Ward, S. E. (1989). Caregiving demands and appraisal of stress among family caregivers. *Cancer Nursing, 12,* 209–215.

Pakenham, K. I. (2001). Application of a stress and coping model to caregiving in multiple sclerosis. *Psychology, Health, and Medicine, 6,* 13–27.

Perkinson, M. A., La Vesser, P., Morgan, K., & Perlmutter, M. (2004). Therapeutic partnerships: Caregiving in the home setting. In C. H. Christiansen & K. M. Matuska (Eds.), *Ways of living: Adaptive strategies for special needs* (3rd ed., pp. 445–461). Bethesda, MD: AOTA Press.

Poulshock, S. W., & Deimling, G. (1984). Families caring for elders in residence: Issues in the measurement of burden. *Journal of Gerontology, 39,* 230–239.

Riley, G. A. (2007). Stress and depression in family carers following traumatic brain injury: The influence of beliefs about difficult behaviors. *Clinical Rehabilitation, 21,* 82–88.

Sachs, D., & Labovitz, D. R. (2004). Range of human activity: Care of others. In J. Hinojosa & M. Blount (Eds.), *Texture of life: Purposeful activities in occupational therapy* (2nd ed., pp. 414–436). Bethesda, MD: AOTA Press.

Sarkisian, N., Gerena, M., & Gerstel, M. (2007). Extended family integration among Euro and Mexican Americans: Ethnicity, gender and class. *Journal of Marriage and Family, 69,* 40–54.

Schumacher, K. L., Beidler, S. M., Beeber, A. S., & Gambino, P. (2006). A transactional model of cancer family caregiving skill. *Advances in Nursing Science, 29,* 271–286.

Schumacher, K. L., Stewart, B. J., Archbol, P. G., Dodd, M. J., & Dibble, S. L. (2000). Family caregiving skill: Development of the concept. *Research in Nursing and Health, 23,* 191–203.

Sellick, J. (2005). *Traditions: Improving quality of life in caregiving.* State College, PA: Venture.

Social Care Institute for Excellence. (2007). *The adult services resource guide 9: Working together to support disabled parents.* London: Author.

Sorensen, S., & Pinquart, M. (2005). Racial and ethnic differences in the relationship of caregiving stressors, resources, and sociodemographic variables to caregiver depression and perceived physical health. *Aging and Mental Health, 9,* 482–495.

Sorkhabi, N. (2005). Applicability of Baumrind's parent typology to collective cultures: Analysis of cultural explanations of parent socialization effects. *International Journal of Behavior Development, 29,* 552–563.

Upton, N., & Reed, V. (2006). The influence of social support on caregiver coping. *International Journal of Psychiatric Nursing Research, 11,* 1256–1267.

U.S. Department of Health and Human Services. (2001). *The characteristics of long-term care users.* Rockville, MD: Agency for Healthcare Research and Quality.

U.S. Department of Health and Human Services, Office of the Assistant Secretary for Planning and Evaluation; Centers for Medicare and Medicaid Services; Health Resources and Services Administration; & U.S. Department of Labor, Office of the Assistant Secretary for Policy, Bureau of Labor Statistics, and Employment and Training Administration. (2003).*The future supply of long-term care workers in relation to the aging baby-boom generation: Report to Congress.* Washington, DC: Author.

Vellone, E., Piras, G., Talucci, C., & Cohen, M. Z. (2008). Quality of life for caregivers of people with Alzheimer's disease. *Journal of Advanced Nursing, 61,* 222–231.

Wells, R., Dywan, J., & Dumas, J. (2005). Life satisfaction and distress in family caregivers as related to specific behavioural changes after traumatic brain injury. *Brain Injury, 19,* 1105–1115.

Woolfsen, L., & Grant, E. (2006). Authoritative parenting and parental stress in parents of preschool and older children with developmental disabilities. *Child: Care, Health and Development, 32,* 177–184.

Yarry, S. J., Stevens, E. K., & McCallum, T. J. (2007, Fall). Cultural influences on spousal caregiving. *Generations,* pp. 24–30.

Young, S., & Hawkins, H. (2006). Special parenting and the combined skills model. *Journal of Applied Research in Intellectual Disabilities, 19,* 346–355.

Zeiss, A. M., Gallagher-Thompson, D., Lovett, S., Rose, J., & McKibbin, C. (1999). Self-efficacy as a mediator of caregiver coping: Development and testing of an assessment model. *Journal of Clinical Geropsychology, 5,* 221–230.

Zukewich, N. (2003). *Unpaid informal caregiving. Canadian Social Trends, 70,* 14–18.

17

◈

Activities, Human Occupation, Participation, and Empowerment

Rita P. Fleming-Castaldy, PhD, OT/L, FAOTA

*E*mpowerment is the process by which marginalized people with decreased power gain control over their lives. It gives people a voice and enables their participation so that they can self-determine their lives (Rapp, Shera, & Kisthardt, 1993). The empowerment process extends beyond personal control to include the ability to systemically influence the social, economic, and political structures in which disenfranchised people live (Charlton, 1998; Freire, 1970).

The roots of empowerment are based in the recognition of the oppressive effects of domination that inhibit the fulfillment of human potential (Freire, 1970). The realization of empowerment for people with disabilities began in the 1960s as the independent living movement gained momentum and people with disabilities self-organized to engage in civil disobedience and confront endemic societal inequities (Fleischer & Zames, 2001). These efforts, inspired by the civil rights movement, eventually succeeded in bringing about substantive legislative initiatives that established the rights of people with disabilities to participate in society (Cottrell, 2005). The Rehabilitation Act of 1973, the Education for All Handicapped Children Act of 1975, the Individuals With Disabilities Education Act of 1990, and the Americans With Disabilities Act (ADA) of 1990 have advanced the inclusion of people with disabilities into education, work, and community contexts (Fleischer & Zames, 2001). Disability rights activists, however, still hold that the improvement of the legal rights of people with disabilities is not sufficient to enable their full participation in society (Fleischer & Zames, 2001; see Figure 17.1). A complete alteration of how society views disability is necessary for real change.

The Social Model of Disability put forth by disability scholars, for example, proposes that disability is not a personal attribute but a societal problem resulting from a complex collection of conditions created by the social environment, such as inaccessible environments, stigma, and prejudice (Shakespeare & Watson, 1997). The World Health Organization's (WHO's; 2007) definition of *disability* in the *International Classification of Function, Disability and Health*

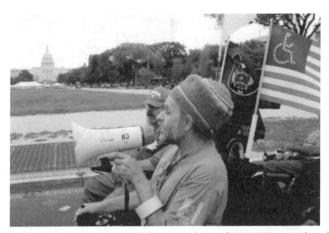

Figure 17.1. Disability rights activists, including members of ADAPT, actively rally against and assertively confront social and political barriers to full participation.

Note. Photograph by Tom Olin. ADAPT Protest, September 13, 2006, Washington, DC. Reprinted with permission.

(*ICF*) also bears the mark of the disability rights movement. The *ICF* does not equate disability with the presence of diagnosis or condition; rather, it is "impairment, activity limitation or participation restriction" (WHO, 2007, p. 3) that is disabling. The *ICF* also emphasizes the consideration of social factors, attitudes, and physical environmental factors that hinder or facilitate a person's performance of desired activities and participation in social roles.

The inherent congruence between the *ICF* definition and occupational therapy is evident. *The Guide to Occupational Therapy Practice* (Moyers & Dale, 2007) and the *Occupational Therapy Practice Framework: Domain and Process* (2nd ed.; *Framework–II*) put forth by the American Occupational Therapy Association (AOTA; 2008) are strongly influenced by WHO's position that all people (including people with disabilities) can be healthy. Health and well-being are attained through participation in meaningful occupations in environments of choice that support full inclusion (AOTA, 2008; Moyers & Dale; WHO, 2007). These documents also assert that occupational therapy's unique purpose as a profession is "facilitating participation of people of all ages in their chosen occupations and activities [and] designing contexts, environments, and policies for individuals and communities that recognize and support differences in opportunities for participation" (Moyers & Dale, 2007, p. 1).

The core values and fundamental beliefs of occupational therapy further affirm the person's freedom to engage in purposeful activities and meaningful occupations; demonstrate independence, self-direction, and autonomy; and attain full and equal societal membership (AOTA, 1993). Occupational therapists believe that people are capable of choice and have the right to make decisions on the basis of their personal preferences. Moreover, they believe that all can and should be active participants in the therapeutic process. Table 17.1 outlines the relationship between key attributes of occupational therapy's ethical principles and empowerment.

Table 17.1. *AOTA Code of Ethics* and Empowerment

Ethical Principle and Key Attributes	Principle's Bridge to Empowerment
Beneficence: Concern for the well-being of service recipients, concerted advocacy for needed services.	Well-being is attained when people have choice and control over their lives; advocating for services and policies that enable self-directed lives for all is expected.
Nonmaleficence: The imposition or infliction of harm to service recipients must be avoided.	Harm is imposed and inflicted when people are deprived of free choice, receive insufficient services, or are given prescriptive options; confronting policies and practices that demean people and deny basic human rights is required.
Autonomy: Respect for service recipients' personal values, beliefs, preferences, and ⸴decisions.	Independence is realized through collaborative partnerships as led by the person; policies and practices that enable autonomous self-direction and honor people's rights to self-determination (e.g., Individuals With Disabilities Education Act [1990]) are necessary.
Duty: The competence of practitioners must be attained and maintained. A commitment to lifelong learning is a mandate.	Empowering practice requires the development of proficiencies beyond professional specialization; the assertive pursuit of knowledge about policies and practices that support people's empowerment and the development of advocacy skills are vital.
Justice: Compliance with laws and AOTA policies ensure that professional services are rendered equitably, objectively, fairly, and truthfully.	The just rendering of services compels practitioners to be astute about all laws and policies that support empowerment; ignorance of the law does not excuse disempowering practices (e.g., poor transition planning).
Veracity: Practitioners must accurately represent themselves and their services to ensure public trust.	Truthful practice, which enables trust, requires informed awareness and honest acknowledgment of personal, professional, institutional, social, or political biases.
Fidelity: All practitioners are responsible for the ethical provision of services; questionable practices must be discouraged, and ethical breeches must be confronted.	Ethical practice requires a shared and unwavering commitment to moral action; being silent when observing or learning of disempowering practices is the same as personally engaging in unethical practice.

Note. From "Occupational Therapy Code of Ethics," by American Occupational Therapy Association, 2005, *American Journal of Occupational Therapy, 59*, pp. 639–642. Copyright © 2005, by American Occupational Therapy Association. Reprinted with permission.

EXERCISE 17.1: THE EMPOWERING APPLICATION OF PROFESSIONAL ETHICS

Reflect honestly and thoughtfully on the links provided in Table 17.1. In what way do you think the identified attributes of occupational therapy's ethical principles support empowering practices? What additional supports and resources may be needed to realize the empowering potential of this ethical code? Do you have any concerns regarding your ability to abide by this Code of Ethics to confront disempowering practices and make possible empowering ones? What actions can you take to develop the knowledge, skills, and attitudes needed to use these ethical principles to facilitate empowerment?

Occupational therapists and occupational therapy assistants can effectively apply their ethical principles, professional knowledge, and skills to attain the goal of full community participation for all people with disabilities (AOTA, 2008; Moyers & Dale, 2007). If practitioners, however, consider only the person's independent activity performance and do not consider the disempowering effects and empowering possibilities of the physical, social, cultural, virtual, and political contexts on occupations, the efficacy of these efforts is questionable (AOTA, 2008; Baum & Law, 1997; Grady, 1995). Authentic occupational therapy can take place only when people become their own "agent of competency via occupation" (Yerxa, 1967, p. 614). Empowerment Theory can thus provide an effective conceptual framework to guide occupational therapists and occupational therapy assistants in their work; it can help them support people with disabilities in becoming active agents in their lives. Practitioners can allow themselves to be led by a person in need of empowerment to advance and facilitate the empowerment process.

Thus, occupational therapists and occupational therapy assistants must become articulate in Empowerment Theory (Taylor, 2001). In this chapter, I provide foundational information to help current and future occupational therapists and occupational therapy assistants understand the theoretical intersection between empowerment and the practice of occupational therapy. I examine the relationships between empowering practices, the therapeutic use of purposeful activity, and the engagement in meaningful occupations that enable participation. My focus is on the empowerment of people with disabilities because practitioners most typically work with these people (AOTA, 2006). This emphasis on people with disabilities is solely because of space constraints and is not meant to imply that practitioners cannot engage in empowering practices with other oppressed groups, such as people who are unemployed, illiterate, impoverished, homeless, imprisoned, or refugees or survivors of war and natural disasters (Kronenberg & Pollard, 2006; Moyers & Dale, 2007).

The information I present can and should be applied to those who are disempowered by a diverse range of internal and external contextual factors. I examine disempowering policies and practices and confront practitioners' acquiescence, historical and continued, with using models that are inconsistent with empowering approaches. Because real challenges to the adoption of empowering practices exist, I make specific suggestions to promote the empowerment of all who engage in occupational therapy services throughout our domain of practice. I emphasize giving voice to the lived reality of people with disabilities who experience empowerment, disempowerment, or both every day. A key source informing my examples will be my brother Kevin, who was diagnosed with Friedreich's ataxia when we were children.

Because we were only 2 years apart in age, I often walked beside Kevin during his lifelong journey in dealing with the ravages of a progressive neuromuscular disease. As a result, my understanding of the disempowerment of people with disabilities began at an early age (although I did not know it at the time) as I observed my brother's "rehabilitation" being limited to the periodic evaluation of his deteriorating physical capabilities. Because Kevin's disorder was rare, these examinations were typically performed with Kevin (wearing only his briefs) in front of an audience of physicians, residents, interns, and nurses who observed the leading physiatrist demonstrate my brother's abnormal reflexes and trace his scoliatic spine to many *oh*s and *ah*s from the enlightened crowd. Things did not improve after Kevin dressed for his "therapy." His treatment sessions were dominated by activities (e.g., bean bag tossing) to purportedly develop his eye–hand coordination. Although the reality that my brother was never going to accurately hit the target seemed blatantly obvious after the first attempt, Kevin's therapists urged him to "try harder." As children, we both knew this was not right. Until my search to find something to help my brother, however, led me to the field of occupational therapy, the possibility that Kevin was more than his disability was never a consideration.

Once I became an occupational therapy student, I quickly applied what I was learning to help maximize Kevin's abilities and compensate for his functional limitations. These efforts worked, and he began to envision possibilities beyond the four walls of his bedroom. Unfortunately, the rehabilitation services he continued to receive did not support the self-determination of goals, and the disempowering practices of Kevin's childhood continued. Although many of his therapists were kind and well intentioned, the reality was that their practice was based on a reductionist medical model, not an empowerment one. As a result, Kevin's functional deficits were the sole focus of occupational therapy interventions, and his desired roles of student, author, music lover, friend, and home maintainer continued to be ignored. Fortunately, I was able to serve as Kevin's de facto therapist. We successfully collaborated to enable him to attain his goals of attending college and living on his own. A self-directed, meaningful life evolved to replace the denigrating existence of being objectified as a diagnosis.

In the 2 decades since Kevin lost his battle with Friedreich's ataxia, the occupational therapy literature has been replete with writings that challenge the medical model that dominated his rehabilitation. *Client-centered* and *family-centered practice* have become widely accepted terms in our profession's lexicon (Kyler, 2008), but social, cultural, political, and economic barriers remain that hinder the translation of this language into empowering practices (Cottrell, 2005, 2007; Kronenberg & Pollard, 2006). Although the empowering potential of activity and occupation is consistently emphasized in the occupational therapy literature, this promise is not always actualized in daily practice (AOTA, 2008; Honey, 1999). Therefore, I include in this chapter various learning activities to raise consciousness about disempowering practices and to develop the knowledge, skills, and attitudes to work with people in an empowering manner.

Occupational Therapy and Empowerment: A Very Brief History

The relationships among empowerment, activity, occupation, and social participation can be traced to occupational therapy's philosophical roots in *moral treatment,* which is based on respect for individuality and the acknowledgment of every person's right to engage in purposeful and meaningful activities with others (Bockoven, 1971; Kielhofner & Burke, 1977; Peloquin, 1989). Participation in the communal work of the institution and daily life regimens (made up of routine habits, domestic chores, creative crafts, and recreational activities) were believed to contribute to health and well-being. Kindness and appeals to rational thought replaced the restraints and punishments that had been used to treat mental illness (Bockoven, 1971; Peloquin, 1989).

Although multiple factors contributed to the demise of moral treatment, the founders of occupational therapy subsequently applied these humane beliefs to the new profession (Kielhofner & Burke, 1977; Peloquin, 1989). Early occupational therapists considered the people they worked with to be "unique individuals with fears, hopes, and aspirations, but most of all people with needs to understand . . . the role they play in life" (Bockoven, 1971, p. 224). The concepts of *individuality, personal choice, autonomy, purposefulness,* and *meaningfulness*—all of which are assumed in *empowerment*—are evident in the profession's early literature on the therapeutic power of *occupation* (Kielhofner & Burke, 1977). Consistent with these concepts, Adolf Meyer (1922/2005) described how the therapeutic use of activities contributed to pleasurable achievements, which motivated patients far more effectively than "exhortations to cheer up and to behave according to abstract or repressive rules" (p. 26). A holistic approach that viewed the person as an autonomous coparticipant was used (Hemphill-Pearson & Hunter, 1997). The therapist provided "opportunities, rather than prescriptions" (Meyer, 1922/2005, p. 27) and used occupations matched to the person's experience, interests, and aspirations (Kielhofner & Burke, 1977).

This *person-centered approach* to the therapeutic use of occupation was effective in enabling choice, developing personal control, and increasing self-efficacy. These are all important components of empowerment. These empowering practices, however, rarely extended beyond the person to implementing the systemic changes that are essential for true empowerment to occur.

The empowering potential of occupational therapy was further constrained when the profession aligned itself with the medical model (Kielhofner & Burke, 1977; Shannon, 1977). This model views disability as a deficit resulting from an undesirable health condition, disease, or trauma that requires professional intervention (Shakespeare & Watson, 1997; WHO, 2007). The professional is the expert who directs the care of the person with disabilities to cure the underlying cause of the disability, to prescriptively intervene to manage symptoms and enable adaptation to functional limitations, or both (Shannon, 1977; WHO, 2007). Although embracing the medical model increased occupational therapy's scientific base and practitioners' understanding of diagnoses (Colman, 1992), it stalled the acquisition of knowledge about occupation and derailed the use of occupation as a tool of personal empowerment (Kielhofner & Burke, 1977; Shannon, 1977). Reflecting on the consequences of this reductionist period for the profession, Reilly (1971) observed that "occupational therapists could stand accused by history of reducing the richness of their humanistic mandates to an ADL self-care list" (p. 244). Other leaders expressed similar concerns about the departure of occupational therapy from its holistic roots and urged the profession to find a way to merge science and occupation to support equal opportunities for health and participation of all people in their communities (West, 1968; Yerxa, 1967).

Mary Reilly (1971) envisioned a project of modernization for occupational therapy that would increase understanding and knowledge about the issues of *human aspiration, personal achievement, occupational choice,* and *quality of life.* This newly strengthened conceptualization of human *occupation* would enable the profession to move away from the medical model and join with social models more compatible with the founding principles and core values of occupational therapy. Over time, alternatives to the medical model did evolve to support therapeutic approaches and practice models that are congruent with the heritage of occupational therapy and empowerment. These include the Social Model of Disability (Shakespeare & Watson, 1997), consumer direction (Kosciulek, 1999), the Strengths-Based Model (Blundo, 2001), self-determination (Wehmeyer, 2005), the Recovery Model (Bishop, 2001), and client-centered and family-centered practices (Baum & Law, 1997; Kyler, 2008).

It is important to recognize that when occupational therapy was struggling to maintain its identity in an era dominated by reductionism, several exemplary practitioners did forge the way toward empowerment. For example, Beatrice Wade collaborated with formerly institutionalized people to organize an association "to instill in these patients a philosophy toward their own rehabilitation" (Wade, 1971, as cited in Bing, 1981, p. 513); Lela Llorens consulted with a community-based children's project to address cultural differences in the delivery of services and the availability of resources in diverse communities. Consistent with empowering practices, Llorens strongly advocated for occupational therapists to recognize the impact of environmental factors and social disparities on children's development (Shortridge & Walker, 1993). Despite the efforts of these exemplary models and the initiation of empowerment models in many venues, the vestiges of reductionism are evident in current practice settings (Kyler, 2008). As a result, the application of empowering practices in occupational therapy remains constrained. I explore these barriers to empowerment and provide strategies to counter their disempowering characteristics later in this chapter.

Although the challenges to empowering practices cannot be ignored, a review of the occupational therapy literature of the past two decades provides hope that disempowering practices may be nearing their demise. Numerous theoretical frameworks and practice examples consistent with the idea of empowerment exist (AOTA, 2008). These include Christiansen's (1999) conceptualization of *occupational identity*, Grady's (1995) call for *inclusive communities*, the Canadian perspective of *enabling occupation* (Townsend, 2003), and Pierce's (2001) *occupational design process*. Others have adopted and adapted many of the core concepts of empowerment, social justice, and the Social Model of Disability to propose the construct of occupational justice (AOTA, 2008; Kronenberg & Pollard, 2006). According to Townsend and Wilcock (2004), *occupational justice* is the fulfillment of the human

> right to experience occupation as meaningful and enriching, the right to develop through participation in occupations for health and social inclusion, the right to exert individual or population autonomy through choice in occupations, and the right to benefit from fair privileges for diverse participation in occupations. (p. 80)

When these rights are restricted because of external factors that the person cannot control (i.e., social, cultural, political, economic constraints), occupational injustice occurs (Kronenberg & Pollard, 2006; Townsend & Wilcock, 2004). Gupta and Walloch (2006) proposed that the concept of *justice* should be infused into practice to assist people in transcending social and occupational barriers and to "enhance their social participation, health, and well-being" (p. 1).

Finally, as occupational therapists move into nonmedical settings and deliver services to disenfranchised populations, they are more consistently framing their practices to be deeply embedded with the profession's core values (Thibeault, 2006). Moreover, a call for committing to and advocating for social and political changes that enable empowerment has become more persistent in the literature (Cottrell, 2005, 2007; Kronenberg & Pollard, 2006; Lohman, Gabriel, & Furlong, 2004).

Empowerment: Definitions and Foundational Concepts

Empowerment has been defined by many authors in diverse but philosophically coherent ways. Rapp et al. (1993) characterized *empowerment* as a process that increases power on an individual, social, or political level so that people can act to improve their quality of life. Similarly, Dunst and Trivette (1996) defined *empowerment* as "reorienting policy and clinical practice so as to have competency-enhancing rather than dependency-forming consequences" (p. 334). Although most definitions and conceptualizations of empowerment include empowering social policy and institutional practices, in this section I focus on concepts related to personal empowerment. I explore issues associated with systemic empowerment in greater depth in later sections.

Prevalent in definitions of empowerment are the interrelated concepts of *autonomy, control, locus of control, self-determination, self-efficacy,* and *self-management.* I now define these concepts (which are sometimes used interchangeably) and discuss their relationship to empowerment.

Autonomy is expressed as free will and independence in setting one's personal agenda. Becoming empowered contributes to increased autonomy (Tengland, 2007).

Control is the ability to exercise free choice over life decisions (Hammell, 2004). *Control* can also be defined as the exertion of "direction and restraint over others with a focus on dominating them and achieving mastery over them" (Fidler, 1993, p. 583). The latter definition has dominated the history of disenfranchised people, including people with disabilities, whereas the former definition is the desired personal outcome of empowerment (Charlton, 1998).

Locus of control proposes that a person's beliefs about the consequences of life events can be internally or externally based. This viewpoint drives people's behaviors (Bandura, 1977). People with an internal locus of control believe they control their own fate. Consequently, they set goals and engage in behaviors to achieve these goals (Kosciulek, 1999). These actions enable empowerment. Conversely, people with an external locus of control may have difficulty setting goals and working to alter their situations because they perceive their efforts as futile. When people are treated in a manner that marginalizes their ability to control their lives, an external locus of control is fostered, and disempowerment occurs.

Self-determination refers to people's inherent right and innate capacity to assume responsibility for, exert control over, and autonomously direct their lives (Wehmeyer, 2005). Empowering practices facilitate and support self-determination.

Self-efficacy is the perception of the ability to perform a given behavior or task to successfully attain a desired outcome (Bandura, 1977). In empowerment, self-efficacy is the factor that explains the difference between people's innate abilities and their actual performance. When people's actions are ineffective because of forces beyond their control, they may internalize this futility even though they may have the inherent capability to succeed (Honey, 1999; Kosciulek, 1999).

Self-management is the ability to exert personal control over services by independently determining when, how, and by whom services are provided (National Council on Disability [NCD], 2004). People who self-manage their services autonomously use free choice on a daily basis. Self-management is a core principle of the disability rights movement and is embodied in the rallying cry of "Nothing about us without us" (Charlton, 1998).

Integrating these concepts with the *ICF* and the *Framework–II,* I propose this behavioral description of empowerment: Empowered people have an internal locus of control and a positive sense of self-efficacy that enable them to self-direct their lives and self-manage their services. These empowering characteristics make it possible for people to autonomously engage in meaningful activities and valued occupations and participate in environments of choice.

Disempowerment of People With Disabilities

Many people with disabilities possess the characteristics just described as inherent to an empowered life. People with disabilities, however, also disproportionately share major disempowering characteristics with other marginalized groups (Kielhofner, 2005). These factors contribute to their disempowerment and include the following:

- *Unemployment:* Fewer than half (46%) of people ages 21 to 64 with a disability are employed, compared with 84% of people in this age group without a disability (U.S. Census Bureau, 2008). The employment–population ratio (i.e., the proportion of the noninstitutionalized civilian population older than age 16 that is employed) for people with disabilities is substantially lower than that for people without disabilities (20% vs. 65%, respectively; U.S. Bureau of Labor Statistics, 2009).
- *Inadequate education:* The high school graduation rate for students with disabilities is only 57% (U.S. Department of Education, 2008). Furthermore, transition planning and transition services are often inadequate in preparing students for their postsecondary school lives (Wehmeyer, 2005).
- *Poverty:* People with disabilities have lower incomes and are more impoverished than people without disabilities. Adults with severe disabilities have a poverty rate of 26%, which is more than three times that of adults without disabilities, who have a poverty rate of 7.7% (Steinmetz, 2002).
- *Limited housing options:* Accessible housing in the United States is scarce. Moreover, the average rent for a modest one-bedroom apartment is higher than the entire monthly income provided to people with disabilities by Supplemental Security Income. Consequently, it is virtually impossible for people with disabilities to obtain adequate, accessible, and affordable housing in the community (O'Hara & Cooper, 2005).

MYTHS ABOUT DISABILITY

Having a disability can be disempowering because of prevailing myths about disability. In the following sections, I present and debunk some major false beliefs that contribute to the disempowerment of people with disabilities.

DISABILITY IS AN ABNORMAL PATHOLOGY

The view of disability as pathological and abnormal has a longstanding history, with one of the most disturbing examples being the display of people with disabilities as freaks in circus sideshows (Longmere & Umansky, 2001). Although these public displays are obsolete, the common view that disability is a digression from the norm still prevails. This stance denies the reality that more than 54.4 million Americans (19% of the population) have a disability (U.S. Census Bureau, 2008). This large population is the one minority group that potentially anyone can join. Can a characteristic truly be considered abnormal when almost one in five people share it and when any person can develop the trait at any moment in time?

DISABILITY IS A PERSONAL TRAGEDY

The perspective that people with disabilities are to be pitied is firmly established in Western culture. Charles Dickens's portrayal of Tiny Tim, the 1960s telethon parades of children with muscular dystrophy struggling to walk while strapped to full leg braces, and biographies and movies produced to evoke sympathy have all contributed to the view of disability as a misfortune (Kielhofner, 2005; Shakespeare & Watkins, 1997; Snow, 2006). Contrary to this atmosphere of pity, disability rights activists celebrate differences and affirm that the personal attributes of people with disabilities are not innately disabling. They challenge people without disabilities to stop feeling sorry for those with them and instead call them to join the fight against social inequality and inaccurate stereotypes that are the true source of disability (Shakespeare & Watkins, 1997; Snow, 2006). In the narration to his award-winning short film titled "Thumbs Down to Pity" (Snow, 2006), an independent young adult with cerebral palsy named Benjamin Snow confronted Hollywood's "pity portrayals" of people with disabilities. He described his daily life as productive, satisfying, and "nothing like" Hollywood typecasting.

DISABILITY IS TO BE FEARED

The possibility of incurring a disability is frightening to many. This fear is manifested in prenatal testing for conditions such as spina bifida and Down syndrome. Although the exploration of the moral complexity of these practices is beyond the scope of this chapter, Neville-Jan (2005), an occupational therapist with spina bifida who was born before these technological advances, raised thought-provoking questions. She wondered, "Would I exist today? Is there a value to having spina bifida?" (p. 528). These questions have been raised by many disability rights activists (Longmere & Umansky, 2001).

When dealing with intellectual disorders and mental illness, the devaluing of life with disability often escalates to fear. The mainstream media often equate these disorders with irrational thought, impulsivity, and violence, and as a result stigmatizing fear reigns. The disempowering impact of fear extends beyond the individual person to the community level: Communities that do not confront stigma fail to protect the rights of people with disabilities or provide opportunities for participation (Corrigan, 2002).

TO HAVE A SATISFACTORY LIFE, PEOPLE WITH DISABILITIES MUST RISE ABOVE THEIR LIMITATIONS

Typically, people with disabilities who are portrayed as successful in the mainstream media are those who have achieved extraordinary goals (e.g., a person with paraplegia climbing a mountain, a wheelchair user completing a marathon). Those living a more routine life are often viewed as having an unsatisfying life because of their disability. Yet people without disabilities are not expected to attain extraordinary success to have a satisfying life. The perception that quality of life is compromised by the limitations imposed by disability is false and disempowering. Contrary to this myth, even people with significant disabilities who require assistance to complete daily tasks can be satisfied with their quality of life, if they perceive that they can self-direct their lives regardless of their functional abilities or limitations (Conneeley, 2003; Fleming-Castaldy, 2009). Disability rights activists have contended that having choice, control, and autonomy in the management of service delivery results in participants' increased power over their lives, thereby increasing their quality of life (Morris, 1997; NCD, 2004; see Figure 17.2). Living a self-determined life (even one considered quite ordinary) can be as satisfying to a person with disability as it is to a person without one.

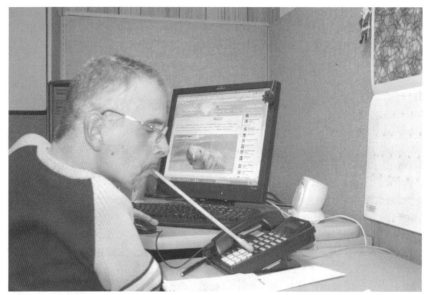

Figure 17.2. Keith Williams, community organizer for the Northeast Pennsylvania Center for Independent Living, asserts, "Contrary to popular belief, people with disabilities multitask like everyone else." Basic adaptive equipment and community-based personal care assistance enable Keith (who has arthrogryposis) to live, work, and play where he chooses. Photographer Nicole Spaldo has worked with Keith as his personal care attendant for 5 years.

THE INTELLIGENCE AND RATIONAL DECISION-MAKING CAPACITY OF PEOPLE WITH CERTAIN DISABILITIES SHOULD ALWAYS BE QUESTIONED

This myth remains prevalent in the approaches used with people with mental health, cognitive, or developmental disabilities. It is erroneous to assume that people who have disabilities that hinder them from learning in a typical manner are not intelligent. Likewise, asserting that all decisions that differ from professional opinion are symptomatic is biased (Honey, 1999). Also erroneous is diagnosing communication deficits, which can result from developmental disabilities such as autism or cerebral palsy, as being indicative of mental retardation (Schoener, Kinnealey, & Koenig, 2008). The impact of these invalid assumptions and diagnoses is beyond disempowering. It is harmful. As poignantly described by David, a teen assumed to be mentally retarded, misdiagnosis can result in never daring to have dreams (Schoener et al., 2008).

PROFESSIONALS HOLD THE KEY TO A PERSON'S RECOVERY FROM DISABILITY

Recovery has been described as the ability to live a satisfying life of choice while managing the impact of illness on life (Corrigan, 2006). Although professional services can support and facilitate recovery, the assumption that a person is incapable of recovery without these services is false. This belief is inherently disempowering because it removes agency from the person with the disability (Bishop, 2001). People with diabilities can and do recover without (and in some cases in spite of) professional intervention. Consumer-operated services can effectively enable recovery and empowerment (Corrigan, 2006). Moreover, children with developmental delays can progress, even if families decide not to implement all the suggested professional interventions (Holzmueller, 2005).

THE DESIRED AND ANTICIPATED OUTCOME OF REHABILITATION IS THE ACQUISITION OF SKILLS TO PERFORM ACTIVITIES THAT ENABLE THE CONTINUATION OF A PREDISABILITY LIFE

Although some people with disabilities can and do attain this goal, most cannot attain the full resumption of previous life activities (Toal-Sullivan & Henderson, 2004). Consequently, if a person perceives that the sole expected outcome of rehabilitation is the resumption of a former lifestyle, unrealistic expectations are perpetuated. When the reality sets in that previous levels of functioning cannot be achieved, emotional distress can occur that may impede the transition to and development of a successful postdisability life.

Feelings of personal helplessness and dissatisfaction with life may be fostered by the unanticipated dependency that occurs when people with significant disabilities must rely on others to complete daily activities (Charlton, 1998). How people with disabilities perceive their dependence on others can influence their quality of life, for example, whether they view the need for services as a sign of their personal inefficacy or as a way to contribute to their independence and personal empowerment (Fleming-Castaldy, 2009; Morris, 1997). Thus, the desired outcome of rehabilitation should not be the independent resumption of activities because this focus is innately disempowering (Charlton, 1998; Toal-Sullivan & Henderson, 2004). Rather, consistent with the *Framework–II* (AOTA, 2008), the outcome of occupational therapy should be active engagement in meaningful and desired occupations in a personally satisfying and self-determined manner. I discuss methods to achieve this outcome in a later section.

PEOPLE WITH SIGNIFICANT DISABILITIES CANNOT LIVE INDEPENDENTLY

The significant functional limitations associated with many disabilities often result in a need for assistance to complete many tasks. Yet independence is not reliant on activity performance. People are independent when they self-determine how and when their desired activities are performed (AOTA, 2008; Charlton, 1998; Hinojosa, 2002). Society's adherence to the myth that disability makes independent living impossible has historically resulted in the institutionalization of people with disabilities. Currently, public funding significantly limits the availability of community-based personal care assistance, leading to the prolonged or permanent institutionalization of people with disabilities in skilled nursing facilities (Cottrell, 2005; NCD, 2004). Institutionalization hinders participation in life and further increases dependency. The resulting diminished autonomy and decreased quality of life is disempowering (Kosciulek, 1999; Magasi & Hammel, 2009; NCD, 2004).

It is important to recognize that the provision of personal care assistance in the community does not ensure that the care recipient's independence is acknowledged, respected, or facilitated. Many community-based programs adhere to the belief that adequate personal care assistance requires professional supervision and agency staff management. Paternalistic policies and practices can disempower people with disabilities by restricting their choice of services and limiting their control over service delivery, thereby fostering a personal identity that is dependent (Bishop, 2005; Mitchell & Kemp, 2000). Charmaz (1983) described the disempowering experience of "being bathed and dressed by strangers with rough hands and patronizing attitudes" (p. 186). He concluded that arrangements made to "aid" the person with disabilities can "underscore fears of incapacity or incompetence" (p. 186) when they are not self-determined. Conversely, the provision of community resources that enable people with disabilities to self-select and self-direct their services results in a more satisfactory life and increased autonomy (Fleming-Castaldy, 2009; NCD, 2004). These effects enable independent living outcomes that are highly congruent with empowerment (Kosciulek, 1999).

IMPACT OF DISEMPOWERING MYTHS ON REHABILITATION PRACTICE

The perpetuation of these myths contributes to the prevalence of disempowering practices among rehabilitation professionals (Kielhofner, 2005). Stigmatization and fear of disability undermine the formation of trusting collaborative relationships (Corrigan, 2002) that are the foundation of empowering practices. Similarly, when professionals pity people with disabilities, they typically adopt a maternal protective approach that makes the formation of an empowering partnership impossible. When a person is not given the opportunity to take chances, not given the right to fail, and not allowed to make mistakes, unhealthy dependence is fostered. The person is also infantilized because personal growth, maturity, and resilience (essential characteristics for empowerment) are developed through such experiences of attempt, failure, and recovery.

Professionals who believe that they are essential for recovery place themselves in the role of expert. Consequently, they do not seek the opinions of people with disabilities about their preferred life course (Honey, 1999). A disturbing example of this is Johnson and Sharpe's (2000) finding that 92% of the special education administrators they surveyed would be least likely to facilitate a student-led individualized education program meeting. When personal goals are expressed, professional feedback is often tokenistic, unsupportive, demeaning, or all of these (Knox, Parmenter, Atkinson, & Yazbeck, 2000). People with disabilities (and their families) are often told by rehabilitation professionals that successful adaptation requires giving up many aspirations perceived as unrealistic (Holzmueller, 2005; Wehmeyer, 2005).

For example, my brother was told by many that attending college was a waste of time because his Friedreich's ataxia was progressive. They could not envision what Kevin could possibly hope to gain from the experience. Kevin's resistance to accepting these imposed limitations was consistently viewed as maladaptive and clear evidence of his denial of the terminal nature of Friedreich's ataxia. Fortunately, one vocational counselor partnered with Kevin to achieve his goal of attending college. The benefits derived from the empowering nature of the experience were far greater than the bachelor's and master's degrees Kevin earned. For many years, attending college provided him with a satisfying, self-directed life made up of meaningful activities and valued occupations, including partying during spring break.

Practitioners who view themselves as experts further undermine the autonomy and control of people with disabilities when they adopt paternalistic approaches (Charlton, 1998). These disempowering practices diminish the self-efficacy and perceived capabilities of people with disabilities. People need to believe that their efforts have the potential to be successful (Bandura, 1977). Therefore, when people with disabilities are treated in a manner that diminishes their internal locus of control, they may have difficulty seeing the point of any efforts to alter their situation. The resulting inability to self-determine desired goals and engage in self-directed behaviors is the hallmark of disempowerment (Fleischer & Zames, 2001).

EXERCISE 17.2: SETTING THE STAGE FOR EMPOWERING PARTNERSHIPS

Consider how you approach an initial session with people with whom you will be working in occupational therapy. Is your approach empowering or disempowering? Compose two to three sentences that you would use in the practice scenarios provided in Table 17.2 to introduce yourself as a practitioner who is willing to partner with a client (or his or her caregiver) to facilitate self-directed participation.

Even if a practitioner does not adopt a paternal or expert stance, the very nature of being a professional automatically establishes a separation from nonprofessionals and infers a hierarchical relationship (Gaitskell, 1998). By definition, a professional has unique specialized expertise (Costello, 1990). This expert status establishes an inherent imbalance of power in the therapeutic relationship and can generate feelings of disempowerment from the person's initial introduction to services (Franits, 2005). Occupational therapists and occupational therapy assistants can be particularly disempowering without even realizing it (Abberley, 1995). As Taylor (2001) observed, occupational therapists often perceive themselves as helpers who fix functional limitations. When occupational therapy education, both academic and fieldwork, emphasizes the attainment of functional independence in performance as the profession's main focus, the disempowering nature of occupational therapy is further reinforced.

Empowerment Theory, the Empowerment Process, and Disability

Empowerment theory integrates theories of control and personal identity with an understanding of sociopolitical contexts to propose that people with disabilities are competent and can proactively participate in life. It focuses on the involvement of people with disabilities in self-determining and controlling their lives (Charlton, 1998). Zimmerman and Warschausky (1998) proposed that empowerment of a person occurs when he or she has perceived control, collaborates with others to attain goals, and is cognizant of supports and barriers to efforts to self-direct his or her life. They described this personal empowerment according to three dimensions: values, processes, and outcomes.

VALUES

The values underlying Empowerment Theory represent core beliefs governing how people with disabilities work with professionals and vice versa. These values include the belief that disability is not synonymous with illness and

Table 17.2. Practice Considerations for Infusing Empowerment Into Occupational Therapy

Practice Setting	Issues and Concerns That Can Affect Empowerment	Case Example
Early intervention	• Sociocultural stigma of parental responsibility for disability • Parents' grief for an anticipated child • Need to emotionally adjust and chart an alternative story for the family • Professional's emphasis on developmental norms or milestones, not uniqueness of child	The parents of a toddler with significant developmental delays report that they have not initiated several of the practitioner's "homework" suggestions because they are too disruptive to the family's routine. The family includes two older children, ages 4 to 12 years.
School based	• Noncompliant educational systems that do not obtain parents' or students' voices for individualized education and transition plans • Participation restrictions that limit engagement and perpetuate segregation	During a transition planning meeting, a 14-year-old describes goals for his or her postsecondary life, which the parents state are not possible given their child's functional limitations. Several team members concur.
Acute care hospital	• Short lengths of stay limit the focus of rehabilitation to the most critical need • Time-consuming documentation required for reimbursement • Reductionist practices dominate care	A 53-year-old concert pianist incurred a concussion and multiple fractures to her dominant hand. She is a part-time student pursuing a music therapy degree. Length of stay is likely 3 days.
Psychiatric partial hospital	• Staff mistrust of the rational thinking capabilities of people with mental illness and discomfort with relationships based on equality • Stigma limits opportunities for participation in educational, work, leisure, and living environments	A 28-year-old man with an 8-year history of schizophrenia begins his first day at a partial hospitalization program after a 5-day hospitalization. He is living in a proprietary home and is unemployed. He states he wants to move into his own apartment, finish his college degree, and get a job.
Skilled nursing facility	• Residency is most often not a personal choice • Diminished community participation • Loss of control over daily life routines • Restricted occupational roles, limited purposeful activities, and social isolation	An 87-year-old new resident is referred to occupational therapy for poststroke rehabilitation. The resident refuses to participate in the initial evaluation because "life is over" now that his or her home is "lost" and all friends are "gone."

incompetence. Rather, people with disabilities are capable of wellness and competence. Consequently, person-directed collaboration between people with disabilities and professionals is respected and expected (Zimmerman & Warschausky, 1998; see Figure 17.3). These values of empowerment are congruent with occupational therapy's core values of equality, freedom, justice, dignity, and truth (AOTA, 1993). They are evident in the profession of occupational therapy in that practitioners believe that people with disabilities are competent and fully capable of independently self-managing their service delivery.

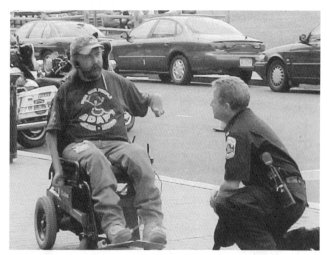

Figure 17.3. Mutual respect is the foundation for empowerment. Michael Auberger talks with an unidentified police officer at an ADAPT rally.

Note. Photo by Kathleen Klienmann. Copyright © 2000, by TRIPIL. Reprinted with permission.

EXERCISE 17.3: SELF-ASSESSMENT OF VALUES REGARDING POWER

Fidler (1993) observed that "the capacity to empower self and others is greatly shaped by our values and beliefs about our self and others" (p. 584). Consequently, examining one's empowering and disempowering personal views and attitudes is essential for self-knowledge and personal growth and to enable efficacy. I provide these questions to prompt self-reflection about your own perspectives that may block or support the implementation of empowerment principles as you practice occupational therapy: What does power mean to you? What is the difference between control and power? Is it acceptable for a professional to be uncertain about a preferred course of action? Consider the cases in Table 17.2. How do you balance the desired empowerment outcome for each person to live a self-determined life with legitimate concerns about the person's realistic chances for success versus failure? Does the person's diagnosis or age influence your perceptions of his or her ability to make decisions to self-direct services?

PROCESSES

Processes are the empowering mechanisms by which people with disabilities work with each other, professionals, agencies, and communities to gain control over their lives. They involve the provision of opportunities to help people with disabilities acquire the knowledge and skills needed to make decisions, self-advocate, and access and manage resources to become self-reliant in the existing sociopolitical environment. Essential empowerment processes include overcoming obstacles that prevent full community participation and changing conditions that present barriers to living a self-directed life (Zimmerman & Warschausky, 1998).

In occupational therapy, these empowering processes begin with ascertaining the person's perspective during evaluation (AOTA, 2008). Subsequent empowering processes include the development of self-determined goals, the provision of person-centered interventions, consumer education and training in personal advocacy skills and effective management of resources, and opportunities to develop and practice leadership skills.

OUTCOMES

The outcomes of empowering processes include increased awareness, control, and participation. People with disabilities who are empowered understand their sociopolitical context. They are motivated to use their acquired knowledge and skills to influence their environment and participate fully in society. They perceive themselves as competent and actively engage in behaviors to exert control over their lives, resulting in an increased sense of autonomy and perceived control (Zimmerman & Warschausky, 1998). At the conclusion of occupational therapy, empowerment outcomes are evident when service recipients have successfully attained self-determined goals for participation, live self-directed lives, and self-advocate to obtain needed services to engage in desired occupations.

Guidelines for Empowering Practices in Occupational Therapy

To counter the disempowering effects of disability and facilitate empowerment, these three general principles should guide occupational therapy practice.

1. *Establish partnership relationships that respect the expertise of each participant.* Client-centered and family-centered approaches grounded in an equitable distribution of power are required for empowering practices (Honey, 1999; Knox et al., 2000; Kyler, 2008). The practitioner should share realistic and accurate information that offers possibilities rather than pathologize the situation (Holzmueller, 2005, Knox et al., 2000; Moghimi, 2007). The person's or caregiver's intimate knowledge of the unique effects of disability on current and envisioned occupational performance, combined with the practitioner's professional competencies, can lead to the attainment of self-determined goals (AOTA, 2008; Wehmeyer, 2005). Moreover, acknowledging the person's expert status

supports his or her autonomy, internal locus of control, and self-efficacy, which are essential characteristics for empowerment (Franits, 2005).

2. *Presume intelligence and the potential for competence.* Schoener et al. (2008) described the experience of David, who was presumed to have an intellectual deficit because of his inability to communicate verbally. The validity of this assumption was not discredited until David was 14, when his professional team used an approach that respected him as an individual and trusted his capacity to learn. The comprehensive, nonjudgmental occupational therapy evaluation provided an accurate determination of David's capabilities, and he subsequently acquired effective communication that he said "Freed my little voice to be heard" (Schoener et al., 2008, p. 547). David's vivid and insightful description of living with autism spectrum disorder provides a most powerful and highly intelligent voice that gives testament to the importance of assuming the intellectual capability of all people with disabilities.

3. *Apply all types of clinical reasoning.* Rogers (1983) identified clinical reasoning as essential for helping people with disabilities live the "good life." Occupational therapists use these complex mental processes to think about the individual; the disability; the uniqueness of the situation; and the personal, social, and cultural meanings the person gives to the disability (Fleming, 1991). Novice practitioners tend to emphasize procedural reasoning because it is concrete (Gaitskell, 1998). Although procedural reasoning is required to identify abilities and challenges to performance, its technical emphasis can be disempowering, especially if it is used exclusively. Practitioners must put procedures into the context of the person's valued roles and meaningful occupations.

Going beyond the singular use of procedural reasoning can serve as an opportunity to initiate an empowering process. Interactive reasoning can be used to develop a collaborative and trusting therapeutic relationship; conditional reasoning can be used to consider the unique developmental, social, and cultural aspects of a person's life (Fleming, 1991); and narrative reasoning can be used to listen to an envisioned story (Mattingly, 1991). These processes can have the desired empowerment outcome of enabling the person to engage in a self-determined intervention program. Pragmatic reasoning can ensure that the practitioner considers the influence of personal and practical constraints on service delivery (Schell & Cervero, 1993). To facilitate empowerment, the practitioner must first acknowledge that neither disability nor its resulting functional limitations are inherently disempowering. Rather, external factors are the cause of the disempowerment of people with disabilities and other marginalized groups (Abberley, 1995). Consequently, the conscious application of pragmatic reasoning is needed to help occupational therapists and occupational therapy assistants understand the social, political, and economic realities of practice and negotiate the pragmatic contextual issues that can hinder or facilitate empowerment.

EXERCISE 17.4: EMPOWERING APPLICATION OF CLINICAL REASONING

Review the case examples outlined in Table 17.2. Identify the evaluation methods and intervention approaches typically used in these practice situations. Reflect on the technical explanations of these methods and approaches (procedural reasoning). Describe how you can explain these procedures to the person (or his or her caregiver) to engage him or her in the occupational therapy process (interactive reasoning) while considering the uniqueness of the person's situation (conditional reasoning). How can you proactively deal with each setting's challenges and pragmatic constraints to facilitate empowering practices? Identify resources and supports that can be used to address existing barriers to empowerment (pragmatic reasoning).

EVALUATION GUIDELINES

Established standards emphasize the consideration of the person's occupational roles, concerns, perspectives, and expectations in occupational therapy evaluation and in the choice of tools (AOTA, 2008; Moyers & Dale, 2007). These fundamental principles enable empowering practices. Moreover, engaging the person and his or her caregiver in an open discussion about the evaluation process and its outcomes can facilitate rapport and the development of a collaborative therapeutic relationship (Hinojosa, Kramer, & Crist, 2005; Moghimi, 2007). This evaluation outcome is essential if an empowering partnership with the person receiving services is to be forged. Conversely, when the core principles of collaboration, self-determination, client-centered practice, or family-centered practice are not applied during occupational therapy evaluation, disempowerment occurs.

The occupational profile has been put forth as the gold standard for person-centered occupational therapy evaluation (AOTA, 2008). However, practical constraints may preclude the use of the profile, such as in an acute care setting with a short length of stay or when the need to relieve pain dominates the situation (Gutman, Mortera, Hinojosa, & Kramer, 2007). Consequently, the use of pragmatic reasoning to select and use person-centered approaches and tools is critical to empowering practices. Hinojosa et al. (2005) proposed that when practical realities constrain the completion of a full occupational profile, the process aspects of this evaluation should be emphasized. Limiting the occupational profile to an initial evaluation is not the most effective use of this tool. Rather, the occupational profile should be used throughout occupational therapy service delivery to inform treatment (AOTA, 2008; Hinojosa et al., 2007). The ongoing collaboration that results in the latter case can ensure that the therapist is engaging with the person (an empowering stance) rather than doing things to or for the person (a disempowering approach).

In addition to the occupational therapy profile, many measures are available to support the integration of empowerment principles into the evaluation process (Law, Baum, & Dunn, 2005). These include the Canadian Occupational Performance Measure, the Coping Inventory, the Occupational Self-Assessment, the Role Checklist, and the Test of Playfulness (Law et al., 2005). The occupational therapy reflective staircase described in chapter 10 also supports an empowering evaluation process. Evaluation tools from other fields (e.g., the Consumer Constructed Empowerment Scale [Rogers, Chamberlin, Ellison, & Crean, 1997] and the Quality of Life Inventory [Frisch, 1994]) can also illuminate the client's perspectives to aid in the establishment of an empowering intervention plan. When using any measurement tool, practitioners must be careful not to let the task-oriented nature of the evaluation process hinder their ability to hear the person's story (Merryman & Riegel, 2007). Active listening to discern the meaning of disability to the person is essential for empowering practice (Franits, 2005).

INTERVENTION GUIDELINES

The *Framework–II* delineates five approaches for use in occupational therapy intervention. Table 17.3 highlights the empowering characteristics of each approach and provides guidelines for using them in an empowering manner.

When implementing these intervention approaches, the application of the core principles of collaboration, self-determination, client-centered practice, and family-centered practice facilitates empowerment. Empowering interventions provide experiences based on choice that facilitate meaningful involvement (AOTA, 2008; Honey, 1999). To be truly empowering, however, occupational therapy interventions must focus on outcomes beyond the walls of the clinic, home, or schoolroom. Occupational therapists can contribute to the empowerment of people with disabilities by providing learning opportunities to help them become self-determined and participate fully in their desired environments. In other words, intervention must move beyond simulated activities in clinical settings to real, in vivo activities.

Interventions that are, or work toward, a match between the person's abilities and expectations are also needed. To ensure that the person is provided with the "just-right" challenge to achieve desired goals, occupational therapists can apply their activity and occupational performance analysis and synthesis skills (AOTA, 2008). Without analyzing clients' performance in activities, practitioners cannot effectively help people develop meaningful occupational roles (Gutman et al., 2007).

The use of activities can provide a context in which people learn what they are capable of achieving. Moreover, if the therapeutic use of occupations is naturalized so that interventions are performed in people's own environments, they are afforded the opportunity to identify barriers and experience challenges that may not be evident in a simulated experience (Pierce, 2001). Using this knowledge, the practitioner and client can problem solve to find

Table 17.3. Empowerment Guidelines for Occupational Therapy Intervention

Intervention Approach and Empowering Characteristics	Empowerment Guidelines
Health promotion • Does not assume disability • Focuses on natural contexts • Aims to create and promote enriched experiences	• Consider all persons as capable of health and wellness, even those with a diagnosed condition • Provide multiple in vivo opportunities for performance of desired activities and meaningful occupations • Create equal opportunities for people with disabilities to engage in natural activities for health and wellness (e.g., wheelchair yoga classes for stress reduction, play groups for new parents and their children)
Remediation/Restoration • Addresses limitations that hinder performance • Develops and restores new or impaired skills and abilities	• Collaborate to determine person's priorities for skill development • Provide interventions to develop the abilities needed to engage in desired occupational roles (e.g., driver rehabilitation to enable resumption of "soccer mom" role; strength, endurance, and mobility training to facilitate assumption of the new role of quad rugby player)
Compensation/Adaptation • Modifies the demands or context of activity to enable performance in natural contexts	• Partner with people to establish their priorities for activity performance • Provide adaptations and compensations that enable performance of the person's desired activities in their natural settings (e.g., adaptive play equipment in a barrier-free playground, palm pilot programmed to give cues that help organize work and school tasks)
Maintenance • Provides supports that enable the retention of performance abilities • Focuses on meeting occupational needs to preserve quality of life	• Recognize the disempowering effect of limited supports and scant resources for maintaining persons with disabilities in their environments of choice • Network with available services to provide needed and desired supports (e.g., service coordination services to enable a young adult with an intellectual disability to live independently in his or her own apartment)
Disability prevention • Addresses risk factors for difficulties in occupational performance • Prevents the development of contextual barriers to occupation	• Assess the person's contexts to identify risks for disempowering disability (e.g., poor ergonomics at work, unrelenting stress due to intense caregiving demands) • Provide consultation and referrals to prevent risks from leading to dysfunction (e.g., consult to ergonomically adapt worksites, refer the parent of an infant with multiple complex medical needs to a home-based family care respite program)

Note. Adapted from "Occupational Therapy Practice Framework: Domain and Process, 2nd ed.," by American Occupational Therapy Association, 2008, *American Journal of Occupational Therapy, 62*, pp. 625–683. Copyright © 2008, by American Occupational Therapy Association. Adapted with permission.

solutions that will enable desired occupational performance in the person's typical contexts.

Educating people with disabilities, their caregivers, and their family members in the principles and methods of activity and environmental analysis, gradation, and modification can also provide effective strategies that enable the postrehabilitation performance of desired activities and meaningful occupations in diverse settings (AOTA, 2008). Knowing how to handle future situations can strengthen the family's control, which sustains them as a family (Knox et al., 2000).

Finally, throughout the occupational therapy process, the development of self-advocacy skills should permeate all interventions. Practitioners can support the person's confident identification of assets, limitations, aspirations, legal rights, and personal responsibilities. If needed, skills training in communication, assertiveness, and personnel management can help people become effective self-advocates for living life as they choose (AOTA, 2008; Hinojosa, 2002).

DEVELOPMENTAL CONSIDERATIONS FOR EMPOWERING PRACTICE

All of these evaluation principles and intervention approaches can be applied across the developmental continuum. Their effective implementation, however, requires an understanding of developmental issues. Failure to consider the person's or caregiver's life stage can contribute to disempowerment. For example, when working with infants and young children, occupational therapists typically support the child's development but are often not cognizant of the impact they have on the unfolding identity of both the child and the family (Holzmueller, 2005). To balance disempowering messages of a hopeless future, occupational therapists and occupational therapy assistants can examine the possibilities unique to the child's evolving story and provide pragmatic advice when hope stagnates. Standardized developmental assessments should be accompanied by measures that ascertain the child's and family's perspectives on their strengths and limitations.

When children reach adolescence, the practitioner can facilitate the transition of decision-making power from the parents to the child. Occupational therapy can help adolescents develop the knowledge, skills, and attitudes needed for self-determined independent living, postsecondary education, employment in adult life, or all of these (Wehmeyer, 2005). Key components of effective transition planning include active collaboration with parents, especially because they may have difficulty seeing their disabled child assuming adult roles and self-selected occupations (Brollier, Shepherd, & Markley, 1994). Supporting the self-determination of adolescents can result in more positive outcomes in adult life (Wehmeyer, 2005). To accomplish this, practitioners must critique the models of practice they use to ensure that the approaches implemented are effectively meeting the person's goals for living a self-directed life. For example, school-based practice traditionally emphasizes the use of sensorimotor and developmental models. These are insufficient, however, for the development of the living skills needed to live a self-determined life after high school (Brollier et al., 1994). Adolescents need interventions that help them negotiate the multiple changes that occur during this life stage, develop a positive, stable role identity, acquire self-efficacy, learn essential life skills, and achieve autonomy (Chinman & Linney, 1998).

When working with adults, the disempowering effects of the medical model must be countered with the implementation of person-directed approaches to ensure that the person's life stage is considered when formulating a self-directed intervention plan (e.g., is the person beginning a career, establishing a household, raising a family?). To facilitate the empowerment of older adults, stereotypical and ageist views that equate age with incompetence and loss of control must be confronted (Loft, McWilliams, McWilliams, & Ward-Griffin, 2003). The disempowering structures that are often inherent in long-term-care facilities (e.g., in nursing homes) must be recognized, and concerted efforts must be made to engage the resident, family members, and primary care providers (e.g., nurses' aides) in service care planning (Ingersoll-Dayton, Schroepfer, Pryce, & Waarala, 2003).

Challenges to Empowering Practice

Although concepts congruent with empowerment permeate the literature of occupational therapy and infuse the profession's theoretical frameworks, evidence that these beliefs have infused actual practice has not been documented. By contrast, the literature on practice realities has identified many constraints to the implementation of empowerment in occupational therapy practice (Honey, 1999; Kyler, 2008; Redick, McClain, & Brown, 2000). Anecdotal information received from students postfieldwork also reflects a lack of integration of these values and beliefs into daily practice. In the following sections, I identify several of the major challenges to empowering practices and describe strategies to address these challenges in a manner that facilitates empowerment.

BUDGET CUTBACKS AND CAPPED REIMBURSEMENT

Economic constraints often result in decreased services and fewer intervention sessions, which in turn limits the opportunities for the voiced opinions of people with disabilities to be solicited, heard, and acted on. Consequently, empowerment is often given a low priority in the rehabilitation process (Redick et al., 2000). A partnership relationship is essential for a person to view acute care as the first step in his or her rehabilitation (Belice & McGovern-Denk, 2002). By implementing evaluations focused on the person's goals, investment in the rehabilitation process is enhanced. Educating people with disabilities, their caregivers, and their family members in the self-management of their postrehabilitation life facilitates recovery (Belice & McGovern-Denk, 2002; Loft et al., 2003; Merryman & Riegel, 2007).

PERSONAL ADJUSTMENT AND IDENTITY CONCERNS

People who have a newly acquired disability may require time to adjust to the reality of their altered lives. They may share many of the stigmatizing myths of disability discussed earlier in this chapter. As a result, a disempowering personal identity may limit their ability to engage in rehabilitation (Kielhofner, 2005; Merryman & Riegel, 2007). The occupational therapist and occupational therapy assistant must take care to avoid labeling this disengagement as evidence of poor motivation. Rather, practitioners should partner with people to identify the social, cultural, physical, economic, and political obstacles to their engagement (Abberley, 1995). Intervention should focus on the removal of these barriers and the provision of supports that enable people to develop a positive self-identity as a person with a disability who is capable of living a full and satisfying life (Kielhofner, 2005). Moreover, the practitioner should endorse the person's potential for recovery (Corrigan, 2002). The development of positive self-efficacy can mediate the disempowering effects of stigma (Vauth, Klein, Wirtz, & Corrigan, 2008).

Lack of Faith or Trust

Many people with disabilities have extensive histories of disempowerment. They are often the recipients of services that offer them little choice or control. Consequently, they may consider attempts to self-direct their services to be futile because experience has taught them that they will not be listened to and nothing will change (Honey, 1999; Merryman & Riegel, 2007). Consistent delivery of the promised approach to partner with the person in an honest and respectful collaboration can renew faith and build trust in the idea that the therapist's desire for the person's participation is not "just talk" (Honey, 1999, p. 264). Interactive reasoning can be used to actively seek the person's voice and establish the practitioner's view of the person as the expert who is capable of self-determination.

Residual Symptoms and Functional Limitations

Careful consideration of the person's capabilities may be needed when there are concerns for the person's safety. Peer advocates and support networks can provide a balance between autonomy and safety (Honey, 1999). Moreover, an important point in recovery is recognizing that the symptoms of mental illness typically require systemic monitoring and planned management for their relief and elimination (Copeland, 2001; Merryman & Riegel, 2007). Programs such as the Wellness Recovery Action Plan can effectively promote wellness, but symptoms can still persist to the point that rational independent decision making is compromised. If this potential reality is recognized, the person can put in place an advance directive regarding his or her wishes for treatment and can designate a health proxy who would make decisions should the person not be capable himself or herself. This action acknowledges diagnostic realities without disempowering the person (Copeland, 2001).

It is important to recognize that people may differ in their inclination for control over different aspects of life and their desire to assert this power (Fleming-Castaldy, 2009; Honey, 1999; Loft et al., 2003). This lack of desire to assert power should not be interpreted as symptomatic of a deficit in motivation or a weakness in will. The person's desire for control and level of comfort with self-direction should be determined and respected. Resources (e.g., a peer advocate, a service coordinator) can be provided to support self-determination at the person's comfort level (Gaitskell, 1998; Honey, 1999).

PRACTITIONERS' ATTITUDES

The vestiges of myths of disability, discussed previously, often influence how professionals approach people with disabilities. Hesitancy to share power, paternalistic or maternalistic approaches, and stereotyped expectations may result (Kielhofner, 2005; Merryman & Riegel, 2007). These disempowering attitudes must be confronted with active self-reflection, honest self-critique, proactive use of supervision, and open dialogue with peers and people receiving services. Assertive use of the resources listed in the next section can help practitioners develop the attitudes needed to effectively infuse empowerment into their practice.

Resources and Supports for Empowerment

Occupational therapists and occupational therapy assistants who hope to enact empowering practices must recognize that support from multiple sources is needed to counter the challenges presented in the preceding section. Pragmatically, an individual practitioner cannot feasibly meet all of a person's needs. Referrals to community-based and national resources, however, can facilitate goal attainment and enable participation. I strongly believe that acquiring knowledge about empowerment and the active pursuit of resources that facilitate empowerment are ethical responsibilities for all practitioners. In the following sections, I briefly discuss key resources and supports that make possible empowering practices.

DISABILITY RIGHTS AND PROFESSIONAL LITERATURE

Reading the history of the disability rights movement can provide occupational therapists and occupational therapy assistants with a deeper appreciation of the longstanding disempowerment of people with disabilities. This appreciation can promote a commitment to advocating for enduring societal changes to prevent history from repeating itself.

First-person narratives of living with a disability can help enhance practitioners' understanding of the uniqueness of people with disabilities (Franits, 2005) and the impact of empowering and disempowering practices and policies (Kielhofner, 2005). A growing body of work in the occupational therapy literature does in fact give voice to the occupational experiences of people with disabilities (Kielhofner, 2005). Integrating the knowledge gained from these readings with the latest professional literature on effective evaluation methods and intervention approaches enables practitioners to provide service that values the person's subjective experience (Franits, 2005). Sharing current information with service recipients provides an empowering level of control because it is the essential foundation for informed decision making (Knox et al., 2000).

PROFESSIONAL NETWORK

Joining with professional colleagues to listen to concerns, share challenges, and celebrate successes can facilitate network participants' personal and professional growth (Metropolitan New York District [MNYD], 2009a). Empowering practices require openness to diverse opinions, a commitment to innovation, and the attainment and maintenance of excellence. An exemplar of the empowering effects of a professional network is the Mental Health Task Force (MNYD, 2009a), whose regular meetings have provided its participants with these benefits.

DISABILITY RIGHTS AND CONSUMER-DRIVEN ORGANIZATIONS

Expanding one's professional networks to include organizations specifically committed to the full participation of people with disabilities is essential for empowering practices. Partnering with members of disability rights organizations (e.g., the National Alliance for the Mentally Ill [NAMI], the American Association of People With Disabilities [AAPD]) and parent, caregiver, and consumer groups (e.g., members of a clubhouse) can help practitioners move from an insular view of the effects of disability on participation to gain a broader perspective of living with a disability. Similarly, practitioners who establish these partnerships can share their expertise on the empowering effects of occupation to enable participation. Together, practitioners and nonpractitioners can work toward producing the societal changes that are needed for participation. For example, members of the MNYD task force described earlier have partnered with a mental health consumer group to present an annual conference focused on recovery. MNYD members have also partnered with the local chapter of NAMI to provide programs supportive of the annual NAMI antistigma empowerment walk (MNYD, 2009a, 2009b). These partnership activities clearly epitomize the values and realize the goals of empowerment.

In addition to the benefits accrued to professionals from these partnerships, practitioners should encourage those receiving their services to join these empowering organizations. For example, Centers for Independent Living (CIL) are primary empowerment sources for people with all types of disabilities because they can provide links to multiple services that enable empowerment (e.g., peer advocates, no-interest and low-interest loans for home modifications). Membership in CIL and other disability rights and consumer-driven organizations introduces the person to an empowerment culture that can foster his or her positive identity as a disabled person (Kielhofner, 2005). Clubhouse programs based on the Recovery Model are particularly empowering for people with mental illness because they do not distinguish between professional staff and nonprofessional consumer members (Bledsoe, 2001). Both CIL and clubhouses provide self- and peer advocacy training that can further support personal empowerment.

ONLINE RESOURCES

All of the national disability rights organizations, and many local ones, maintain excellent Web sites dedicated to the empowerment of people with disabilities. Several of these send free e-blasts to inform subscribers about current issues, practices, and policies that support empowerment (e.g., NAMI stigma buster alerts and AAPD Justice for All Network dispatches). Practitioners should share these resources with all service recipients because "information equals power" (Honey, 1999, p. 262). The power of information technology should be harnessed to disseminate knowledge, build partnerships, and advocate for societal change (Baker, 2000; Cottrell, 2005).

The disempowering effects of practices that do not use available resources versus the outcomes of empowering practices that integrate clinical reasoning with additional supports became strongly evident during my doctoral research. I conducted a study of the quality of life of people with disabilities who use personal care assistants. The information I gathered from almost all participants who had received or were currently receiving occupational therapy services reflected that their occupational therapists had not informed them of key resources (Fleming-Castaldy, 2009). For example, Jim, a young adult who incurred a cerebral vascular accident at age 19, stated he was not informed of any resources that would support his return to college and independent living. His rehabilitation focused solely on clinic-based interventions to facilitate return of sensorimotor function and independent performance of basic activities of daily living (BADLs). Jim did not attain complete sensorimotor return and remained dependent in several BADLs. He was discharged home to live with his family and receive BADL assistance from aides employed by a home health agency. As a result, he "felt like a baby," felt "all dressed up with nowhere to go," and "spent a lot of time thinking about how much life sucks."

He lived this "nonexistence" until his second stroke at the age of 22 "saved his life." Although the second rehabilitation period did not have a very different functional outcome from the first, the quality of life that Jim subsequently achieved was the polar opposite of that after the first. Although Jim continued to require assistance for BADLs, he reported that he was highly satisfied with his life. To assist him in tasks, Jim hired people he likes "who can adapt their schedule around mine" and "who know I'm not an idiot just 'cause I need help." He is a senior in college, lives independently in an off-campus apartment ("I felt too old for a dorm"), and works as a peer advocate. He is also deciding which graduate program best suits his interests and whether he should first take time off to travel Europe with friends. As Jim summed it up, "Life is good."

What enabled Jim to move from a life of despondency to one of satisfaction and hope? Jim attributed this substantial change to his new occupational therapist. This therapist used the Role Checklist to identify his past, present, and future valued roles. Together they discussed the depressing reality that Jim could not identify any valued role beyond family member (which Jim stated was not good because he felt like a burden) and that he saw no future role performance for himself. The therapist asked Jim to envision and describe his optimal future. Subsequent to this evaluation, the therapist and Jim collaboratively identified goals for the resumption of his valued roles. All occupational therapy sessions (even those that were focused on the return of sensorimotor function) were structured toward the acquisition of Jim's desired roles. Multiple sessions focused on developing his ability to self-direct his personal care and improve his self-advocacy skills. On discharge, the therapist provided Jim with a referral to his area CIL. Although this center was an hour's drive from his home, Jim was able to partner with CIL staff via the Internet and targeted in-person meetings to obtain consumer-directed personal care assistance and vocational services. These services enabled him to attain the future he had imagined with his therapist. By using all types of clinical reasoning and by looking beyond the clinic walls, this practitioner provided Jim with the knowledge, skills, and attitudes he needed to live an empowered life of his own choosing.

Sadly, Jim's experience with an occupational therapist committed to empowering practices was unique in my research. More often than not, people typically reported disempowering practices. These people included a woman with multiple sclerosis who reported that her life was not as satisfying as it had been in the past. Her declining vision made reading too difficult, and she stated that her therapist had advised her to use Books on Tape®, which she could not afford. Sadly, this woman was not aware (and apparently neither was her therapist) that a public library would loan these free of charge and that the Library of Congress has a free home-delivery program with thousands of Books on Tape for people who have a visual impairment or a physical disability. Similarly, an uninformed occupational therapist did not tell a person who sorely missed driving that programs were available to support automobile adaptations. A parent, frustrated by his inability to have home care agency aides provide assistance to enable him to attend his children's school functions, never learned that consumer-directed services were available to give him this desired control. Such findings troubled me greatly because I knew that supports external to traditional occupational therapy services could empower these people to lead self-directed lives, participate in meaningful activities, and engage in desired occupations.

EXERCISE 17.5: COMMUNITY RESOURCES FOR EMPOWERMENT

Find out what resources are available in your local community to support the empowerment of people with disabilities and other disenfranchised groups. Key resources to track down are CIL; adult education programs, One-Stop Career Centers; and consumer, family, and caregiver support and advocacy groups. Identify national resources that can be accessed to supplement local ones. Because it is important to determine the efficacy of services before recommending them, contact each resource as a potential consumer. Critique the resource's policies, service usefulness, and availability, and contact personnel to assess whether community resources are congruent with empowering practices.

Ensuring Future Empowering Practices in Occupational Therapy

For occupational therapy to become a profession recognized as one of empowerment, its practitioners must individually and collectively articulate the relationship between the use of occupation and the ability to lead a self-determined life. Empowering practices must infuse the process of occupational therapy across the developmental continuum and in all practice settings. Occupational therapists and occupational therapy assistants committed to the empowerment of disenfranchised people must also recognize that the attainment of subjective empowerment is not synonymous with the achievement of objective power. Objective power occurs when structures, systems, and policies exist that enable and support subjective empowerment (Charlton, 1998; Honey, 1999). Thus, people may have the capacity to self-direct their lives, but their efforts may be thwarted by systemic barriers (e.g., lack of transportation to get to their desired work). Consequently, practitioners must proactively and assertively work with others outside the profession to ensure that all can fully participate in society as they choose. To help make this elusive aim a reality, I propose that practitioners take these actions:

- *Revitalize a commitment to the founding principles and core values of occupational therapy.* The ethos of occupational therapy is inherently congruent with empowerment (Peloquin, 2005). Steadfast dedication to this heritage and enduring spirit strongly supports practitioners' engagement in empowering practices.
- *Use the* AOTA Code of Ethics (AOTA, 2005) *as the bridge from disempowering practices to empowering ones.* The ethical code of occupational therapy provides an effective moral guide for rejecting disempowerment and working vigilantly toward the empowerment of all. Table 17.1 de-

scribes how key attributes of occupational therapy's ethical principles can provide a conceptual bridge to empowering practices. Consistent and honest personal reflection is required to ensure the actualization of these connections in daily practice.

- *Design research projects that are fully inclusive of people with disabilities or other marginalized groups throughout the research process.* Research based on empowering practices recognizes the validity of the disability rights mantra "Nothing about us without us." Research should not be focused on the objective examination of disenfranchised people. Rather, the aim of empowerment research is to learn from participants. Therefore, researchers must actively seek out people to be the primary informants of their lived experiences (International Disability Research Centre, 2006). In putting forward research priorities for occupational therapy, Gutman (2008) proposed that occupational therapy research should address concerns that the people with whom practitioners work identify as most important. Consequently, the examination of the impact of disability experiences on participation should be a research priority (Gutman, 2008). To examine participation, participatory action research and participatory intervention research can be used (International Disability Research Centre, 2006; Knox et al., 2000). These research approaches assertively apply empowering practices to both research design and implementation. Multiple participatory action and participatory intervention research exemplars exist to guide occupational therapy researchers in their development of research projects that are inclusive of the voice of people with disabilities and their caregivers; sensitive to social, cultural, and political contexts; improve the quality of life of disenfranchised groups as a community and as individuals; and achieve "a shared vision for social change" (International Disability Research Centre, 2006, p. 5).
- *Integrate empowerment theory into occupational therapy educational curricula.* To help future occupational therapists and occupational therapy assistants develop the knowledge, skills, and attitudes needed for empowering practice, occupational therapy curricula must broaden their scope to include the disability rights perspective. The desired outcome of occupational therapy must be firmly established as the person's ability to lead a self-directed, occupationally meaningful life, not merely to perform activities independently. Moreover, students need to become more astute about the economic, social, and political barriers to full community participation faced by marginalized populations. Thibeault (2006) urged occupational therapy educators to stop training students in "a vacuum, a vacuum of the rich" and to "train students to be responsible global citizens" (p. 160). Confronting students' attitudes about disability, power, control, choice, and independence may contribute to producing reflective practitioners committed to empowering practices (Taylor, 2001).
- *Partner with disability rights organizations and other activists representing disenfranchised groups.* Occupational therapists and occupational

therapy assistants can join with advocates, policymakers, and lobbyists to remove social, economic, and political barriers to participation (Cottrell, 2005; Lohman et al., 2004). I believe that we have a moral obligation to confront social inequities that disempower people because to not act is to acquiesce (Lohman et al., 2004).

- *Inform participants in occupational therapy about empowering options for their lives.* The *Framework–II* includes self-advocacy and occupational justice as outcomes of occupational therapy (AOTA, 2008). If, however, people are not cognizant of the supports and resources available to them, these goals may be difficult (or impossible) to achieve. Consistent with my research, Magasi and Hammel (2009) described the disempowerment of adult women forced to live in nursing homes because they were unaware of community-based living alternatives. Redick et al. (2000) found that few occupational therapists used available resources to inform service recipients about the ADA Title III even though the vast majority (90%) acknowledged the importance of these mandates for the participation of people with disabilities. Only 1% to 5% reported implementing ADA-related activities with their clients, and only 14% used a CIL as an ADA resource. Practitioners may assert their commitment to participation, but many do not actualize their viewpoints. Practitioners must move beyond token statements of support for participation to actually serve as informational and organizational liaisons to people with disabilities. Increasing knowledge about choices that enable self-determination and participation is essential for the achievement of empowerment (Magasi & Hammel, 2009; Redick et al., 2000; Wehmeyer, 2005).

Summary

It was not my intention in this chapter (nor was it feasible) to describe the full range of ideas, theoretical principles, and actions that make up empowerment. Rather, it is my hope that the chapter will increase awareness

---

EXERCISE 17.6: ADVOCATING FOR EMPOWERMENT

Reflect on the challenges to empowering practices in the different practice situations described in Table 17.2. What policy changes are needed to remediate societal barriers to empowerment? Conduct an Internet search to identify a professional association (e.g., AOTA) or disability rights organization (e.g., ADAPT) that is actively working to change disempowering policies. Review the advocacy options available. Identify those that you can act on to further their efforts to enact empowering policies (e.g., write a letter to your state or federal representative, participate in the NAMI walk, join a rally).

of the potential for occupational therapy to serve as a vehicle for empowerment. The congruence between empowerment and the foundational principles, core values, and ethical code of occupational therapy is clear, yet occupational therapists and occupational therapy assistants must realize that beliefs alone cannot empower. They must recognize the multifaceted nature of people and the complexities of their contexts to acknowledge that the real gains made in occupational therapy are often stymied by external disempowering barriers. Consequently, practitioners must be prepared to confront the myths, services, and policies that limit rather than promote empowerment. I hope that the learning exercises provided in this chapter spark active reflection, raise critical consciousness, and engender a personal commitment to the development and promotion of empowering practices and policies.

By partnering with people with disabilities and other marginalized people, their families, and their caregivers, practitioners can help service recipients develop the knowledge, skills, and attitudes needed to enable subjective power and to advocate for the systemic changes required for objective power. These empowerment outcomes, combined with the empowering potential of purposeful activity and meaningful occupation, can enable participation long after occupational therapy services have ceased. This result empowers people to be their own agents of change and to live a self-determined life in environments of their own choosing and fulfills the envisioned purpose of occupational therapy to enable participation for all.

Acknowledgments

My deep appreciation is extended to Allison Amole, Allison Kearney, Colleen Scannell, Lauren Siconolfi, and Nicole Spaldo for their significant contributions to this chapter. These members of my University of Scranton graduate faculty–mentored research group completed annotated literature reviews related to empowerment across the developmental continuum, engaged in stimulating discussions about the actualization of empowering practices in occupational therapy, and provided honest and helpful editorial critiques. Their recognition of the relevance and importance of empowerment to their roles as future practitioners affirmed my faith in the power of occupation as a method of empowerment. I thank Jenna Osborn, University of Scranton graduate assistant, for her assistance with specific editorial tasks.

Dedication

This work is dedicated to my brother, Kevin Michael Fleming (1954–1989). Although Kevin could not win his battle with Friedreich's ataxia, his tenacious fight to live a self-directed life remains my inspiration.

References

Abberley, P. (1995). Disabling ideology in health and welfare: The case of occupational therapy. *Disability and Society, 10,* 221–232.

American Occupational Therapy Association. (1993). Core values and attitudes of occupational therapy practice. *American Journal of Occupational Therapy, 47,* 1085–1086.

American Occupational Therapy Association. (2005). Occupational Therapy Code of Ethics (2005). *American Journal of Occupational Therapy, 59,* 639–642.

American Occupational Therapy Association. (2006). *2006 AOTA workforce and compensation survey.* Bethesda, MD: Author.

American Occupational Therapy Association. (2008). Occupational therapy practice framework: Domain and process (2nd ed.). *American Journal of Occupational Therapy, 62,* 625–688.

Americans With Disabilities Act of 1990, P.L. 101–336, 42 U.S.C. § 12101.

Baker, M. (2000). Modernising the NHS: Patient care (empowerment): The view from a national society. *British Medical Journal, 320,* 1660–1662.

Bandura, A. (1977). Self-efficacy: Toward a unifying theory of behavioral change. *Psychological Review, 84,* 191–215.

Baum, C., & Law, M. (1997). Occupational therapy: Focusing on occupational performance. *American Journal of Occupational Therapy, 51,* 278–288.

Belice, P., & McGovern-Denk, M. (2002). Reframing occupational therapy in acute care. *OT Practice, 7*(8), 21–22, 24–26.

Bing, R. (1981). Occupational therapy revisited: A paraphrastic journey [Eleanor Clarke Slagle Lecture]. *American Journal of Occupational Therapy, 35,* 499–518.

Bishop, M. (2001). The recovery process and chronic illness and disability: Applications and implications. *Journal of Vocational Rehabilitation, 16,* 47–52.

Bishop, M. (2005). Quality of life and psychosocial adaptation to chronic illness and acquired disability: A conceptual and theoretical synthesis. *Journal of Rehabilitation, 71,* 5–14.

Bledsoe, C. (2001). Unique eyes and different windows of opportunity: The consumer provider perspective. *Occupational Therapy in Mental Health, 17*(3/4), 23–42.

Blundo, R. (2001). New Frames of Reference—Learning strengths-based practice: Challenging our personal and professional frames. *Family in Society, 82,* 296–305.

Bockoven, J. S. (1971). Occupational therapy—A historical perspective: Legacy of moral treatment—1800s to 1910. *American Journal of Occupational Therapy, 25,* 223–225.

Brollier, C., Shepherd, J., & Markley, K. (1994). Transition from school to community living. *American Journal of Occupational Therapy, 48,* 346–353.

Charlton, J. (1998). *Nothing about us without us.* Berkeley: University of California.

Charmaz, K. (1983). Loss of self: A fundamental form of suffering in the chronically ill. *Sociology of Health and Illness, 5,* 168–195.

Chinman, M., & Linney, J. (1998). Toward a model of adolescent empowerment: Theoretical and empirical evidence. *Journal of Primary Prevention, 18,* 393–413.

Christiansen, C. (1999). Defining lives: Occupation as identity: An essay on competence, coherence, and the creation of meaning [Eleanor Clarke Slagle Lecture]. *American Journal of Occupational Therapy, 53,* 547–558.

Colman, W. (1992). Maintaining autonomy: The struggle between occupational therapy and physical medicine. *American Journal of Occupational Therapy, 46,* 63–70.

Conneeley, A. (2003). Quality of life and traumatic brain injury: A one-year longitudinal qualitative study. *British Journal of Occupational Therapy, 66,* 440–446.

Copeland, M. (2001). Wellness Recovery Action Plan (WRAP): A system for monitoring, reducing, and eliminating uncomfortable or dangerous physical symptoms and emotional feelings. *Occupational Therapy in Mental Health, 17*(3/4), 127–150.

Corrigan, P. (2002). Empowerment and serious mental illness: Treatment partnerships and community opportunities. *Psychiatric Quarterly, 73*(2), 217–228.

Corrigan, P. (2006). Impact of consumer-operated services on empowerment and recovery of people with psychiatric disabilities. *Psychiatric Services, 57,* 1493–1498.

Costello, R. (Ed.). (1990). *Random House Webster's college dictionary.* New York: Random House.

Cottrell, R. P. (2005). The Olmstead decision: Landmark opportunity or platform for rhetoric? Our collective responsibility for full community participation. *American Journal of Occupational Therapy, 59,* 561–567.

Cottrell, R. P. (2007). The New Freedom Initiative—Transforming mental health care: Will OT be at the table? *Occupational Therapy in Mental Health, 23*(2), 1–24.

Dunst, C., & Trivette, C. (1996). Empowerment, effective helpgiving practices, and family-centered care. *Pediatric Nursing, 22,* 344–337.

Education for All Handicapped Children Act of 1975, P.L. 94–142, 20 U.S.C. § 1400 *et seq.*

Fidler, G. (1993). Nationally Speaking—The quest for efficacy. *American Journal of Occupational Therapy, 47,* 583–587.

Fleischer, D., & Zames, F. (2001). *The disability rights movement: From charity to confrontation.* Philadelphia: Temple University Press.

Fleming, M. (1991). The therapist with the three-track mind. *American Journal of Occupational Therapy, 45,* 341–349.

Fleming-Castaldy, R. (2009).*Consumer-directed personal care assistance and quality of life for persons with physical disabilities.* Unpublished doctoral dissertation, New York University. (ProQuest Dissertation and Theses Full Text Database Publication No. 3295337)

Franits, L. (2005). The Issue Is—Nothing about us without us: Searching for the narrative of disability. *American Journal of Occupational Therapy, 59,* 577–579.

Freire, P. (1970). *Pedagogy of the oppressed.* New York: Continuum.

Frisch, M. B. (1994). *QOLI: Quality of Life Inventory.* Minneapolis, MN: Pearson Assessments.

Gaitskell, S. (1998). Professional accountability and service user empowerment: Issues in community mental health. *British Journal of Occupational Therapy, 61,* 221–222.

Grady, A. (1995). Building inclusive communities: A challenge for occupational therapy [Eleanor Clarke Slagle Lecture]. *American Journal of Occupational Therapy, 45,* 300–310.

Gupta, J., & Walloch, C. (2006, August 28). Process of infusing social justice into the *Practice Framework:* A case study. *OT Practice, 11*(15), CE1–CE7.

Gutman, S. (2008). From the desk of the editor: Research priorities of the profession. *American Journal of Occupational Therapy, 62,* 499–501.

Gutman, S., Mortera, M., Hinojosa, J., & Kramer, P. (2007). The Issue Is—Revision of the *Occupational Therapy Practice Framework. American Journal of Occupational Therapy, 61,* 119–126.

Hammell, K. W. (2004). Dimensions of meaning in the occupations of daily life. *Canadian Journal of Occupational Therapy, 71,* 296–304.

Hemphill-Pearson, B., & Hunter, M. (1997). Holism in mental health practice. *Occupational Therapy in Mental Health, 13*(2), 35–47.

Hinojosa, J. (2002). Position Paper—Broadening the construct of independence. *American Journal of Occupational Therapy, 56,* 660.

Hinojosa, J., Kramer, P., & Crist, P. (2005). *Evaluation: Obtaining and interpreting data* (2nd ed.). Bethesda, MD: AOTA Press.

Holzmueller, R. (2005). Case Report—Therapists I have known and (mostly loved). *American Journal of Occupational Therapy, 59,* 580–587.

Honey, A. (1999). Empowerment versus power: Consumer participation in mental health services. *Occupational Therapy International, 6*(4), 257–276.

Individuals With Disabilities Education Act of 1990, P.L. 101–476, 20 U.S.C., Ch 33.

Ingersoll-Dayton, B., Schroepfer, T., Pryce, J., & Waarala, C. (2003). Enhancing relationships in nursing homes through empowerment. *Social Work, 48,* 420–424.

International Disability Research Centre on Social and Economic Innovation. (2006). Participatory intervention research with a disability community: A practical guide to practice. *International Journal of Disability, Community, and Rehabilitation, 5*(1), Article 1. Retrieved April 14, 2009, from www.ijdcr.ca/VOL05_01_CAN/articles/block.shtml

Johnson, D., & Sharpe, M. (2000). Results of a national survey on the implementation of the transition service requirements of IDEA. *Journal of Special Education Leadership, 13*(2), 15–26.

Kielhofner, G. (2005). Rethinking disability and what to do about it: Disabilities studies and its implications for occupational therapy, *American Journal of Occupational Therapy, 59,* 487–496.

Kielhofner, G., & Burke, J. (1977). Occupational therapy after 60 years: An account of changing identity and knowledge. *American Journal of Occupational Therapy, 31,* 657–689.

Knox, M., Parmenter, T. R., Atkinson, N., & Yazbeck, M. (2000). Family control: The views of families who have a child with an intellectual disability, *Journal of Applied Research in Intellectual Disabilities, 13,* 17–28.

Kosciulek, J. (1999). The consumer-directed theory of empowerment. *Rehabilitation Counseling Bulletin, 42,* 196–212.

Kronenberg, F., & Pollard, N. (2006). Political dimensions of occupation and the roles of occupational therapy. *American Journal of Occupational Therapy, 60,* 617–625.

Kyler, P. (2008). Client-centered and family-centered care: Refinement of the concepts. *Occupational Therapy in Mental Health, 24*(2), 100–120.

Law, M., Baum, C., & Dunn, W. (2005). *Measuring occupational performance: Supporting best practice in occupational therapy.* Thorofare, NJ: Slack.

Loft, M., McWilliams, M., McWilliams, C., & Ward-Griffin, C. (2003). Patient empowerment after total hip and knee replacement. *Orthopaedic Nursing, 22,* 42–47.

Lohman, H., Gabriel, L., & Furlong, B. (2004). The Issue Is—The bridge from ethics to public policy: Implications for occupational therapy practitioners. *American Journal of Occupational Therapy, 58,* 109–112.

Longmere, P., & Umansky, L. (2001). *The new disability history: American perspectives.* New York: New York University Press.

Magasi, S., & Hammel, J. (2009). Women with disabilities' experiences in long-term care: A case for social justice. *American Journal of Occupational Therapy, 63,* 35–45.

Mattingly, C. (1991). The narrative nature of clinical reasoning. *American Journal of Occupational Therapy, 45,* 998–1005.

Merryman, M., & Riegel, S. (2007). The recovery process and people with serious mental illness living in the community: An occupational therapy perspective. *Occupational Therapy in Mental Health, 32*(2), 51–73.

Metropolitan New York District. (2009a, January). MNYD Mental Health Task Force. *NYSOTA News,* p. 12.

Metropolitan New York District. (2009b, January). NAMI NYC—Metro Walk May 9, 2009. *NYSOTA News*, p. 13.

Meyer, A. (2005). The philosophy of occupational therapy. In R. P. Cottell (Ed.), *Perspectives for occupation-based practice: Foundation and future of occupational therapy* (pp. 25–28). Bethesda, MD: AOTA Press. (Original work published 1922)

Mitchell, J. M., & Kemp, B. J. (2000). Quality of life in assisted living homes: A multidimensional analysis. *Psychological Sciences, 55*(2), 117–127.

Moghimi, C. (2007). Issues in caregiving: The role of occupational therapy in caregiver training. *Topics in Geriatric Rehabilitation, 23*(3), 269–279.

Morris, J. (1997). Care or empowerment? A disability rights perspective. *Social Policy and Administration, 31*(1), 54–60.

Moyers, P., & Dale, L. (2007). *The guide to occupational therapy practice.* Bethesda, MD: AOTA Press.

National Council on Disability. (2004). *Livable communities for adults with disabilities.* Washington, DC: Author.

Neville-Jan, A. (2005). The problem with prevention: The case of spina bifida. *American Journal of Occupational Therapy, 59,* 527–539.

O'Hara, A., & Cooper, E. (2005). *Priced out in 2004: The housing crisis for people with disabilities.* Boston: Technical Assistance Collaborative.

Peloquin, S. M. (1989). Moral treatment: Contexts considered. *American Journal of Occupational Therapy, 43,* 537–544.

Peloquin, S. M. (2005). Embracing our ethos, reclaiming our heart [Eleanor Clarke Slagle Lecture]. *American Journal of Occupational Therapy, 59,* 611–625.

Pierce, D. (2001). Occupation by design: Dimensions, therapeutic power, and creative process. *American Journal of Occupational Therapy, 55,* 249–259.

Rapp, C., Shera, W., & Kisthardt, W. (1993). Research strategies for consumer empowerment of people with serious disabilities. *Social Work, 93,* 727–735.

Redick, M., McClain, L., & Brown, C. (2000). Consumer empowerment through occupational therapy: The Americans With Disabilities Act Title III. *American Journal of Occupational Therapy, 54,* 207–213.

Rehabilitation Act of 1973, P.L. 93–112, 29 U.S.C. § 701 *et seq.*

Reilly, M. (1971). Occupational therapy—A historical perspective: The modernization of occupational therapy. *American Journal of Occupational Therapy, 25,* 243–246.

Rogers, E., Chamberlin, J., Ellison, M., & Crean, T. (1997). A consumer-constructed scale to measure empowerment among users of mental health services. *Psychiatric Services, 48,* 1042–1047.

Rogers, J. C. (1983). Clinical reasoning: The ethics, science, and art [Eleanor Clarke Slagle Lecture]. *American Journal of Occupational Therapy, 37,* 601–616.

Schell, B., & Cervero, R. (1993). Clinical reasoning in occupational therapy: An integrative approach. *American Journal of Occupational Therapy, 47,* 605–610.

Schoener, R., Kinnealey, M., & Koenig, K. (2008). You can know me now if you listen: Sensory, motor, and communication issues in a nonverbal person with autism. *American Journal of Occupational Therapy, 62,* 547–553.

Shakespeare, T., & Watson, N. (1997). Defending the social model. *Disability and Society, 12,* 293–300.

Shannon, P. (1977). The derailment of occupational therapy. *American Journal of Occupational Therapy, 31,* 229–234.

Shortridge, S. D., & Walker, K. F. (1993). Lela A. Llorens. In R. J. Miller & K.F. Walker (Eds.), *Perspectives on theory for the practice of occupational therapy* (pp. 65–90). Gaithersburg, MD: Aspen.

Snow, B. (2006). *Thumbs down to pity.* Retrieved February 18, 2009, from www. disabilityisnatural.com/index-ben.htm

Steinmetz, E (2002). *Americans with disabilities, 2002.* Washington, DC: U.S. Census Bureau.

Taylor, M. (2001). Independence and empowerment: Evidence from the student perspective. *British Journal of Occupational Therapy, 64,* 245–252.

Tengland, P. (2007). Empowerment: A goal or a means for health promotion? *Medicine, Health Care, and Philosophy, 10,* 197–207.

Thibeault, R. (2006). Globalization, universities, and the future of occupational therapy: Dispatches for the majority of the world. *Australian Occupational Therapy Journal, 53,* 159–165.

Toal-Sullivan, D., & Henderson, P. (2004). Client-oriented role evaluation (CORE): The development of a clinical rehabilitation instrument to assess role change associated with disability. *American Journal of Occupational Therapy, 58,* 211–220.

Townsend, E. (2003). Reflections on power and justice in enabling occupation. *Canadian Journal of Occupational Therapy, 70,* 74–87.

Townsend, E., & Wilcock, A. (2004). Occupational justice and client-centered practice: A dialogue in progress. *American Journal of Occupational Therapy, 71,* 75–87.

U.S. Bureau of Labor Statistics. (2009). *New monthly data series on the employment status of people with disability.* Retrieved February 23, 2009, from http://data.bls.gov/cgi-bin/print.pl/cps/cpsdisability.htm

U.S. Census Bureau. (2008). *Number of Americans with a disability reaches 54.4 million.* Retrieved February 28, 2009, from www.census.gov/Press-Release/www/releases/archives/income_wealth/013041.html

U.S. Department of Education, Institute of Educational Sciences, National Center for Educational Statistics. (2008). *Students with disabilities exiting high school with a regular diploma.* Retrieved February 28, 2009, from http://nces.ed.gov/programs/coe/2008/section3/indicator22.asp

Vauth, R., Klein, B., Wirtz, M., & Corrigan, P. (2008). Self-efficacy and empowerment as outcomes of self-stigmatizing and coping in schizophrenia. *Psychiatry Research, 150,* 71–80.

Wehmeyer, M. (2005). Self-determination and the empowerment of people with disabilities. *American Rehabilitation, 28*(1), 22–29.

West, W. (1968). Professional responsibility in times of change [Eleanor Clarke Slagle Lecture]. *American Journal of Occupational Therapy, 52,* 9–15.

World Health Organization. (2007). *International classification of functioning, disability and health* (10th ed.). Geneva, Switzerland: Author.

Yerxa, E. (1967). Authentic occupational therapy [Eleanor Clarke Slagle Lecture]. *American Journal of Occupational Therapy, 21,* 155–173.

Zimmerman, M. A., & Warschausky, S. (1998). Empowerment theory for rehabilitation research: Conceptual and methodological issues. *Rehabilitation Psychology, 43,* 3–16.

18

Preparing for the Future: How Activities Relate to Human Occupation

Marie-Louise Blount, AM, OT, FAOTA
Jim Hinojosa, PhD, OT, FAOTA
Paula Kramer, PhD, OTR, FAOTA

In this chapter, we discuss research that supports the therapeutic use of activities and occupation, and we discuss the implications of this scholarly work on the future of the profession. Our objective is to link this work with our vision for the profession into the next decade. The profession's valuing of and perspectives on activity and occupation will shape future occupational therapy research and practice.

During the past 10 years, the profession has frequently used the term *occupation* without having one specific, accepted definition of the term. During this same period, the term *purposeful activity* has not been frequently used, yet it is one of the basic tenets of the profession, having been equated with *occupation* for years (American Occupational Therapy Association [AOTA], 1979). As noted in Chapter 1, the *Occupational Therapy Practice Framework: Domain and Process* (2nd ed., or *Framework–II*; AOTA, 2008) uses the terms *occupation* and *activity* interchangeably. The profession predominantly uses *occupation*, and yet the World Health Organization (2001) uses the terms *activity* and *participation*. We believe that occupational therapy must reconcile its language with that of the rest of the world and of the layperson, to aim at understanding and recognition of occupational therapy. We suggest that although as a profession, occupational therapy continues to use the term *occupation,* the term *activity* is more understandable to others. Using more common language will lead to greater understanding of occupational therapy.

Some questions we asked to begin this process of analyzing research and scholarly publications included whether purposeful activity and occupation should be examined as two separate constructs. If so, we would have to have clear and precise definitions. Would it be best to examine activities and occupation as legitimate tools used by practitioners to bring about change, referring here to the means of intervention? Would it be better to examine purposeful activity and occupation from an "ends" perspective as the outcome of intervention? Because each of these questions appeared essential to understanding how activities relate to human occupation, we used them to provide a framework for our discussion. We have not attempted to critique all the research related to occupational therapy. In fact, we have carefully selected publications to illustrate these questions and provide basic information that you can use to develop and refine your own ideas.

Examining Purposeful Activity and Occupation as Distinct Concepts

Although occupational therapy scholars have proposed that *purposeful activities* and *occupation* are two distinct concepts, their definitions in publications and research studies are not precise. In fact, confusion is often evident when authors claim that the two concepts are similar. As stated in the *Framework–II*, "Sometimes occupational therapy practitioners use the terms *occupation* and *activity* interchangeably to describe participation in daily life pursuits. . . . In the *Framework*, the term occupation encompasses activity" (AOTA, 2008, p. 629). This statement would imply that occupation is a broader-level concept than activity. As discussed in chapter 1, however, the philosophical base of occupational therapy (AOTA, 1979) uses *occupation* and *activity* interchangeably.

Occupational therapists and occupational therapy assistants are ultimately concerned with human occupation. Occupations are grounded in personal meaning, are goal directed, are personally satisfying, and reflect practitioners' cultural background (Hinojosa, Kramer, Royeen, & Luebben, 2003). Practitioners must recognize that occupations are made up of activities and tasks. Some activities are purposeful because they are meaningful or have a meaningful outcome for the person engaged in the activity. Other activities occupy time and may not have personal meaning; they just need to be done.

Therefore, we propose that occupational therapists and occupational therapy assistants use the language most appropriate for the situation and what they are trying to communicate. The attachment of the word *occupation* to other concepts does not strengthen practitioners' commitment to the construct of occupation. In fact, to the outsider, this attachment may be confusing and limit practitioners' ability to communicate effectively.

Purposeful Activity and Occupation as a Means

Many occupational therapists and occupational therapy assistants believe that occupation can be both the means and the ends of occupational therapy. These practitioners believe that they can use occupations in their interventions with clients to bring about change. They also believe that the outcome of intervention is the client's ability to engage in his or her occupations. In this book, we have proposed that occupations can be defined only by the person who is engaged in them. Occupational synthesis takes place when the client who has received occupational therapy spontaneously and unconsciously engages in activities that are personally meaningful and support his or her ability to function. From our perspective, occupational therapists and occupational therapy assistants use activities. When possible, they use purposeful activities. The goal of intervention and the outcome is that the client integrates these purposeful activities into his or her occupations and continues to engage in them as part of everyday life. The engagement in activities within the context of intervention is activity as a means. When the client integrates purposeful activities into his or her daily occupations, it becomes occupations as an end (see Chapter 6).

Qualitative basic research has begun to produce a body of theoretical information about occupation (Gewurtz, Stergiou-Kita, Shaw, Kirsh, & Rappolt, 2008). This work should be continued with increased focus on establishing a sound body of theoretical knowledge about the construct of occupation as it relates to people and society. However, confusion about how to study purposeful activity appears to exist.

Establishing the effectiveness of specific occupational therapy interventions requires that practitioners examine the treatment modalities they use within the context of a frame of reference or guidelines for intervention that specify their application. Applied research must examine treatment guidelines within the theoretical rationale that underlies them and is concerned with practical answers about whether a theoretically based intervention (e.g., frame of reference, conceptual model of practice, guidelines for intervention) has the outcome that it predicts (Mosey, 1996). From this perspective, activities are one tool that occupational therapists and occupational therapy assistants use to bring about change. As a tool, activities must be examined within their theoretical context. For example, dressing activities may be used with children to develop body awareness, imaginary play skills, or activities of daily living (ADL) skills. For an adult, dressing may be an activity used to develop socially appropriate self-care skills. When providing occupational therapy, one therapeutic tool is rarely used alone. Most often, on the basis of the intervention's theoretical base, several tools are used in specified manners as therapeutic media.

Although we suggest examining the use of activities within the context of the frame of reference used, much occupational therapy research has focused on establishing the efficacy of using activity. In these studies, purposeful activities or occupations are the independent or treatment variable (e.g., cause, treatment, controlled factor, manipulated variable). Many of these studies have supported the basic belief that therapeutic activities are more effective if they have meaning to the person (Gewurtz et al., 2008; Lyons, Orozovic, Davis, & Newman, 2002; Yoder, Nelson, & Smith, 1989).

Importance of Meaning

While writing Chapter 4 on activity analysis, Karen A. Buckley raised the following questions with the editors: Is meaning the important dimension of an activity that makes it purposeful to the person participating in it? Is meaning adequately addressed in discussions of purposeful activities and occupation? These questions led to a provocative conversation about the importance of meanings in determining whether an activity was purposeful. By definition, all occupations have meaning to the person engaged in them. The subjective meaning that a person gives to an activity determines whether it is an occupation. As Hasselkus (2002) observed, occupations are a source of meanings and give meaning to people's lives.

Hammell (2004) wrote, "Doing of self-care, productive and leisure activities is inadequate to address issues of meaning in people's lives" (p. 296). *Meaning* is the essence of what makes an activity purposeful. Although therapists often give more attention to the goal directedness of a purposeful activity, the activity's meaning to the participant is probably more important. We should note that this meaning is not always positive. For example, a person may find an activity humiliating (Hammell, 2004). Examples might be using stacking cones as a treatment activity when the person does not see any meaning in stacking cones or having an engineer used to working with complex machinery screwing nuts onto bolts. Perhaps in the end, the meaning an activity has for a person will determine its therapeutic potential. If a person realizes that participating in an activity he or she thinks is boring or useless may result in improvement, then the person's thoughts about the activity might change. When he or she adds subjective meaning to the activity, the activity then becomes meaningful. The issue of meaning requires further research and philosophical examination.

Published Research Based on the Question(s) That Underlie the Study

Many occupational therapists and occupational therapy assistants may think they do not need to learn about research because they are interested only in being clinicians. Evidence-based practice, however, demands that all practitioners have a basic understanding of research and its influence on practice. With support from research literature, occupational therapists and occupational therapy assistants can provide better services. When practitioners read published research, it is important that they first understand the research questions that are the foundation of that research. Identifying research questions is the first step to conducting useful research. Before selecting appropriate research methods, the researcher needs to answer the question "What exactly do you want to find out?" (Punch, 1998). Once the researcher has a clear research question, she or he then needs to determine the kind of data necessary to answer the question and how the data can be collected and analyzed.

Students often ask where research questions come from. As intelligent creatures, people constantly ask questions and search for the answers. Researchers use systematic methods to investigate questions to explain behavior and understand people's lives. In fact, finding interesting research questions is not difficult; they emerge as practitioners observe their environment and actions. Questions come from therapists' practice, everyday observations, and reading. In this section, we present only a few examples to illustrate how research is based on research questions.

Occupational therapists often ask questions related to their daily practice, such as "Are the activities selected effective for achieving the goals?" For example, Paul and Ramsey (1998) asked whether music-making activity as a form of occupationally embedded exercise could improve active shoulder flexion and elbow extension in people with hemiplegia. Practitioners need to add to their understanding about the meaning of occupation. To improve the quality of services, some people may ask what the nature of occupations is for their clients. Lyons et al. (2002) investigated what the occupational experiences of people with life-threatening illness are while they are attending a day hospice program. Other therapists have examined the relationships between purposeful activities and performances and behaviors. For example, Yoder et al. (1989) conducted a randomized group experiment to examine whether differences are elicited by the purposefulness of activities when applied to elderly female nursing home residents as they compared the duration and frequency of rotatory arm movement. Recently, Bravi and Stoykov (2007) examined the use of an upper-limb training protocol that involved task-oriented training. Research questions such as these determine what research is done in occupational therapy, and most important, these questions and their answers eventually determine what practitioners learn.

Although many occupational therapy researchers have collected much information about the application of purposeful activities and occupations, more research to substantiate practice is still greatly needed. According to Gutman (2009), editor of the *American Journal of Occupational Therapy,* the profession's research priority is conducting research related to occupational therapy interventions. She argued that a need for applied research exists.

In an earlier editorial, Gutman (2008) noted that

> The *Centennial Vision* . . . urges the profession to provide evidence supporting the efficacy of occupational therapy in six broad practice areas: (1) children and youth; (2) productive aging; (3) mental health; (4) health and wellness; (5) work and industry; and (6) rehabilitation, disability, and participation. . . . In accordance with occupational therapy's societal contract and in an effort to fulfill the mission of the *Centennial Vision,* the profession must strive to meet five specific research priorities:

1. Provide evidence for the efficacy of clinical practice
2. Test the reliability and validity of our assessment instruments
3. Examine how engagement in occupation can promote developmental milestones, health and wellness throughout the lifespan, and productive aging
4. Provide fundamental or basic research information regarding how specific disability experiences affect community and social participation—with the intent to ultimately use this information to develop clinical guidelines that can be tested for efficacy
5. Explore topical questions (i.e., current issues) whose answers will provide direction for the profession's continued growth and evolution. (p. 499)

This list provides directions for researchers to ask questions concerning different aspects of occupational therapy practice, from specific factors to broad models and from the individual level to the societal level.

Just asking questions is not enough, however. Occupational therapy researchers need to ask important, relevant, and answerable questions, clearly stated in straightforward manner. Occupational therapists and occupational therapy assistants work in many different settings by applying various therapeutic modalities with a wide range of populations. The potential for research is unlimited. With an increased demand for practitioners to provide evidence and to grow bodies of knowledge to support practice, occupational therapy researchers should focus on investigating occupational therapy effectiveness and developing theories about the nature of human occupations and relationships between health and occupation (Gillette, 1991). Once a person has a research question, he or she needs to develop a comprehensive outline that describes the implementation of the study.

Published Research Based on Research Methodology

Occupational therapy has moved from an earlier emphasis on quantitative research methods to the now widespread use of qualitative research methods; however, both qualitative and quantitative research methods appear to be important in occupational therapy research. Choosing to use either a qualitative approach or a quantitative approach does not make research good or bad. However, whether a study uses the most appropriate approach to investigate the problem under study is crucial. The approach is what makes the research valuable or not (Plante, Kiernan, & Betts, 1994).

Specific research questions dictate the best approach, and different research questions will lead to different methods (Plante et al., 1994; Punch, 1998). In this section, our intention is not to educate readers about the details of qualitative and quantitative methods but to provide a few examples of each method to illustrate how they can be used in occupational therapy research.

QUANTITATIVE

Briefly stated, a quantitative approach focuses on examining preselected variables that have been thought to be pertinent, on the basis of either existing theoretical statements or the researcher's own interpretation, to determine measurable and causal relationships among them. The investigators manipulate the numerical data through statistical analysis to seek an explanation of the causes and determinants of the phenomenon (Creswell, 1998: Tamhane, 2009; Velleman & Bock, 2008).

An occupational therapy researcher who uses quantitative designs typically uses experimental, quasi-experimental, or nonexperimental (i.e., descriptive or single subject) designs or identifies and isolates specific variables and then uses specific measurement instruments to collect information on these variables. To support and justify therapeutic use of purposeful activities, occupational therapy researchers have been greatly concerned with proving occupational therapy's value to society by presenting the efficacy of occupational therapy intervention. Nelson (1993) believed that with experimental analysis of occupational therapy practice, occupational therapists will be led to clear definitions of terms and precise statements about relationships between concepts. In addition, studies with quantitative research designs can be replicated to verify the findings and add them to the existing knowledge. For example, Lin, Wu, Tickle-Degnen, and Coster (1997) conducted a meta-analysis including 17 quantitative studies to examine the relationship between an activity's purposefulness and motor performance. With the presentation of quantitative data, the results reinforce the advantage of activities with added purpose over nonpurposeful exercises.

Moreover, some researchers have suggested that quantitative research methods provide better communication with other professions in the scientific community. With numerical comparisons, quantitative research findings can strengthen the evidence for the efficacy of occupational therapy intervention. Clark et al. (1997) evaluated the effectiveness of occupational therapy preventive services for well elderly people in a randomized controlled trial. With 361 participants, they compared the differences in several outcome measurements elicited by the occupational therapy group, the social activity control group, and the nontreatment control group. Clark et al. reported statistically significant findings across various domains, providing strong support for the effectiveness of preventive occupational therapy services. This publication, along with another from the same group on this topic (Hay et al., 2002) and one by Doris Pierce (2001) on occupation and activity, are among the most frequently cited in the field. In 2007, Legg et al. did a systematic review to assess whether occupational therapy focused explicitly on personal ADLs enhances recovery for patients after stroke. On the basis of inclusion criteria, they identified nine randomized controlled trials with a total of 1,258 participants and concluded that occupational therapy can improve performance and reduce the risk of deterioration.

Although manipulating independent variables and obtaining a control group is difficult, many occupational therapy researchers choose to approach their questions by using descriptive or one-group design. In 1999, Dolecheck and Schkade examined 6 elderly participants' performance in dynamic standing endurance when they engaged in different types of tasks. Although the sample was small, with a repeated measures design they found a statistically significant increase in standing time with personally meaningful activities versus nonmeaningful tasks. White, Mulligan, Merrill, and Wright (2007) used a quasi-experimental design to determine whether 68 children with possible sensory-processing deficits performed less well on an occupational performance measure. They found statistically significant differences and concluded that children who have been identified with sensory-processing deficits are likely to experience some challenges in performing everyday occupations.

With limited sources of samples, many researchers use single-subject or case study designs. Single-subject designs compare each individual's performance across a time line under different conditions. Such designs enable researchers to examine the efficacy of intervention with people with some specific characteristics. Through careful inspection of data, they can provide information about why an intervention is effective for one client but not for others (Dunn, 1993). Melchert-McKearnan, Deitz, Engel, and White (2000) designed a single-subject, randomized, multiple-treatment design to compare the effects of two conditions, purposeful activity (play) and rote exercise, on performance with 2 burn-injured children. The results suggested that the use of a play activity in comparison to rote exercise yielded better outcomes. The data, however, implied that there might be a point later in the rehabilitation process when rote exercise may be as effective as play activities in meeting therapeutic goals, and further replication of this study was suggested. In another single-subject study, Dickerson and Brown (2007) investigated the use of constraint-induced movement therapy for a 24-month-old child with hemiparesis. Daily measures of hand use on eight gross and fine motor activities supported the finding that improvements were maintained after completion of the treatment and postsplinting phases.

QUALITATIVE

A researcher chooses to use a qualitative approach when exploration and participant-centered detail concerning the phenomenon is needed. The approach is holistic in its context. Qualitative research helps researchers to obtain a better understanding of a social phenomenon from the participants' perspective (Creswell, 1998). Therefore, qualitative data are useful for developing theories and understanding natural behaviors.

Qualitative research methods can be used to develop theories by generating a systematic knowledge base and understanding concerning participation in occupations. They can also be used to investigate the effect of occupational therapy intervention on the quality of life, health, and wellness. Qualitative researchers believe that a focus on participants' perspectives and experiences and what these experiences mean to them provides the most meaningful data. Moreover, many researchers believe that qualitative research methods have a goodness of fit with searching for viable information about clients' performance in a natural context (Dunn, 1993; Yerxa, 1991).

Many qualitative approaches can be applied in occupational therapy research. They provide new knowledge to the profession by exploring complex, multilevel human qualities (Yerxa, 1991). In a qualitative study, Price-Lackey and Cashman (1996) used a narrative approach with life history interviews to discover the life experience of one woman with a traumatic head injury. This study illustrates the usefulness of gaining clients' perspective as occupational beings by gathering life histories with a focus on occupation, the importance of collaborative patient–therapist goal setting, and the necessity of considering both the doing and the meaning aspects of occupation. It supports the belief that the therapeutic relationship may be enhanced through the use of life history interviewing in practice.

As another example, Perrins-Margalis, Rugletic, Schepis, Stepanski, and Walsh (2000) conducted a qualitative study to investigate the effects of purposeful activity on the performance of people with chronic mental illness. On the basis of their interpretation of a horticulture experience from the participants' perspective, these authors gained a more in-depth understanding of the effect of horticulture as a group-based activity on quality of life, which was a composition of life satisfaction, well-being, and self-concept. Carin-Levy, Kendall, Young, and Mead (2009) used a qualitative paradigm to see whether exercise and relaxation classes motivated participants to take part in other purposeful activities. They found that participants continued to use what they learned and perceived improvement in their own quality of life.

Recently, Reynolds, Vivat, and Prior (2008) studied 10 women with chronic fatigue syndrome or myalgic encephalopathy, using interviews and written narratives to learn about the meanings of art-making. They determined that art-making occurred as part of a broader acceptance and adjustment process. Isaksson, Josephsson, Lexell, and Skar (2007) used in-depth interviews of 13 women with spinal cord injuries to learn about their encounters in occupations. Results supported the finding that change for these women was complex because they struggled but were able to regain participation in occupations.

Future Research on Activities, Purposeful Activities, and Occupation as Means and End

The health care delivery system and associated reimbursement structures have a direct influence on practitioners' attention to and use of activities, purposeful activities, and occupations. Although we believe that the critical outcome of occupational therapy should be the client's ability to engage in occupations, occupational therapists and occupational therapy assistants successfully use a wide range of interventions, all of which are important and should be examined for their efficacy and effectiveness in creating environments in which clients' performance skills and behaviors change in a positive direction. Activity, purposeful activity, and occupation as a means are only three unique therapeutic modalities used by practitioners. Other modalities, beyond the scope of this text, include conscious use of self, use of the nonhuman environment, the teaching–learning process, activity groups, sensory stimulation, and physical agent modalities, and whenever using any of these modalities, practitioners must keep in mind the central concern—occupation as an end.

Recognizing the importance of activities, purposeful activities, and occupation as a means, it is critical that practitioners understand how and why they must examine these therapeutic tools within the context of occupational therapy. Each is important in its own way.

Sometimes occupational therapy must provide the most cost-effective intervention. In these cases, clients' occupation may take second place, and the most cost-effective intervention may be activities. At times, if addressing a performance deficit, the occupational therapist may need to provide an activity that must be accomplished or practice a task that is necessary to complete an activity.

Occupational therapists and occupational therapy assistants find purposeful activities essential because they are the building blocks for occupation—the end goal. Practitioners learn to select, adapt, modify, grade, and create activities that meet their clients' therapeutic needs. They understand that if the client understands the activities' purpose and focuses attention on their completion, performance improves or behaviors change. When this happens, the client is able to synthesize or incorporate his or her performance and behaviors into daily life occupations.

Occupations should be studied in the context of the body of knowledge that underlies this fundamental construct. Occupational science leadership identifies the importance of developing a discipline. Although developing a discipline is important, practitioners need to balance research to support the emerging discipline along with research to support occupational therapy. Occupational therapy involves the use of a wide range of theoretical approaches and tools to bring about change. Occupational therapy scholars and researchers must provide a body of knowledge that supports the practice of the profession.

Creating Our Future

Many practitioners are interested in predicting and understanding what the future will hold. The course of life often prompts them to speculate about what lies ahead for them as individuals. In a larger sense, practitioners would like to know the shape of the future for those close to them, for the profession, for the nation, and for the world. Some project this curiosity well beyond the immediate sphere to the universe at large and try to tie their course to long-term celestial change. Contemplating the future also leads many to speculate about matters of religion and ultimate fate. This chapter, however, has a more mundane intent. Namely, we set out to look at the future of human activity and how it may affect occupational therapy. We begin with some notions about change at the societal level to put our thoughts into some context and provide them with some shape.

CHANGE AT THE SOCIETAL LEVEL

The future, as an unknown terrain, may seem inviting. One may anticipate the people, places, and events of the future with joy. The future may also seem fearsome, inhabited by unwanted changes, anticipated losses, and debility. That people's view of future events will vary by age, circumstances, health, and system of belief is clear. People sometimes seek knowledge and understanding in a vain effort to control the future or at least make it less uncertain.

Media depictions of the future have long been inhabited by sleek young people wearing body-conforming suits (and never wearing winter coats or carrying umbrellas) who stand near glossy, curved rocket ships or missile-like automobiles. These people of the future have ultramodern, uncluttered homes, set against a backdrop of soaring highways and flyovers. People can see some of these elements in the world today. Yet the world they inhabit is also very different from space-age fantasies. It is more accurately a juxtaposition of startlingly new and strikingly innovative changes with the familiar, traditional, tried-and-true aspects of life.

Of course, people have no way to actually predict what will happen tomorrow, next week, next year, or in 2100. They do live with certain indicators of direction and possibility such as knowledge of past and present human affairs, the acceleration of technological change, information about population trends, and data regarding acid rain and global warming. On some of these indicators, we discuss some of the areas of the most significant change. We explore how these changes are affecting human activity, but only as we can see them now, from our vantage point. We note that sudden and trans-

---

EXERCISE 18.1: PERSONAL REFLECTION

Answer each of the following questions in three sentences or fewer: (1) Who am I? (2) Who would I like to be? (3) What are the similarities between the person I perceive myself to be and the person I would like to be? (4) What are the differences? (5) What conclusions can I draw from this assignment? (Insel & Roth, 1985, p. 74)

forming change may be less likely than incremental change but remember that it too can occur and possibly render all careful study of trends futile.

Media and Communication

Some of the most rapid changes during the mid- to late 20th century have been in the modes and means of communication, as well as the content of people's communications. Recent writing (Standage, 1998) has suggested that the introduction of telegraphy was seen to be as transforming in its day as computer technology is perceived at present. Since the introduction of the telegraph, however, the world has seen the development of all sorts of radio and wireless communications (including wireless telephones), global print media circulated by wireless communication and rapid transportation systems, and television and video recording in rapidly proliferating forms. Computer technology spawns new applications, wonders, and intrusions into people's lives every day. "The Information Age" is indeed upon us and has already had interesting effects on the way in which people incorporate activity into their lives.

People now commonly have access to high-definition television with many channels, a wide range of radio stations of varying types, and online news with chat options. These sources of information and entertainment have transformed people's lives in a very short span of time. Yet it is still common to hear people say that they are bored or that there is nothing on television or radio. Changes in media and modes of communication have also transformed people's activity-driven lives. A few of these effects on human activity are that many people spend a good part of their workday sitting at a monitor and keyboard; watching television and other sedentary activities rather than physical activities fill leisure hours; knowing which buttons to push, and when, not only operates the stereo, VCR, and DVD player but also controls many household appliances, cars, and jet aircraft. A current hot topic is widespread obesity related to these changing activity patterns and the importance of food in people's lives, as discussed in Chapter 3. The use of exercise equipment, yet another technology, is one way of balancing human activity because contemporary lives have overall become much more sedentary.

The ways in which people use their hands to accomplish tasks have radically changed. Technology has freed people from many manual tasks. For example, instead of writing letters and going to the post office to mail them, people send e-mails or text messages. Programs now allow one to talk into the computer rather than typing. In some cases, however, technological changes have created the need for more complex fine motor skills. The trends just described are likely to continue through the coming decades.

Other Technological Change

Although communication technology has a primary effect on people's lives, one can see even from the preceding discussion that general technological change affects many aspects of people's existence. These changes are primarily influencing the lives of people in the so-called "developed world." Indeed, places still exist where it would be difficult to find a telephone, where many people cannot read, and where hand tools take the foreground in the home, leisure, and work environments. How technological changes will move to new populations in the future is, in itself, a challenging issue to consider.

With rapidly developing and increasingly available technological devices and equipment, people have developed new ways of interacting with both the devices and each other. Today, many people have special skills to operate stereos and videocameras, digital satellite television, and many household appliances; they learn the special skills and knowledge needed to operate modern cars; and even more expertise, training, and experience are needed to control the advanced equipment involved in flying a jet or in information processing.

Now and in the future, changing technology will affect every aspect of people's lives, from high-powered toothbrushes to food processors (Hafner, 1999), to color copiers, to magnetic resonance imaging, to robotics, to mood- and activity-enhancing drugs, just to name a few. Technological change and new products will affect not only people's knowledge and interactions but also their bodies, how and why they move, and what they think and desire. "We have always been empowered—yet oddly constrained—by the vocabulary of the moment" (Hall, 1999, p. 128). In effect, this changing technology will lead to transformations in people's daily activities. Occupational therapists and occupational therapy assistants will have an increased need to understand and analyze these changes and new activity patterns. Exploring them with clients whose own lives will display altered activity patterns, newly emerging interests, and restructured circumstances will be critical. Practitioners must also analyze how age and generation influence activity and activity choices, even before taking into account the influence of disability and possible new limitations on the lives of clients.

Technological change will add to the resources available in the rehabilitation process and may, like other societal changes, affect both the need for occupational therapy services and the way in which those services are offered. Technological change affects how practitioners carry out their daily activities, the way they feel about the things that they do, and the tools they use.

CHANGES IN HEALTH AND ILLNESS

In the developed world, increasing attention is paid to the maintenance and promotion of health. Attention to people's personal habits (e.g., smoking) and environmental factors (e.g., food additives) has led to changes in practices for some people and to legislation and social restriction in other cases. How people will define healthy practice and healthy living in the future remains to be seen, but occupational therapists and other health care practitioners are likely to continue giving attention to preventive measures and health-promoting activities.

Other recent health and illness trends that will probably extend into the future include the realization that newer, frequently more virulent communicable diseases often spread rapidly around the world because of increased international travel. The notion that a disease might be restricted to one community, one region, one nation, or even one continent is an illusion. Along with greater concern about the spread of such diseases, more attention will probably be paid to international public health measures.

In the United States, another notable health trend that is likely to extend into the future is the increasing use of pharmaceuticals in medicine. This development has already had a significant impact on the health care system. How the growth of pharmaceutical treatments will influence the future structure and practice of health care is still a matter of speculation but will no doubt have an effect on how health care is delivered.

CHANGING RESOURCES

Recent history has indicated that the way in which money, goods, and other resources are generated, traded, and used in the world has also changed. People can be sure that such change will continue, and they can be fairly sure that all quarters of society will experience economic booms and busts and consequent adjustments. People seeking to improve their circumstances and to find solutions for their own personal dilemmas will have difficulty doing so when the economy is faltering and will have more opportunities to meet their goals in prosperous times. In the United States, fluctuating resources and no guaranteed health care coverage suggest that some types of health care may not be available to some portion of society. In turn, economic uncertainty and resulting shortages of services will lead to segments of society being unable to fulfill their personal goals for well-being, leading to social unrest and to anomie. In good times, more possibilities exist for addressing social ills and shortages, but the choices made will never address all social inequities present in society.

Occupational therapists will have to take issues of resources and their effects on people's lives into consideration when planning interventions, perhaps even more so than they do currently. Creativity and ingenuity will particularly be called for with those who have fewer resources and pressing needs. Yet at the same time, perhaps, other clients may require knowledge of how to invest online or how to use the latest sophisticated adapted equipment. Thus, as much as practitioners need to be prepared to work in a world in which technology will be ever-changing and continually more demanding, they will also need to give more attention to their own adaptive skills and knowledge of the simplest and most rudimentary ways to solve problems of living and doing. They will need to address their willingness to offer services pro bono when that is required to provide those services in a more equitable fashion.

Tradition: The Pull of the Familiar

Most people would not be satisfied with form-fitting spacesuits and barren landscapes filled only with objects constructed by people, objects that emphasize efficiency over other features. Within most people stirs a desire for the asymmetric, the familiar, even the traditional. As one of the authors, Marie-Louise Blount, was writing these words, she was influenced by the landscape surrounding her. She observed that she was distracted by the goldfinches and the wildflowers as she sat outdoors and wrote. The natural beauty all around her reinforced the obverse of the electronic world at her fingertips. Yes, electricity, telephones, and a computer were nearby, but her world, and everyone's worlds, are also shaped by family, expected behaviors, familiar foods, joys of work, and beautiful objects.

Most people enjoy a world that combines the new and startling with the established and familiar (Friedman, 1999). Sociologists have called the fireplaces in people's homes, the oatmeal they eat for breakfast, and the flowers in their window boxes by the name *rural survivals*. There is every reason to believe that the good and bad of people's past and present activity lives will follow them in some form into the future. Occupational therapists and occupational therapy assistants who emphasize the importance of arts and crafts in their reserve of purposeful activities remind people that the drive to make things with their hands and to shape beauty are human impulses that will not be lost to practitioners or their clients in the future.

Consequences of Change

Looking at people's daily activities, both the mundane and the special, that adaptation to change is a requirement of the human condition is clear. This requirement is true for the little child trying to overcome difficulties of movement, for the young adult coping with a devastating injury, and for the senior citizen dealing with the physical and mental changes caused by aging. Human beings hold some aspects of their futures in their heads and hands. As stated earlier, some roads of the future have already been paved by past actions; one can foresee some developments by careful reading of current trends; most people make choices that shape their futures in clear ways. Nations, too, plan educational, transportation, and communication systems and relationships with other nations, thus influencing their futures.

Much, however, of what occurs in people's lives and in the larger world is unplanned and indeed unplannable. Moreover, most actions have unintended consequences. In the past, for example, the link between smoking tobacco and lung cancer was not known. Likewise, discernible but unintended connections exist among World Wars I and II and developments in the Balkans, and the history of European and U.S. relationships with the peoples of the Middle East has led to upheavals in the world today. People's efforts to lead healthy lives do not invariably lead them to the outcomes that they anticipate. Serendipity and tragedy can surprise and shock one at any moment. These observations serve to remind us as occupational therapists that a good future is always uncharted and that even the best treatment plans need reconsideration.

THE LIFE COURSE

One scientific avenue that provides practitioners with reports from time to time is the approach to human development that promotes the extension of the healthy human life span. For some people, the living environment has become cleaner over the past few centuries. It has also provided better nutrition, safer childbirth, fewer children per family, and the diminution of some diseases. Definitions and configurations of families also have changed, and they are expected to change more in the future (Collins, 2008). Some of these factors have permitted an extended lifespan for many human beings. The conscious plan and intent by some to move further in this direction holds tantalizing prospects of even longer and more successful lives.

Nonetheless, one major concern of occupational therapists and occupational therapy assistants (within their emphasis on normal and therapeutic activity) must be enhancing and fulfilling an already extended life course. Practitioners must continue to attend to all the issues of human development, both healthy and deleterious, that they have made their focus. In the future, the promise of increased longevity, the issues of human development and aging, and the intersection of these factors with purposeful activities and occupation will continue to be a central theme. In doing so, practitioners should not over- or under-emphasize either end of the life cycle, nor should they neglect adolescence, young adulthood, or middle adulthood, no matter to what numerical ages these periods correspond. The transitions of life and aging, as normal and inexorable processes, will always color a person's activities and interests and will therefore color the way in which practitioners apply activities therapeutically.

BELIEF SYSTEMS AND HUMAN ACTIONS

Predictions of the future and generalizations about outcomes cannot fail to take into account how ideology, convictions, and political actions affect human behavior. Neat plans not only become messy because of unintended consequences but also become complicated because the choices people make are dependent on their particular interpretations of the world. That is, they are sometimes based on fervently held beliefs, religious traditions, political opinions, or ideological conditioning. A portion of what makes the future unpredictable are those very belief systems that lead people to wage war, to demand conformity with the tenets of their religion, to promote new educational systems, to fear change, or to engage in new individual or shared activities (just to name a few possibilities). As a result, practitioners truly cannot know what the future will hold for occupational therapy. Still, it is their responsibility to stand for, promulgate, and adapt the tenets of the profession to the climate of the belief systems that develop. Moreover, those who have been engaged in this process must pave the way for occupational therapists of the future to draw from the knowledge and achievements of the past, to avoid the pitfalls that experience has revealed, and to trace indicators of how purposeful activities are changing. In doing so, practitioners will be as prepared as they can be to assist those who need such assistance to lead fuller and more satisfying lives in the future.

GENETIC ENGINEERING

One area of knowledge that is bound to influence not only people's activities but also the very nature of their beings is the burgeoning science of genetics. Work to increase knowledge in this area has already been wildly successful and will no doubt continue in this direction. Alterations to the gene pool to treat illnesses and disabilities, to promote fertility, or to vary heritability are highly likely to affect the practice of occupational therapy and even who its clients will be. For example, future practice will no doubt include more twins and triplets. More complex multiple pregnancies and low birth weights will produce children in need of intervention. In the future, the profession will continue to see a changing human landscape resulting from increased knowledge and success in enhancing fertility. Changes in the field of fertility intervention are already garnering attention, but some commentators believe that they will affect a relatively small proportion of the population. Nonetheless, occupational therapists specializing in pediatrics will probably see many representatives of this portion of the population.

Cloning, efforts to modify genetic impairment, and even selective eugenics will be discussed and used by some to control reproduction, to inform reproductive choices, and to deal with heritable disease. As with other predictions for the future, one can be sure that some of these advances will have unintended consequences. Possibilities for new and as yet unimagined developments in the areas of genetics and reproductive technology probably form the most revolutionary changes in the society of the future. These developments will affect people's notions about family and definitions of human beings and relationships and will certainly affect occupational therapy practice.

FUTURE PRACTICE

As described in the chapters of this book, occupational therapy practice is based on the use of purposeful activities with the ultimate goal that clients will engage successfully in occupations. Occupational therapists and occupational therapy assistants believe in the importance of activities and occupations. In the real world, however, many practitioners are often unable, unwilling, or reluctant to use activities as part of their daily interventions. Why is this? When practitioners are asked what they do in practice, they often answer by describing specific intervention strategies or techniques. Many also describe specific hands-on manipulations or exercises that are performed during treatment sessions. Some state or infer that devising an activity with a client takes more time than just giving that client an exercise to do. The focus is on the result of the exercise rather than its meaningfulness. These kinds of answers reinforce the belief that the techniques for treatments are more important than the performance of the specific activity itself, even when the ability to perform that activity may be the goal the client is trying to achieve.

However, occupational therapists and occupational therapy assistants are ultimately concerned with the client's ability to engage in occupations. Engagement in occupations requires that clients be able to perform the many purposeful activities that are foundational to the specific occupations of their lives. Therefore, practitioners should be comfortable explaining the outcomes of intervention in terms of the client's ability to engage in occupations.

Activities are used in treatment because they are the foundations for engaging in occupations. Thus, practitioners' measures of success are really the clients' ability to perform the specific activities so that they can ultimately engage in occupations. Occupational therapy practitioners need to reaffirm the importance of the person's ability to perform occupations.

Demonstrating Occupational Therapy's Value

The future of occupational therapy is rich as society focuses on function—the person's ability to engage in meaningful tasks. The challenge for practitioners is to move forward and yet be true to the roots of the profession. Practitioners must value clients' personal needs and desires and remember what is meaningful to them. They have to put aside their expectations of the client and focus on the client's expectations of himself or herself. Practitioners need to learn about their clients' culture and work with them to identify meaningful activities and occupations consistent with their values and their heritage. Focusing on the client's will, not on the practitioner's desires, is the art of occupational therapy practice. Once practitioners have mastered artful practice that is true to the profession, they then have to move forward in the world of science. Moving forward involves documenting what occupational therapists and occupational therapy assistants do, explaining how valuable it is to the person, and conducting research to demonstrate the value of occupational therapy in a scientific manner. Once the importance of occupation to the individual person is recognized, the value of occupation to society becomes immediately apparent. Society can benefit from people who are willing and able to engage in meaningful occupations through the effective use of occupational therapy.

Occupational therapy's concern with a person's ability to perform purposeful activities and occupations is grounded in functional outcomes. In the therapeutic process, the therapist first establishes functional goals—goals that are meaningful to the client and will help him or her perform activities and occupations successfully. To determine whether the intervention has been effective, occupational therapists need to have clearly identified functional outcomes. Inherent in functional outcomes is the client's ability to perform purposeful activities so that he or she can engage in occupations. *Functional performance* implies that a person is able to perform specific activities that allow him or her to perform occupations and, thus, be a more functional human being. What could be more functional than dressing oneself, feeding oneself, or being able to take care of one's children? In our view, occupational therapy is based on a concern for developing optimal and independent function. The foci of future practice will be the measurement of an intervention's success through the demonstration of functional outcomes and the refinement of occupational therapy's theoretical base through the determination of which frames of reference or types of interventions are most efficacious for clients. Highlighting the person's ability to do something valued as the result of occupational therapy's interventions will demonstrate its value to society.

Practitioners' concern for the person's needs must be broadened to involve the context of the person's life. Practitioners can no longer focus only on the person's needs and physical environment because activities occur in a much broader framework. A person's meaningful activities often involve other people. Thus, families and communities (and other social contexts) must be included in interventions. Currently, occupational therapists include families and communities in a limited manner. For example, children are treated with family-centered care, and inpatient units have seen a push to involve clients' families. The conceptual expansion described earlier will bring interventions out of a clinical setting, making the activity more meaningful to the client and other significant people in his or her life. It will also bring the practice of occupational therapy into contact with a larger population and demonstrate its value to a broader public.

Another possible change in practice will be attending to both groups and individuals. Currently, practitioners use groups in intervention; however, the broader conceptualization of groups as target populations holds great potential. Currently, practitioners treat people with repetitive motion injuries. In the future, however, more attention may be directed toward the prevention of such injuries by intervening with groups who may be prone to such problems. Occupational therapists might be involved in changing the environment, or they might try to change the way in which specific activities are carried out. Prevention is just a small part of occupational therapy practice today, but it should become more significant in the future. The increasing aging population will demand practitioners' attention to help them adapt their activities so that they can continue to be vitally involved in their chosen occupations. The adaptation of activities on a larger and broader scale will become an essential component of practice.

Reflecting on future practice, we realize that the future is always unpredictable, sometimes exciting, and often threatening. Although we cannot predict what the future actually holds, we can reflect on whether occupational therapy has a sound foundation from which it can evolve. Shifts in the practice sites and service delivery models are becoming evident in all areas of practice. Since the 1990s, occupational therapy services have shifted from clinic settings to more integrated community, classroom, and home settings. Today, occupational therapy has the potential to become a prominent profession in the 21st century. Yet, its potential prominence will only become a reality if practitioners provide interventions that are responsive to societal change. Occupational therapy's strength has always been its practitioners' willingness and ability to adapt and change in response to society. If occupational therapy is to continue to be viable, practitioners must continue to examine their interventions in the light of a changing society; they must examine society to set their intervention priorities and to select the most appropriate tools for interventions. What activities do people value? What activities do people desire and need to engage in? How can occupational therapists and occupational therapy assistants use activities therapeutically if they do not know what activities are foundational to society's occupations? In addition, practitioners need to have an expanded appreciation of society that includes understanding the needs of minority, poor, chronically ill, and elderly people. Whether and how occupational therapy addresses these issues may determine how viable it will be in the next decade.

Occupational therapists and occupational therapy assistants must also become familiar with changes in the health care and education systems as they evolve. Moreover, they cannot afford to continue to passively watch and attempt to respond to changes; rather, they must actively shape newly emerging systems. Moving beyond direct services, practitioners must advocate for the concerns of the individual client within managed services, and they must begin to create new service delivery models that ensure quality care in natural environments.

Summary

Many things in the world move in cycles; ideas come in and out of fashion just as skirt lengths and hairstyles do. As professions grow and develop over time, they too experience a fluctuation of ideas. They respond to societal changes, or they become obsolete. When the profession of occupational therapy was founded, its basis was occupation, and it stressed the importance of engaging in occupation for a healthy and productive life. People may have used the term *occupation* differently then; however, they clearly recognized its importance to daily life. The term *occupation* has gone in and out of fashion in the profession and is currently widely used, with a renewed recognized focal importance.

Although little agreement exists among scholars on the definitions of *occupation* and *purposeful activity,* they do agree that these concepts are basic to occupational therapy. Discussions of the meanings of these terms to occupational therapists has consumed much attention in several countries (Canadian Association of Occupational Therapists, 2002; Christiansen, Baum, & Bass-Haugen, 2005; Golledge, 1998; Reed & Sanderson, 1999). The profession adopted a hierarchy (Hinojosa & Kramer, 1997) in which *occupation* is the umbrella term, with *purposeful activities* being an important component under that umbrella. It is critical that our profession continue to explore these terms, defining them and debating their relationship both to each other and to the practice of occupational therapy.

The challenge facing educators in the future is to encourage the exploration of these concepts, to debate their meanings, and to identify how they relate to practice. Students need to learn to think about the relationship among activity, purposeful activity, and occupation and how these concepts apply to intervention and to the profession as a whole. These concepts are the cornerstone of the profession and need our attention. Although the profession has grown extensively, it has also come full circle, moving closer to its roots. It is critical that we clarify the meaning and importance of *occupation* and *purposeful activities,* and through this explain and describe both what we do and how it is important to society.

In 1961, Mary Reilly claimed that "occupational therapy can be one of the greatest ideas of 20th century medicine" (Reilly, 1962, p. 1). As we move into the 21st century, despite changes in society and technology, occupational therapy continues to provide a valuable service to people and society. It has changed and grown, just as society has changed and grown, and practitioners still provide a fundamental and meaningful service to people by helping them maintain control of their lives through participation in occupations and activities that are meaningful to them. The future will provide the practice of occupational therapy with many challenges, yet behind each challenge lies an opportunity to promote the importance of human activity and occupation.

References

American Occupational Therapy Association. (1979). The philosophical base of occupational therapy. *American Journal of Occupational Therapy, 33,* 785.

American Occupational Therapy Association. (2008). Occupational therapy practice framework: Domain and process (2nd ed.). *American Journal of Occupational Therapy, 62,* 625–683.

Bravi, L., & Stoykov, M. E. (2007). New directions in occupational therapy: Implementation of the task-oriented approach in conjunction with cortical stimulation after stroke. *Topics in Stroke Rehabilitation, 14*(6), 68–73.

Canadian Association of Occupational Therapists. (2002). *Enabling occupation. An occupational therapy perspective* (rev. ed.). Ottawa, ON: CAOT Publications ACE.

Carin-Levy, G., Kendall, M., Young, A., & Mead, G. (2009). The psychosocial effects of exercise and relaxation classes for persons surviving a stroke. *Canadian Journal of Occupational Therapy, 76*(2), 73–80.

Christiansen, C. H., Baum, C. M., & Bass-Haugen, J. (Eds.). (2005). *Occupational therapy: Performance, participation, and well-being* (3rd ed.). Thorofare, NJ: Slack.

Clark, F., Azen, S. P., Zemke, R., Jackson, J., Carlson, M., Mandel, D., et al. (1997). Occupational therapy for independent-living older adults: A randomized controlled trial. *JAMA, 278*, 1321–1326.

Collins, G. (2008, July 17). Las Vegas envy. *The New York Times,* p. A21.

Creswell, J. (1998). *Qualitative inquiry and research design: Choosing among five traditions.* Thousand Oaks, CA: Sage.

Dickerson, A. E., & Brown, L. E. (2007). Pediatric constraint-induced movement therapy in a young child with minimal active arm movement. *American Journal of Occupational Therapy, 61*, 563–573.

Dolecheck, J. R., & Schkade, J. K. (1999). The extent dynamic standing endurance is effected when CVA subjects perform personally meaningful activities rather than nonmeaningful tasks. *OTJR: Occupation, Participation and Health, 19*, 40–54.

Dunn, W. (1993). Useful research strategies for studying service provision in real life contexts. *Developmental Disabilities Special Interest Section Newsletter, 16*(2), 1–3.

Friedman, T. L. (1999). *The Lexus and the olive tree: Understanding globalization.* New York: Farrar, Straus & Giroux.

Gewurtz, R., Stergiou-Kita, M., Shaw, L., Kirsh, B., & Rappolt, S. (2008). Qualitative meta-synthesis: Reflections on the utility and challenges in occupational therapy. *Canadian Journal of Occupational Therapy, 75*(5), 301–308.

Gillette, N. (1991). The Issue Is—The challenge of research in occupational therapy. *American Journal of Occupational Therapy, 45*, 660–662.

Golledge, J. (1998). Distinguishing between occupation and purposeful activity, part 2: Why is the distinction important? *British Journal of Occupational Therapy, 61*(4), 157–160.

Gutman, S. A. (2008). From the Desk of the Editor—Research priorities of the profession. *American Journal of Occupational Therapy, 62*, 499–501.

Gutman, S. A. (2009). From the Desk of the Editor—How to appraise research: Elements of sound applied design. *American Journal of Occupational Therapy, 63*, 123–125.

Hafner, K. (1999, May 27). Honey, I programmed the blanket: The omnipresent chip has invaded everything from dishwashers to dogs. *The New York Times,* p. G125.

Hall, S. S. (1999, June 6). Journey to the center of my mind. *The New York Times Magazine,* pp. 122–128.

Hammel, K. W. (2004). Dimensions of meaning in the occupations of daily life. *Canadian Journal of Occupational Therapy, 71*, 296–305.

Hasselkus, B. R. (2002). *The meaning of everyday occupation.* Thorofare, NJ: Slack.

Hay, J., LaBree, L., Luo, R., Clark, F., Carlson, M., Mandel, D., et al. (2002). Cost-effectiveness of preventive occupational therapy for independent-living older adults. *Journal of the American Geriatrics Society, 50*(8), 1381–1388.

Hinojosa, J., & Kramer, P. (1997). Statement—Fundamental concepts of occupational therapy: Occupation, purposeful activity, and function. *American Journal of Occupational Therapy, 51*, 864–866.

Hinojosa, J., Kramer, P., Royeen, C. B., & Luebben, A. (2003). The core concept of occupation. In P. Kramer, J. Hinojosa, & C. B. Royeen (Eds.), *Perspectives in human occupation: Participation in life* (1–17). Philadelphia: Lippincott Williams & Wilkins.

Insel, G. M., & Roth W. T. (1985). *Core concepts in health* (4th ed.). Palo Alto, CA: Mayfield.

Isaksson, G., Josephsson, S., Lexell, J., & Skar, L. (2007). To regain participation in occupations through human encounters: Narratives from women with spinal cord injury. *Journal of Head Trauma Rehabilitation, 22*(4), 229–233.

Legg, L., Drummond, A., Leonardi-Bee, J., Gladman, J. R., Corr, S., Donkervoort, M., et al. (2007). Occupational therapy for patients with problems in personal activities of daily living after stroke: Systematic review of randomised trials. *British Medical Journal, 335*(7626), 922–930.

Lin, K., Wu, C., Tickle-Degnen, L., & Coster, W. (1997). Enhancing occupational performance through occupationally embedded exercise: A meta-analytic review. *OTJR: Occupation, Participation and Health, 17*, 25–47.

Lyons, M., Orozovic, N., Davis, J., & Newman, J. (2002). Doing–being–becoming: Occupational experiences of persons with life-threatening illnesses. *American Journal of Occupational Therapy, 56*, 285–295.

Melchert-McKearnan, K., Deitz, J., Engel, J. M., & White, O. (2000). Children with burn injuries: Purposeful activity versus rote exercise. *American Journal of Occupational Therapy, 54*, 381–390.

Mosey, A. C. (1996). *Applied scientific inquiry in the health professions: An epistemological orientation* (2nd ed.). Bethesda, MD: American Occupational Therapy Association.

Nelson, D. L. (1993). The experimental analysis of therapeutic occupation. *Developmental Disabilities Special Interest Section Newsletter, 16*(2), 7–8.

Paul, S., & Ramsey, D. (1998). The effects of electronic music-making as a therapeutic activity for improving upper extremity active range of motion. *Occupational Therapy International, 5*, 223–237.

Perrins-Margalis, N. M., Rugletic, J., Schepis, N. M., Stepanski, H. R., & Walsh, M. A. (2000). The immediate effects of a group-based horticulture experience on the quality of life of persons with chronic mental illness. *Occupational Therapy in Mental Health, 16*, 15–32.

Pierce, D. (2001). Untangling occupations and activity. *American Journal of Occupational Therapy, 55*, 138–146.

Plante, E., Kiernan, B., & Betts, J. D. (1994). Method or methodolotry: The qualitative–quantitative debate. *Language Speech and Hearing Services in Schools, 25*, 52–54.

Price-Lackey, P., & Cashman, J. (1996). Jenny's story: Reinventing oneself through occupation and narrative configuration. *American Journal of Occupational Therapy, 50*, 306–314.

Punch, K. F. (1998). *Introduction to social research: Quantitative and qualitative approaches.* Thousand Oaks, CA: Sage.

Reed, K. L., & Sanderson, S. N. (1999). *Concepts of occupational therapy* (4th ed.). Baltimore: Williams & Wilkins.

Reilly, M. (1962). Occupational therapy can be one of the greatest ideas of 20th-century medicine. *American Journal of Occupational Therapy, 16*, 1–9.

Reynolds, F., Vivat, B., & Prior, S. (2008). Women's experiences of increasing subjective well-being in CFS/ME through leisure-based arts and crafts activities: A qualitative study. *Disability and Rehabilitation, 30*(17), 1279–1288.

Standage, T. (1998). *The Victorian Internet: The remarkable story of the telegraph and the nineteenth century's on-line pioneers.* New York: Walker.

Tamhane, A. C. (2009). *Statistical analysis of designed experiments: Theory and applications.* Hoboken, NJ: Wiley.

Velleman, P. F., & Bock, D. E. (2008). *Stats: Data and models* (2nd ed.). Boston: Pearson/Addison-Wesley.

White, B. P., Mulligan, S., Merrill, K., & Wright, J. (2007). An examination of the relationships between motor and process skills and scores on the Sensory Profile. *American Journal of Occupational Therapy, 61,* 154–160.

World Health Organization. (2001). *International classification of functioning, disability and health.* Geneva, Switzerland: Author.

Yerxa, E. J. (1991). Nationally Speaking—Seeking a relevant, ethical, and realistic way of knowing for occupational therapy. *American Journal of Occupational Therapy, 45,* 199–204.

Yoder, R. M., Nelson, D. L., & Smith, D. A. (1989). Added-purpose versus rote exercise in female nursing home residents. *American Journal of Occupational Therapy, 43,* 581–586.

Index

Note. Page numbers followed by *f, t,* or *b* indicate figures, tables, or boxed material, respectively.